Extraordinary

HOW ONE WOMAN'S
BREAST CANCER JOURNEY
INSPIRED A COMMUNITY

*"When you hear that cancer affects so many people,
I always thought that meant so many people got the disease.
But what I now realize is that so many people are moved
to do extraordinary things for others because of cancer.
This is an incredible gift, and perhaps it is God's way
of connecting us to our humanity."*

JEN PAGANI (OCTOBER 8, 2007)

BY JENNIFER BURNETTE PAGANI

ISBN: 978-1-7347075-4-0
Edited by: Alicia Grace

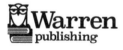

Published by Warren Publishing
Charlotte, NC
www.warrenpublishing.net
Printed in the United States

Dedication

I cannot overstate the tremendous power of all of you who are praying for us, thinking of us, caring for our children, feeding our family, writing notes of inspiration, and sending those positive vibes. Without all of you, I don't know how we would make it through this. Each and every person who has been so kind and giving and thoughtful is a direct contributor to saving Jen's life, and I thank you all. We are so very blessed, and there is not one moment of one day that we forget that fact. When this is behind us, and Jen writes her book, (I really hope she does) the dedication page will have to be its own chapter.

Goodnight and God Bless you all,

JOE PAGANI (FEBRUARY 6, 2008)

Introduction

Jennifer Pagani had a perfect life. She found joy in being a loving mother, wife, daughter, friend, two-time Iron Man competitor, and health aficionado; and she was married to her soulmate, Joe Pagani. Together they had two sons, Rocco and Luca, and were a happy and healthy family. In August of 2007, shortly after the birth of their second son, Jen was diagnosed with HER-2/neu-positive stage 3 breast cancer. After her initial diagnosis, Jen began to post about her journey as a breast cancer warrior on Caring Bridge, an online blogging platform where people share information about their health journeys with friends and family.

Jen had always desired to help others; it was just part of who she was. But as she began to fight her own battle with breast cancer, she developed a passion for advocating for and assisting local women who battled the same disease. In 2009, Jen, with the help of her family and friends, created the Go Jen Go Foundation to support breast cancer patients and survivors.

This book is comprised of entries from Jen's Caring Bridge journal. Along with her sons and the foundation, this book is Jen's legacy, a fulfillment of one of her last wishes. Her family and friends sincerely hope that Jen's words—her genuine, first-person account of fighting such a terrible disease—bring peace, comfort, and understanding to those affected by breast cancer.

Jen wrote often during her six-and-a-half-year journey. Her words are those of a woman who filled important roles and touched the lives of many people, while she endured treatments and struggled with questions about God's plan. Some entries were authored by her husband, Joe, and those entries usually updated Jen's readers about her progress when Jen was unable to write herself.

The first entry in Jen's Caring Bridge journal was written by Joe, and it introduces Jen's family, friends, and readers to the difficulties their family faced in the following years.

THE BEGINNING

August 9, 2007

Our story began shortly after the birth of our second boy, Luca, on May 4, 2007. It was a joyous time! After many challenges with our first son, Luca turned out to be an easy baby and a great breastfeeder. But due to a surgical cyst removal many years prior, Jen was only able to feed Luca from one breast. This caused inflammation and other changes in Jen's non-feeding breast and armpit. Jen and her OB/GYN discussed these and other changes at her six-week postnatal checkup, and both of them thought the complications were related to breastfeeding. However, at eleven-weeks post-delivery, Jen was having rib and arm pain, and her breast was redder and had developed a very large, hard mass. She was concerned and made a doctor appointment.

We went to the OB/GYN on Monday, July 30 and were seen by Dr. Wicker, the doctor who had delivered our first son. He told us "not to be alarmed," but thought we should see a breast specialist that day. He personally called the head of CMC's (Carolina Medical Center's) surgical oncology department, Dr. Richard White, and had us go directly there for an appointment at the Blumenthal Cancer Center. After squeezing us in for an evaluation, Dr. White ordered biopsies and mammograms to be done that day and scheduled a CT scan, bone scan, and an echocardiogram over the next few days. We were terrified, but we still did not think it was cancer.

We met with Dr. White late in the afternoon the very next day, and he told us Jen had an aggressive form of breast cancer with a large tumor in her breast that had spread to the lymph nodes. We were in shock. Jen could not stop shaking. He said there was a possibility of organ or bone metastasis because of the sudden growth of the tumor. If it had spread to the liver, lung, or heart, the prognosis was bleak: two years. If it had only spread to the bone, five years. Dr. White said both of those numbers were raw statistics and meant very little to an individual patient, but it was all we could think about.

Jen had the CT scans, and we waited for more news. During those horrible and dark twenty-four hours, Jen felt pain in her upper abdomen that she was certain was her liver. Despair swept us both up, and we couldn't lift ourselves out. Dr. White's phone call with the news of a clean CT was like a dream. We cried tears of relief for hours.

Next was the bone scan. Again, terrified, Jen thought the pain she had been feeling may be in her ribcage. This time, we had to wait all weekend. It was worse than before. We were either crying or trying not to cry the entire time. The following Monday, we met with Dr. Gary Frenette, the medical oncologist, and he told us the bone scan was clean. He was talking about a cure instead of a number of years. Jen said, "I never thought I could be so happy to hear that I *just* had breast cancer!" We celebrated with our families and prepared for "the fight." We still had the brain scan, but we were hopeful. The brain scan came back negative on the same day Jen started chemo.

Jen's official diagnosis is HER-2/neu-positive, receptor negative, invasive, ductal, stage 3 breast cancer with local lymph involvement. Her treatment will follow the protocol from the National Cancer Institute study B31, with chemotherapy, immunotherapy, surgery, radiation, and continued immunotherapy. This treatment will last a year.

We have a long and difficult road ahead of us, but the outpouring of love and support that Jen has received in this past week has shown us that the path will not be a lonely one. Thank you all for everything you've done, every note you've sent, and every prayer you've said. Jen will continue to rely on her friends and family to push her through to the cure!

Joe

Jen's family is thankful to Caring Bridge for being a wonderful resource during Jen's time of need. For more information about Caring Bridge, visit www.caringbridge.org.

2007
Jen's Story Begins

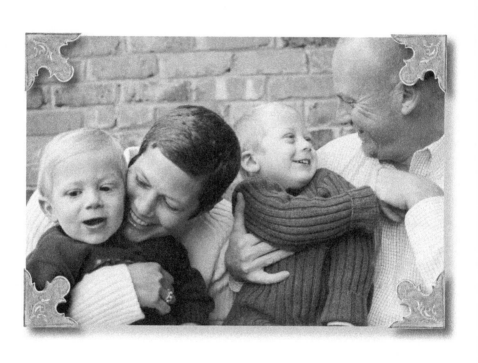

August 11, 2007

*T*he past week and a half has been so overwhelming I am not even sure where to begin ....

It is so true that your life can change in one instant. Two weeks ago, life was about preparing for Rocco's second birthday party and trying to balance the demands of everyday living with two little ones. Then came the diagnosis: *cancer*. Everything since then has been different. Nothing to come will ever be the same.

Chemo: my first opportunity to fight back at this monster inside of me. I am so relieved and thrilled to have begun the fight. I know that I have a long road ahead of me, but I will do whatever it takes to *live*. The suffering will make the success all that much sweeter. And after contemplating my mortality for the past few days, I have realized what a gift from God life truly is.

I want to thank all of you that have already sent such an outpouring of love and support our way. Family and friends will help us get through this. Please continue to pray for us. Thousands of voices sound much louder than one.

August 13, 2007

*T*oday is the fourth day after my first chemo last week. Tomorrow will be exactly two weeks since we got the diagnosis. In that short amount of time, I have been blessed with so many prayers and so much help from all of you. It is making a difference! I am feeling the effects of the chemo but not too badly. As a mom and an athlete, I am used to feeling tired and achy. What is much more tough, though, is trying to spend time resting and meditating rather than playing and caring for my sons. It is incredibly hard, but I am trying to focus on the big picture. My greatest challenges in this are the psychological and emotional ones. The physical one I am up for. Please pray for my family. They need strength and patience too.

AUGUST 14, 2007

5:30 p.m. This same hour, two weeks ago today, I found out I had cancer. It has been the shortest and fastest two weeks of my life. I am totally overwhelmed by all of those reaching out to me. Many of them I do not know well or have not met at all. Your words of hope, faith, and strength inspire me. I meditate on healing and feel the tide of love from God and others wash over me and through me. This must make a difference in the battle for my life. Those of you who know me well may be surprised by these words. But these past days have changed many things about me.

I am still struggling with the unknowns and lack of guarantees that come with this diagnosis. I am trying to take it one day at a time. The "what ifs" could literally kill me. But every time I check this site or hear from a friend, I feel the strength inside me grow, and the doubt recedes a little bit more into nothingness.

AUGUST 16, 2007

GREAT NEWS! The prayers and well wishes are working! The one-week, post-chemo blood work looks "great" (the oncologist's words). We had a bunch of questions and concerns, and he addressed them all. I told him I thought maybe the tumors had gotten smaller, and he said probably not this soon. But then he measured, and they have definitely decreased in size! The oncologist said "sweet!" This is incredible; it means the chemo drugs are working against my type of cancer!

I know this journey is filled with many ups and downs and lots of uncertainty, but this is certainly a victory worth celebrating! Please keep praying for me. It is working!

AUGUST 17, 2007

Words aren't adequate to express how deeply I am touched by all of the support. I am truly inspired by how freely people are opening their hearts up to me. Three weeks ago, I was a fairly private person.

Present circumstances are moving me to be otherwise. Cancer is my chance to become a better person.

AUGUST 19, 2007

Today I woke up and started singing Sinéad O'Connor's "The Last Day of Our Acquaintance" in the shower. It's a beautiful and soulful ballad about her divorce. I, however, was singing to my hair and shampoo. It is funny that both the song and the artist's haircut are appropriate. We have our haircut "party" at noon today. Christopher, Keaton, Kennedy, and I are all getting the number-two buzz cuts. I'm kinda excited and kinda nervous.

Right now, we are on our way to Mass and are going to be a bit late. I promise I won't tear up a picture of the pope while I'm there. :-) (Sinéad O'Connor did this on *Saturday Night Live* in the '90s.)

We will post some pics of my new look later.

AUGUST 20, 2007

Well, the hair is gone. It took forever to come off. Apparently when my hairstylist of many years told me that I had the thickest head of hair she had ever seen, she was not lying. We finally got it down to a number-two cut. I feel like I took off a wool cap. We actually had to reset our thermostat, so the house is now a bit warmer.

AUGUST 21, 2007

I have never been too open with my emotions. I usually find it awkward expressing myself openly, even to my family and dearest friends. I hope that cancer changes this about me. I sense this occurring already, mainly when I am in front of the computer or putting pen to paper. I think the courage to be comfortable talking face to face about my deepest, most sincere feelings will come. In the meantime, know that having such incredible support from my family during this has been a totally amazing experience. From the moment Joe and I first got the diagnosis, we have been surrounded and supported by you every step of the way. From so many of us crying together that first night, to the grandmas basically moving in, to the help getting to appointments and with chores, to driving in town just to sit and spend a few hours with us, to coming over to just to hang out, or to celebrate my new haircut ... all these things mean so much. I think they have galvanized this family and made us all better people, and made us all appreciate each other that much more. Cancer definitely does have an upside.

August 23, 2007

The past two days have been filled with appointments and were quite draining. We took advantage of the Presbyterian Multidisciplinary Clinic to get a second opinion. I was very stressed at the beginning of the day because I just did not know what they were going to tell us about my prognosis and diagnosis. We were seen by two medical oncologists, two surgical oncologists, and two radiation oncologists, plus a genetics counselor, a nutritionist, a social worker, and a survivor/volunteer. This was all provided for free!

Basically, they confirmed the plan of action we are currently on. There are one or two ways we could differ in chemo if I don't continue to respond favorably. We learned new info and also became that much more confident in my current treatment path. This was such a great clinic, and they were very reaffirming! I am so impressed at how the medical community in Charlotte rallies together to meet the needs of its citizens. It seems the care for my well-being extends past family, friends, and neighbors and into the heath organizations themselves. This is eye opening.

I also attended my very first support group meeting. It was quite emotional but a great experience. The group is diverse, and it was very helpful to hear the things I am feeling and going through from such different perspectives. This disease cuts across all age groups, cultures, and social classes, and it was incredible for me to talk with people, with whom I would not think I had anything at all in common (except the obvious: breast cancer), and feel such a connection with their humanity and their emotional struggles. It was definitely a cancer "growing moment."

AUGUST 24, 2007

Sometimes I just sit at the computer and cry. Today is one of those days. When I am scared and struggling to stay positive in the midst of all this uncertainty, I get online and I find things that touch me deeply and give me strength. I know I have to just take things one day at a time, but sometimes that seems so hard to do. I do appreciate every day, and I think I am on my way to staying more present in the moment. It is currently the most difficult thing for me, but I am making headway.

Thank you all.

AUGUST 26, 2007

Well, yesterday was a much better day than the day before! It is a constant battle, and on my way to victory, I am sure to suffer a few defeats.

I must admit, though, that I was feeling a bit frustrated and sorry for myself again this morning because I am having trouble staying asleep. It seems very ironic to me that when you are faced with potentially much less time on this earth than you thought you would have, individual moments can drag on for what seems like eternity. However, when I logged on, I read all of your entries and felt inspired and much better! Thank you!

We go to Duke to get a third opinion on Monday and Tuesday of this week. Then Thursday is the next chemo. YES!

This was a bit rambly, but it is five o'clock in the morning.

AUGUST 27, 2007

We are off today to Duke to get one more perspective, answer more questions, and hopefully confirm our current path. Of course we are a bit nervous about it. Please keep us in your thoughts and prayers! When we get back to town, I anticipate being quite tired. But I have several appointments Wed and then chemo again Thursday. So it might be a while before I can write again ...

Thinking of you all ....

AUGUST 28, 2007

We just got back from Duke a little bit ago. We saw an oncology fellow and a very highly recommended breast cancer specialist, Dr. Marcum. It seems that the original improvement we saw in the tumor has stopped and the other changes we noticed in the breast (I'll spare you details, some things need to stay private) are not good. The cancer has spread on the surface of the breast. Our worst fears have been realized yet again.

Ordinarily they wait for two rounds of chemo before making a change in treatment. We cannot wait that long. This Thursday, they are changing my chemo regimen. It will follow a study done at MD Anderson in Houston, ironically, where my best friend Mindy works doing reconstructive surgery on cancer patients. I will still get Herceptin but now on a different schedule and much more aggressively. Other new drugs will be added in later. The potential side effects of this treatment are serious but worth it. The rest of treatment stays the same: mastectomy and radiation, followed by nine more months of Herceptin (I think—not 100 percent on that last part).

The GOOD news in all this is that this regimen should STOP AND SHRINK the cancer. If this fails, we still have one experimental drug to try. After that we are SOL.

Anyway, I held it together for the entire appointment but then cried all the way to the car and sobbed for quite a while on the drive back. Joe managed to keep it together. I hope he lets some of it out when he is ready.

For whatever reason, in the midst of all that crying, I felt like this was the path to be on. This is the way to the cure. There was and is a calm that is now present in the midst of this storm. I know I will still have some tough moments. But MY INNER VOICE IS SAYING THIS IS MY PATH TO A CURE. I didn't hear that before!

So, I wanted to let you all know where I stand. Please do not tell me you are sorry. I know you mean well, but it does not help. I CAN DO THIS!!!! I AM NOW MOVING FORWARD TO RECOVERY.

Please continue the well wishes, the notes of inspiration, the support for Komen and other breast cancer research, and of course, the prayers. They have helped so much already and will continue to help on my new journey!

P.S. I had gotten used to my GI Jen haircut, but it isn't going to last. My hair is starting to fall out like sprinkling rain. Oh well. Next stop: bald and beautiful.

AUGUST 29, 2007

*A*lso, a VERY BIG THANKS to everyone at CLCC who contributed diapers, wipes, and clothes for both boys! We were overwhelmed and so thankful. It is so hard to manage day to day stuff right now, and this is a huge help. It is also incredible that Rocco is getting a weekly playdate with his buds from school. That continuity is helping him a lot!

I was thinking more about all this last night. I always thought God had given me strong shoulders for swimming, but maybe they are to carry this burden. That being said, I can't wait until tomorrow to start my new drugs and start kicking this cancer in the ass!

AUGUST 31, 2007

*W*e met with my Charlotte medical oncologist, Dr. Frenette (a very intelligent, compassionate, communicative, and funny man) yesterday. We reviewed the info from our Duke visit and discussed at great length how to proceed. We also found out that my tumors and lymph nodes have continued to shrink!! The Duke doc did not measure them because it is done with calipers and must be done by the same doctor over time to achieve consistency. Obviously, this is good news!

After discussing all the most current studies relevant to my situation, we switched my chemo regimen over to that of another highly effective protocol. I am so excited to get the weekly Herceptin now! That is the new drug that is HIGHLY EFFECTIVE on my HER2 positive type cancer. The other good news from the visit is that at the end of this three-month chemo period, I will have two regimen options for the following three months. Big thanks to my best friend Mindy who works at the MD Anderson Cancer Center and who is sending us UP TO THE MINUTE chemo trial results! We are psyched! Does all this sound confusing? Try sitting in on one of these appointments when the docs start throwing all this information around!

AUGUST 31, 2007

*W*e were due to leave for the beach for a week tomorrow. This will be the first year of our lives without seeing the ocean. So much has changed so quickly.

I would like to thank Oak Island Accommodations and the owners of the beautiful house *La Porte de la Mer* for working with us on our rental deposit. Such acts of kindness go a long way, and I am already excited about going next year. I need something fun and non-cancer related to look forward to!

Thank you again, everyone, for doing so much for us! Thanks for my signs, Rob! Have a great Labor Day Weekend, and Go Dawgs!

September 4, 2007

just came in after visiting outside with some neighbors. God it was great to do something so normal! I am happy that the weather is finally changing so that I can get outside a bit more. Despite this website and the calls of many friends, I feel a bit like a bird in a gilded cage. My life now revolves around healing rather than the old, normal stuff, like carting the boys around, school, playdates, and going to the grocery store or the YMCA. I still find myself stunned at how much our lives have changed in the past five weeks, how much "normal" is being redefined.

It did me good to run into everyone like that. I have been focusing a bit too much on the long-term treatment picture (twelve weeks of weekly chemo, four months of chemo every three weeks, surgery, five weeks of radiation, and then nine more months of weekly immunotherapy). Long term is quite daunting and mentally challenging. Then I try to think about when I trained for the Ironman races. Same deal: an overwhelming big picture that I had to break into manageable pieces. I managed to do it then, and I know I'll do it now. I think it just took a bit of normalcy to get my head back on track.

September 6, 2007 10:04 a.m.

oe and I have so much to be thankful for! I never would have imagined that we would have so many people supporting us. It is an incredible gift to see the love and goodness in so many. I did not see that very clearly BC (before cancer). I thank God for this and other lessons this illness will bring.

Does anyone know the Bible verse that goes something like, "Rejoice in this day, God made it"? That comes to mind so often now, and I would like to get it right. I used to see the quote at the outside track at the Harris YMCA. I was always so thankful to be out exercising. That was when I truly felt God's presence and power. Especially when my friend Laura and I were out on our really long bike rides, training for the Ironman races. That was where I worshipped him ... when I was pushing my body and mind and communing with the sun, the wind, the sky, and wide-open spaces. I really miss that now. I have been inside due to sickness, chemo, or the heat for too long. I want to go back outside and be with God.

SEPTEMBER 6, 2007

*T*hanks to everyone who has been on the website and also to those who responded about my Bible verse question! You forwarded many helpful and inspirational verses. The one I was thinking of is Psalms 118:24—"This is the day that the Lord hath made, let us rejoice and be glad in it." If I can keep that in mind each day, everything else will fall into place.

SEPTEMBER 7, 2007

*W*ell, "chemo lite" (slice of lime, no ice) was not too bad at all. I wasn't really sure what to expect, but the only side effect seems to be fatigue. I could not get out of bed today and am ready to go back right now. Other than that, I am doing great.

It has been so good to see some friends and neighbors these past few days! I really miss seeing everyone and doing regular stuff. As my reaction to chemo/managing my low blood counts gets more predictable, I will be back out there in circulation again, and I can't wait!

SEPTEMBER 8, 2007

*W*ell today has been interesting. Rocco has decided to put the Terrible in Twos this morning. He was all set to see Big Mama and Big Daddy and get a pancake breakfast with them. However, they couldn't make it up from Hilton Head due to illness (this whole low white blood cell count thing is tough to deal with), and he has been pretty much inconsolable since. Joe (he is getting the lion share of this difficult behavior) and I are exasperated and frustrated. We took Rocco to Dick's Sporting Goods to cheer him up and let him burn off some of the negative energy. I had another "you know your life has changed when …" moment in the store when I was looking at jackets that would be cute and warm to wear to chemo rather than what would look good on me and wick away sweat. Ah, life on chemo with little kids.

Hopefully my GA Dawgs will crush the Gamecocks tonight!

SEPTEMBER 10, 2007

It has been wonderful to be away! It was great to spend time with Big Mama and Big Daddy, and also get time for just Joe and I.

As I am writing this, I have a view of the tide coming in over the low country. It is so soothing. The colors and the movement are spell binding and have really soothed my soul. Although it is a quick trip, it has been very therapeutic. Sitting under an umbrella on the beach with a good book is a simple pleasure, but a treasured one. It has been great to listen to the surf and feel the ocean breeze. I have also thoroughly enjoyed getting some sun, though I did have to ask Joe and Big Daddy how to manage the rays on my balding head. I must also give some credit to the residents of Hilton Head—no one openly gawked at me as I walked on the beach in a bikini with my new chrome dome. I kind of assumed everyone would stare, but no one really did. It was really nice!

We are getting ready to walk out on Dolphin Point for the sunset. I have been looking forward to it all afternoon. Watching the sky melt with the sea over Skull Creek is such a beautiful sight! I have truly been rejoicing in this day that has God made!

SEPTEMBER 14, 2007

This Caring Bridge website is truly a gift from God! It is incredible to hear from so many people! I log on and instantly feel connected to the love and strength of so many. I can almost feel the power of it all coming right through my keyboard and into my heart and my body. In my mind's eye it is like a flowing mass of white blue light, something I think God looks like (no I am not smoking pot to alleviate chemo nausea).

Is there a Bible verse about God being the Way and the Light? That Light and chemo lite are both working! I can feel a difference in the tumor today, just one day after treatment. It is getting smaller and softer! My breast is starting to feel like a breast again, rather than a breast with a pool ball tucked under the skin.

Here is some cancer irony for you. I actually went to Target to buy some new fall clothes (have to look good for chemo!) since most of my current pants are falling off of me. Who would have thought I could look "skinny" and still weigh 150 pounds?! It was so fabulous to do something that normal and to get to do it with my mom to boot! Anyway, I was trying on some of the new longer cut, slim-fit tops, and my mom and I both noticed that my cancer breast looked much more flattering in the tops than my other, post two-breastfeeding-babies-boob did. Hmmm. Not sure what to make of that. Maybe God has a sense of humor!

SEPTEMBER 16, 2007

Chronologically, I am jumping around a bit. This was the busiest week that I have had in quite a while (mostly in a good way: i.e., not all doctor related appointments). This past Friday was the Komen Survivor luncheon. I was a bit nervous about going because I still cry at the drop of a hat, and as my husband pointed out, "anytime you get that many women together for something, someone is bound to shed a tear or two." There were eight-hundred women there! I wasn't sure whether to feel saddened or joyous about the size of the group.

Mom and I sat at a table with about eight other women. It was a very diverse group. Of course I was the youngest (lucky me) and the most recently diagnosed. Our table was a bit quiet at first, and it was a bit awkward making conversation at the start of the meal. The real icebreaker occurred when one of the women just got up, gave me a hug, and told me it would be okay—I must had the deer-in-the-headlights look being a luncheon newbie. A couple of other women did the same. Then everyone began sharing their stories of hardship and triumph. It was amazing! It filled me with strength and hope. I felt connected to these women through our common bond. I felt, maybe more than ever, that my purpose in surviving will be to serve others. What a fantastic revelation, to feel a calling to fulfill a higher purpose in life! I am somewhat anxious (hopefully I will acquire some patience on this journey, as it is in short supply right now!) about figuring out how to do that, but I think it will be revealed to me in good time.

September 18, 2007

Wow! I have really missed being able to journal. These past few days have been jam-packed with breast cancer events and lots of fun time trying to keep up with Rocco. It has been wonderful to feel up to doing so much, even though afternoon naps are now a must. I have chemo heavy (no ice, no lime, side of steroids and antihistamines and two warm blankets, please) this Thursday, so I am hoping to cram a few more things in before then!

This past Saturday, Joe and I had the honor of attending Serve for the Cure, a high school girl's volleyball tournament at Latin organized by Suzie Pignetti. Suzie is a fellow breast cancer survivor and a real dynamo who has raised thousands of dollars for the cause since her diagnosis and recovery. She found out about me from her son and daughter-in-law, who live in my neighborhood. I had only met Danietta, Suzie's daughter-in-law, a few times and had not yet met her husband or kids before tournament day, so it's amazing that they told Suzie of my story! Suzie donated the proceeds from the money raised at the tournament to Komen on my behalf.

One of the cancer's greatest gifts so far has been to witness this outpouring of love and effort on my behalf from people I don't even know. I was never one to think that people were inherently good hearted. Just watch the news to see bad human behavior or drive in rush hour to see the worst—this means you, guy in the beige SUV, who would not let me merge yesterday despite my blinker and my obviously sickly-looking, balding head! Sure, I thought there were definite good ones among us, but they were the exception rather than the norm. Now, however, I feel differently. The capacity for good must be in us all. Otherwise, how would you explain people like the Pignetti's or the Carson's, or the other people volunteering at the tournament and for Komen who have NO DIRECT CONNECTION to breast cancer?! This generosity of spirit is truly something to celebrate! There are heroes among us and perhaps one in us all.

September 18, 2007

Okay. I am back to relating current events. After a big first half of the day spent outside in this fantastic weather with Mr. Rocco, I was off to a two-hour "Look Good, Feel Better" class at the cancer center run by very nice volunteers with donations from the cosmetic companies! I was not too sure what to expect. Makeup is not really my thing, and I have already decided wigs aren't either. It was really quite interesting and very informative, especially regarding how to minimize your risk of infection from your makeup while your counts are low. I won't bore you with all the details, but ladies, throw out your mascara if it is more than six weeks old!

Being the only one there flaunting my baldness, I became the guinea-pig head for the second half of class: head coverings. The instructor asked who was going to or was already wearing a wig. Everyone's hand went up but mine. She looked at me and said she had me pegged as a non-wig person. What gave it away? My bald head or my righteous studded belt with the huge (everything's bigger in Texas) cross buckle I got while in Houston visiting Mindy? Anyway, I was a good sport (her words) as she put everything from a wig (I looked ridiculous!) to a turban on my head, and the ladies in class "ooh'd" and "ahh'd" like she was doing magic tricks. I, of course, could see what she was doing in a mirror and mainly thought I looked like someone who was bald and was trying to hide it. The one exception was when she wound two shimmery, sequiny scarves on my head. I looked exactly like a fortune teller. Now, she did have a good point when she mentioned that we would all need some good, dressy looks for the holidays. I think I might opt for something in a "dressy" black ball-cap, but who knows?

September 20, 2007

Ahh, the chemo hangover begins. I have to look at the computer with my head slightly turned to the side so I can focus on it. Weird. I got an cocktail of anti-nausea and chemotherapy meds: Benadryl (which is very strong IV and makes me loopy and tired), Decadron (a steroid—maybe I should try out for pro baseball next season), Herceptin (my lifesaving monoclonal antibody), and Taxol. Quite a mix, not too bad. I might be off the journal for a few days while I sleep and deal with my hangover.

Just a quick note to those of you struggling to train (or not training at all) for Komen. My oncology nurse said that a very large study showed that thirty minutes of exercise a day had almost as much of an impact on recurrence rates as did a chemo routine. Wow! Just think what exercise can do for you healthy folks! Get your asses off the couch and get out there!

Sorry for the language, six hours of chemo makes me sassy!

September 21, 2007

So much for sleeping (at night anyway). I have heard a few other chemo patients complaining of this at the infusion center. Apparently, the Decadron is the culprit.

The current chemo physical side effects really are not that bad and are very similar to a case of the flu. It is the mental side effects that are so very difficult for me to deal with. The aches and pains (which are numerous) trick my mind into wondering about whether or not the cancer has spread to other parts of my body. The fact that the entire upper right quadrant of my body hurts in one way or another is very troubling to me! The tumor hurts when it is shrinking, which is very good. But the almost constant pain/ache in my ribs and near my liver is unbelievably distressing! The doctors are not sure what is causing this, and I don't get re-scanned until November. I am struggling mightily not to let this eat away at my mental and emotional fortitude. Speculating on the "what ifs" is like looking into the great abyss. I have to choose to stop letting my mind go in this direction, and I am doing that more frequently now, because it is HELL when I don't.

I read recently in a book that I got at the Komen luncheon that the will to live and the courage and strength to fight are not enough to save your life. YOU HAVE TO BELIEVE THAT YOU WILL LIVE NO MATTER WHAT. I am still struggling with that. I want it more than anything. I know I have the strength and courage to wage this war. BUT HOW DO I ACQUIRE THE BELIEF? My husband has it, my parents have it, JuJu has it, but I am not there yet. I know it takes time, and I know talking about these fears helps, but when will it happen for me? How can I make that so important leap, especially with the constant physical reminders of what might be?

I am not by any means giving up on myself, and I have no plans to wait until my scans come back in November to truly believe. I am working on it now. I am strengthening my will and resolve NOW. It will come in its own time, and that time is drawing near. As Winston Churchill said, "Never, never, never give up."

SEPTEMBER 22, 2007

Well, I had a good night's sleep last night, thank God. That does so much for my attitude. I was quite the grump yesterday, but today is a new day! Thank you to all who sent me messages of inspiration yesterday—they really helped! I am feeling a bit flu-like but went for a walk with Joe around the neighborhood. It did my heart and soul good to see all the pink ribbons. They are very motivating!

A bit of exercise definitely makes me feel better, and I wanted to get outside before the heat and humidity force me in for a few days. Where did our beautiful fall go? I feel like a bird in a gilded cage when the weather drives me in.

SEPTEMBER 24, 2007

Well, we had lots of help this weekend. JuJu had Luca and Gammy and Papa had Rocco. Joe had help from his Uncle Ronnie and from my brother Jeff with projects around the house. They got tons done! I hope it was cathartic for Joe, who has not gotten to do many around-the-house projects he likes because this year has been a mess (kitchen leak and renovation, pregnant wife, cancer diagnosis). He has missed out on his usual guy stuff and has only gone shooting once in the past year or so. He deserves to have some fun!

On another note, it is tough to see how much those around me are sacrificing daily. I see the fatigue on their faces. I sometimes wonder if we will make it to April or May, when I will finally be done with chemo, surgery, and radiation. That seems like so far away. In the meantime, I guess I need to make peace with being so needy. It is just not a role I am very familiar with or like at all but will have to accept to get well. Knowing that I would do the same for others as they are doing for me definitely helps soothe my guilt.

September 25, 2007

*T*rying to do this while Luca is fussing/squirming in my lap ....
I went to a guided imagery class last night. I wasn't sure if I was really feeling up to going, but it definitely helped. I got some great tips on visualization techniques that bridge the gap between the mind and body and have a huge impact on healing and on living.

At one point during the night, we were asked to draw literal or figurative pictures of where we would like to be in six months (duh-cancer free!), where we are now, how we would get there, and what our cancer looks like. Okay, so my last art class was in sixth grade (got an A!), but apparently those skills just don't stick. I just sat for a minute, not sure at all what to draw and wondering how I would pull it off if I knew, while my other experienced classmates immediately began to scribble furiously. Then the final picture just came to me, just as it spontaneously popped into my head a few weeks ago. (Keep in mind that in six months I will just be finishing up chemo and still have a mastectomy, radiation, and nine months of Herceptin immuno-therapy to go.)

My cancer-free place is on top of the Tetons. I can clearly see myself on top, arms stretched to the sky, a 360-degree, transcendental view of me (think of a movie shot where a helicopter camera circles something to catch a complete image), with the high plains and the Elk Refuge in the background. I can see the contrast of the white snow and gray-colored scree (small glacial debris) and the golden hues of the valley below dotted with brown specks (which must be elk and perhaps buffalo). It is real. And while it won't happen in six month's time, it will happen next year. Joe is already working out the details of booking our trip.

September 27, 2007

*O*kay, so I have been a bit grumpy since heavy chemo last week. Right now, I am home alone and reveling in the quiet! I have chemo lite this afternoon. It's no big deal, but I am a bit nervous about seeing Dr. Frenette. The nagging pain in the side of my ribs is now accompanied with a lovely feeling of pressure in my sternum. It kind of hurts a bit to take a big breath, and I'm still struggling with the worries about metastasis. I know it is unlikely with the way the tumor and lymph nodes are shrinking, but dammit, why can't it ache somewhere else in my body! Why does it have to ache around the bad booby? I would love for just my left knee to hurt or maybe even a pinky finger. Somewhere away from the disease site so my mind would not constantly play tricks on me.

I am off to do some meditation/guided imagery to help with these concerns.

SEPTEMBER 29, 2007

Well, I have had some great news to share since my chemo lite appointment on Thursday, but I haven't had a chance to do it until now. We, of course, had our usual litany of questions for Dr. Frenette (he said he has never gotten asked physics, chemistry, and physiology questions in just one office visit before—I just like to make sure he to earned his PhD/MD degrees and didn't just squeak by). I had some major concerns about all the pain around my right breast, ribs, and sternum. He examined me, and we found that the tumor had gone from 9 x 9 cm to 5 x 5 cm! That is almost a two-thirds reduction in size.

We are all very excited! Dr. F also said with that much cancer-cell death going on, he was almost certain that it would cause pain due to inflammation, etc. What great news! He offered to re-scan me now, but after the visit, I opted to wait until my regularly scheduled scans in November. This visit was news that my body is healing, and now my mind can heal some more too! Have a great weekend, everyone!

OCTOBER 1, 2007

I can't sleep. I finally decided to get up since I have been awake since four o'clock in the morning. My body is so incredibly tired (beyond Ironman tired—this is a new level of tired), but I just can't seem to get comfy or let my mind settle down. I'm not really thinking about cancer or anything specific, believe it or not. My body is so tired that I can feel the effort in my arms just from typing. This has been going on for a week or so now, but tonight it is the worst. I tried an Ambien last night, and that did not help at all. So now I am unbelievably tired and feel hungover/fuzzy to boot. Wonderful.

Okay, enough with the complaining. That was pitiful. Get over it, Jen. Nap later.

Let's talk about some good stuff. I can't believe Komen is finally here! I am excited but also a bit nervous too. I know I will want to spend more time with everyone than I will have energy for. Just the thought of it makes me more empathetic with poor Rocco when he is in the middle of doing something really fun and I make him take his afternoon nap or put him down for the evening. Hopefully Joe won't have to drag me off kicking and screaming for my afternoon nap, too.

October 3, 2007

Hope everyone is having a great week and is looking forward to this Friday and Saturday. My whole family is so excited! I can't wait to see everyone and revel in the positive energy not just from our awesome team but from the other survivors and their supporters too! I am so excited but definitely a bit nervous. I have realized this past week that I have a certain amount of gas in my tank and feel great, but then, BAM, I am out of gas and totally pooped. Please forgive me if I can't spend as much time with you all as I would like; I will simply run out of gas at some point and have to rest to recharge my battery, so to speak. I sound like I am married to a mechanic or something, with all these slightly-off car metaphors. Sorry.

I can't wait to see our sea of green and pink and white! Joe had a Go Jen Go flag made, and it looks incredible. We will carry it with us during the 5K walk. I'm excited, but this will be by far the most I will have done in a two-day stretch since starting chemo. I know I will have to pace myself and will need some serious time for naps/quiet time, or I will risk overdoing it, and in my current chemo'd state that might mean getting sick. So, if you see me chatting with someone and notice how tired I look, PLEASE come over and tell me to sit down and shut my yapper!

OCTOBER 3, 2007

his is what I wanted to write yesterday but wasn't able to. I went to my guided imagery class again Monday evening. I changed my centering technique, the time you spend quieting your mind to prepare for the imagery, and it was fabulous. In ten minute's time, I went away from the room I was in to a large place (it made me think of the verse Psalm 118, "I called upon the Lord in distress: the Lord answered me, and set me in a large place …"). I have had this feeling only a few times before. It is really amazing! The lines between my body and my surroundings blur, and I can't tell if I am very large and the center of things, or if I really am not there at all but more of an observer. I can't quite put it to words. It is reminiscent of transcendentalism, but I don't look back down on myself (I may, however, be the "transparent eyeball" of Emerson's that I heard so much about in high school). I am an observer, but I can also act. It is an amazing feeling, and a place where revelations are made. The mind is very powerful! I wish I could go there at will. It is one of things I try to achieve with each session.

I wonder if any of you have had this experience? It is funny how much harder it is for me to train my mind as opposed to my body. But, in order to beat this disease, my mind and my body both have to participate in the battle.

OCTOBER 4, 2007

ust woke up from a little post chemo-lite nap. And I can't believe it, Komen is just two days away! I can't wait to see everyone tomorrow and at the race. It is going to be incredible! I am a bit nervous too, though, since I don't like to be the center of attention. But, as several of you pointed out, there will so much positive energy surrounding me this weekend. And as my friend Brian, who is a bit of a hippie, said to me, "Just surf the waves of love." Coincidentally, I have wanted to learn to surf (not wimpy East Coast surfing but the kind you do in the Pacific with big waves and wet suits) all of my adult life. So, look for me. I'll be the one surfing in a green T-shirt with a big smile on my face.

OCTOBER 8, 2007

*T*he whole race was so inspirational and magical! It started off great when I walked under the overpass and saw our tailgate tents (thanks to the army of people who got that area and all the food and beverages set up!) and all the Go Jen Go shirts. It was early so the light was still soft, and it seemed a bit like a dream. Could all this really be in support of me?

After some encouraging words to those on our team braving the 5K run, Joe and I went to the survivor tent. It was touching to see other women who have each won their fight. I felt strength in their successes. And, by the time we got back to the tailgate area, most of our team had arrived. I was blown away by the sea of green! I can't believe how incredibly lucky I am to have such a large, loving support group. What an amazing feeling to walk with everyone rallying around the Go Jen Go flag! It was one of those magical moments that rank up there with my wedding day and the birth of both of my sons, an event surrounded by an aura of love and an expectation that exceeds anything else. All through the walk, I felt buoyed by our team. I felt the strength and love and determination to win this fight, and I felt it all from you! Not only did our team amaze me, but so did all the participants walking to support others. It made me realize something very important about this disease. Before, when I would hear that cancer affects so many people, I always thought that meant so many people got the disease. But what I now realize is that so many people are moved to do extraordinary things for others because of cancer. This is an incredible gift, and perhaps it is God's way of connecting us to our humanity.

I loved coming back to the tent and talking with everyone afterward. Your presence was such a gift and so inspiring. Thank you all for what you have done for me and my family. I know that is inadequate for all that you have given, but it is truly heartfelt, and I don't think I could say it any other way.

Now that this great event has passed, please continue to keep us and the other women fighting breast cancer in your thoughts and prayers. We have won some very important battles, but the war wages on.

OCTOBER 14, 2007

Well, the past few days have been mentally quite tough. I think it has been a combination of that day-after-Christmas feeling following the end of race weekend, being quite tired from all the festivities/visits, and, of course, heavy-chemo. Good thing Aunt Erin bought us the extra-large boxes of tissues from Costco! This weekend alone would have been worth the cost of membership just in Kleenex! Also, I have been somewhat incommunicado these past few days but am now starting to crawl out of my hole. Please don't fault me for not returning phone calls, saying "hi" if I see you out in the neighborhood, etc. Sometimes I am just a bit too fragile to even open my mouth.

I feel like I am almost done wallowing in my despair. I have tried to shorten the duration of these emotional setbacks when they happen, but they seem to ebb and flow like the tides, and I am tossed about at their mercy until the earth shifts slightly and I am free. Tomorrow is a new day and most certainly will be a brighter one.

OCTOBER 18, 2007

Apparently, my moodiness has been as least in part due to chemo brain. Yesterday morning, I wrote to tell you all that I was doing much better. But the blues must be at least in part to the effects of chemo on my brain, because I forgot to save the entry!

We actually went out for pizza Tuesday night, and it was fantastic to do something so ordinary. We ate outside, and Rocco and I ran around the fountain and laughed and giggled. We also took him to Ben and Jerry's. When we were there, a woman in line noticed my hair (or lack of it) and asked if I was a survivor. We exchanged stories for a minute and said our goodbyes. We were sitting in the store, eating our cones, when the woman walked back in and asked if she could pray for me. I was a bit surprised (BC, before cancer, I would have been very uncomfortable and thought the woman odd), but I said yes. She laid a hand on my shoulder and started praying for my recovery, right there, out loud in the ice cream store. I sat and listened with my eyes closed and felt a stirring in my soul and a warmth in my shoulder where her hand was. I received her love and prayer with an open mind and with hope. I think this is a positive change in me since my diagnosis. Perhaps Jesus, divine physician and healer, visits in mysterious ways. Rocco apparently thought it was rather mysterious too. I did not hear him, as I was focused on the woman's words, but apparently, while he was eating his cone, he kept looking up at the woman and then his Daddy and asking, "Who's that?"

It was a great evening! I have such an appreciation for the little things that I lacked before, and we finally got our money's worth out of Ben and Jerry's!

OCTOBER 20, 2007

What a glorious day! Juju has Luca, and Rocco is with his godparents, who got him all whacked out on chocolate-chip pancakes and then let him skip his nap. He is going to be hell on wheels when he gets home, but I know he had a great day!

Despite the fact that I should stay away from crowds (germs) and Joe is supposed to be resting, we just could not stay in. We went to Keaton's football game for a bit and then went to Trader Joe's, my new favorite store! It was great to be out—mentally rejuvenating! Because Trader Joe's has an incredible selection of organic whole foods AND the prices are good, we bought a bunch of really healthy stuff for me to try to incorporate into my diet (raw seeds, almond milk, stevia, and a few organic prepared foods). I am so excited. The *Crazy Sexy Cancer Tips* book has me delving deeper into the nutrition and healing piece of all this. I am going to check into juicers, wheatgrass/grinders, and raw/organic/whole-foods recipes.

Driving around, we saw people doing the Avon Breast Cancer Walk. We honked and waved at everyone. I considered putting a chair out on Carmel and thanking everyone personally, but it just seemed too emotionally overwhelming at the moment! It was very inspirational! These folks all raised a minimum of $2,000 and then walked thirty miles. WOW! I think this is going to go on my calendar for next October, which is filling up due to Breast Cancer Awareness month. I am really looking forward to being healthy and strong next year, and working my ass off to raise more funds and fun for the cause. Think Pink.

OCTOBER 21, 2007

*T*his morning, Rocco and I had a great walk! I felt pretty good. Taxol gets those lungs burning, though! We came home and put up "spy-webs" and a big scary spider—think of Rocco with his fists clenched and his whole body shaking kind-of-scary. It was great! Then I hopped in the shower and all the other scary stuff popped into my head. (I wish it was something as simple to deal with as a big spider!) The real scary stuff is so frequently with me, lurking just beneath the surface of everything I do. I struggle with the thought of precognition versus fear. Someone wrote on my site weeks ago that you know if it is your time to go. Sometimes I think you do. Is this just fear? There is plenty of it—not really about death itself, rather, fear for those I will leave behind. Or is it precognition? I wonder this often. How do I know?

I think a lot of these thoughts are fueled by the near constant pain in my ribs and chest, and the fact that the damn tumor is still in my breast. Neoadjuvant, chemo before surgery and/or radiation, is tough to deal with sometimes (most women get adjuvant therapy). I know it is for the best, but sometimes I think it fuels my doubts. Lots to think about ....

OCTOBER 25, 2007

*T*hank you, everyone for all the inspiring words, letters, and calls. Every one helps! It helps to hear the perspective of others, even if they have not walked down the same path. And, frequently, something rings so true to my ears that I know the universe intended me to hear it. Wayne Dyer would be so proud of that last statement!

Today, we head off for some lite-chemo and some heavy decisions about my next course of drugs. We are going to go over the pros and cons of the FEC plus Herceptin regimen. It seems like the best choice at the moment, but we need to address that little issue of permanent congestive heart failure as a side effect. Boy, would it be fun to survive cancer but not be able to walk from the bed to the couch without getting winded! Maybe I could get the Ironman people to give me a special circumstances extension to eighteen months on the finish deadline instead of the usual eighteen-hour one.

I am noticing that my cancer humor freaks a few of you out, and you just flat out don't know how to react! See ya later.

October 29, 2007

*A*hhh, I am so glad to be able to sit down and write. These last few days have been a bit nuts, both good and bad. I have quite a bit of catching up to do. Let's start with my oncologist appointment this past Thursday. I had not seen Dr. F in one month (because he was out of town when I would have normally seen him following my last heavy chemo day), which is a very long time considering I only received my diagnosis three months ago! In hindsight, I think the length between appointments really affected my mental state. I need assurance from the big man (talking about Dr. F, not God, but assurance from him is necessary, too!) more than anyone else. After all, he is managing my care. The news from him was good! My tumor is still shrinking, around 3 x 3 cm now! Fantastic! I told him I was still concerned about the rib pain and metastasis. After giving the standard "there are no guarantees" speech, he said he felt confident the scans won't show any metastases. I get re-scanned on November 12 and 14 and will get results with him on that Thursday. I'm still a wee bit nervous about that!

If you are still awake after all that, I'll fill you in on this weekend. We had two Halloween parties, and Big Mama and Big Daddy came to town. Both Rocco-Monkey and Luca-Penguin looked absolutely precious in their Halloween costumes! It was lots of fun, but it totally pooped me out! I go from tired to exhausted (and grumpy) in the blink of an eye. I need one of those shirts that says, "I go from zero to grumpy in six seconds."

Rocco had a blast, even though his nap/sleep times were a bit off due to the festivities and sugar consumption. But yesterday he put the Terrible Twos! We did not help him at all by feeding him chocolate-chip pancakes (a Big Daddy tradition) for breakfast and then double-chocolate cake later. JuJu graciously took both him and Luca last night so Joe and I could get some rest. Thanks, JuJu!

I am very excited about Halloween! Rocco is too! We have the neighborhood party and trick-or-treating still to look forward to! This all works out perfectly with chemo. My next heavy day and last Taxol is Thursday! Talk to you later.

OCTOBER 30, 2007

What a gorgeous fall day. I love the crisp weather and bright blue skies! The contrasts found in nature are what I love about fall. Brilliant skies, bright leaves, cool air—they make me feel alive. Natural contrasts have a deep effect on me. Jackson Hole, which to me is the most mystical, magical place on earth, is full of them. My soul is from there—I knew it the first time I went. It has huge bright or starry skies, sweeping and softly-colored plains dotted with the most fantastic animals (elk, moose, and bison), a meandering, stony river, and a beautiful lake (Jenny Lake, how appropriate) that reflects the gray and white majesty that is the Tetons. Another favorite place of mine, full of such incredible contrast, is the coast of Maine, where our friends the Kelly's (some of you met them at the Komen race) have a house. There you find the deep blue (and very cold) ocean crashing against a brown and rocky coastline with vibrant, green pines. The whole place looks like a postcard or an L.L. Bean catalog cover.

I never really considered how much of an impact contrast has in my life until now. Now that my very life is in peril, I see the impact of contrast everywhere. It both inspires me in nature and challenges me as I move through the highest of highs and the lowest of lows that follow my cancer diagnosis. Mentally, emotionally, and spiritually, the contrast is tough to ride out. But I am realizing this so much better than everything turning to gray and meeting in a blurry middle where I cannot stay present in the moment because of fear for the future. With time and a lot of work (guided imagery especially), I am learning to acknowledge and accept my lows and move on. I still have plenty of work to do, but I have come a long way.

OCTOBER 30, 2007

Apparently, in an effort to experience dramatic highs and lows, my subconscious directed me to eat half of a double-fudge chocolate cake that Big Daddy and Big Mamma left for my birthday. Since my diet has been pretty darn healthy lately, I am sure to be in for a sugar-and-fat roller-coaster ride on this one.

November 1, 2007

Well, we had a big time last night at the Kingswood neighborhood Halloween party and then out trick-or-treating! It was so good to see all the neighbors and thank folks for all they have done for us. Both boys looked precious, and Rocco had a blast! He was so cute and well-mannered while trick-or-treating. When we came home, he did laps around the den and kitchen due to his sugar high. It was great.

I just got home from my very last round of Taxol! Yeah! It did me lots of good, but I am glad to get the first milestone out of the way. I figure it is about the same as getting out of the water after completing the more than two-mile swim in the Ironman. I still have the bike and run to go, but I'm feeling good and am confident I can finish.

Thanks, Dad, not only for taking me but for sitting there with me for hours on end and then sitting in rush hour to drive all the way back to the lake. Thanks to Gammy for taking both boys up there for the next few days as I move through my flu and migraine phase. And another thanks to JuJu for keeping sweet baby Luca for most of this past week.

Time to go lie down.

November 2, 2007

Well, I managed to sleep until five o'clock in the morning. That's not bad considering I never sleep well after the Decadron they give me with heavy chemo. But I'm fighting a headache, grumpiness, weepiness, and the need to be alone while trying not to get too depressed about being by myself. Although I am responding well to the chemo, I am struggling with the bleak nature of my diagnosis. It's very worrisome that the type of cancer I have is "aggressive," likes to spread (metastasize), and is more likely to reoccur. I overheard two other women in chemo yesterday who are dealing with metastases (stage 4 of 4). Scary! The good news is that one of them has had bone metastases for five years now, and it is not spreading. But it's still a very scary thought for someone who would like to live another forty years. I haven't even reached my half-way point yet! I want to be around to see my boys go to high school and college and start dating and get married. And I hope to be around for grandkids, too. I just feel I have so much left to do and desperately hope I am around to do it.

NOVEMBER 5, 2007

What a weekend. I wish I could say it was a good one, but it was tough (it still is tough)! It is a bit ironic that I look forward to the heavy chemo to kill more of the cancer, but my mental state takes a nosedive following the heavy doses. I have heard from other survivors that this is common and is probably more of a drug side effect than anything else. Still, it stinks.

I am REALLY having a tough time right now, and all this crying is hell on my eyelashes, which are falling out at an alarming rate! I guess it all boils down to my upcoming bone scans next Monday, and MRI and CT scans on Wednesday. Thank God I will meet with Dr. Frenette next Thursday to get the results back. My problem with staying positive is the rib/side pain. Without it I feel like I would be very optimistic!

I struggle constantly with the implications of that. On one hand, the pain could have saved (or at least extended) my life by getting me to the doctor in the first place, but on the other hand, it could mean something much more ominous, like metastasis. It could mean a whole lot less time on this planet than I want.

To ease my mind, I went back and listened to the taped meetings of my last appointment with my surgeon and the last two with Dr. Frenette. What a roller-coaster ride! The great news is that I am responding so well to chemo. The big, terrifying question is: what if the blips that showed up on my lung, liver, and bone (which were "probably not metastatic") really are disease? It did not help that I overheard two breast cancer patients in chemo talking about how they were now in stage 4, which means metastasis to brain, liver, lung, or bone.

According to my doctors, I am getting the most aggressive course of therapy now, and "do we really want to do more extensive testing" to determine if it is in those places when "it would not change my treatment?" What a thing to ponder! Do we want to proceed thinking I am doing well, or do we want to find out more conclusively where the disease is and potentially wreck my sense of hope and optimism?

Why are the average life expectancies so low with stage 4 (two to five years)? Does the chemo just not work in those places? Is the most you can hope for stopping the spread of the disease rather than destroying it? I know there are miraculous recoveries from stage 4 out there. What would that mean for the quality of time I would most likely have left? Granted, I know I am not your typical breast cancer patient, and that survival statistics are just that and don't apply to me as an individual, BUT I am still scared shitless at the possibility of it lurking in there somewhere really bad.

Hopefully I will look back on these thoughts at the end of next week and feel such a sense of gratitude and relief that they are behind me. In the meantime, I am just going to do my best to get through this rough patch. It's time to pull myself up by my bootstraps (what does that really even mean? I picture a solider stuck in the mire and blood on the battlefield, struggling to move onward despite horrifying circumstances—or am I remembering the expression wrong?) Digression must be my middle name! And the chemo brain doesn't help one bit!

Well, this has been quite cathartic. Thanks for listening. I think I am done with the "poor me" shit (sorry, Mom and JuJu!) for now. Time to get back to fighting!

November 6, 2007

Thank you all for such inspiring comments when I am struggling! All the different perspectives are so helpful! I feel better than I have in days, although I am still worried about next week's scans. I will be a happy camper when I get good news about the scans next Thursday.

I had an echocardiogram today, and it looks good. So far, my ticker is holding up well to the chemo and is in good shape to start the new drug regimen. I actually knew the cardiologist from my old YMCA days and got to speak to him for like twenty minutes. His wife's family has history with the disease, and he was so informative and compassionate. It really helped settle me down and give me hope.

November 9, 2007

I'm feeling better still. I had some very powerful images come to me while meditating during Herceptin yesterday. I saw Yellowstone through the eyes of an eagle and flew until I came to a huge valley with bison running all through it. It may have been a valley I had the privilege to see in the heart of winter on a snowmobile trip that Joe and I took a few years ago. Yesterday, it was not snow covered but mellowed and yellow like late fall. The bison were moving through the short grass, grazing and rutting. Then

I was no longer the eagle but an incredibly strong, alpha bison running through the valley. I could feel my incredible power, and a connection to time passed; I was in the present and the future. I felt empowered and totally connected to the universe. It was unreal. I must have some Native American in me somewhere, because it seemed so much like what I imagined they must experience on a vision quest. It might bring to mind tacky dream-catcher mirror ornaments and black-velvet paintings with wolves on them when I say that, but it was anything but cheesy!

Anyway, my spirits have been lifted since my time in the valley yesterday. I feel like I have seen the powerful connection I have to the universe and that I am not due to leave it anytime soon. When I can access that purity of existence, which is sometimes a bit hard to do when running about the day to day business of things, I almost feel like I can say with certainty how long I will live, and for those of you wondering how long, I won't leave this body for many, many years from now.

November 11, 2007

It's been kind of a crazy weekend. Right now, I'm feeling calm and at peace with this week's scans even though some anxiety creeps in from time to time. Joe says he is not worried but has been out of sorts for a while now. Tomorrow is the bone scan. I will have the results on Tuesday. I'm going to try to stay busy and distracted until all the results are in on Thursday. This week will be more difficult than usual for everyone.

Just to share a little good news: I was out walking Baby Luca in the neighborhood today and saw a crow. My friend Brian revealed to me years ago that the crow was my totem—yes, I thought the same thing. A crow? How unglamorous. But crows are resourceful, determined, and smart. In my mind I asked the crow if he had anything to tell me, and I thought he said, "Your scans will be okay." I walked on and thought, "Well that was silly. I just made all that up." But then I looked down, and someone had spray-painted "OK" in orange paint (on Tottenham in front of the new construction, for those of you who live in Kingswood and want to look) right on the road under my feet. Hmm. That lends itself to the saying that "coincidences are God's way of letting us know He exists." Off to the edge again ....

November 12, 2007

Well, one scan down. You have got love getting injected with solution that comes in a solid lead container! The tech ("I'm not a radiologist") said he did not see anything. We will get the official word tomorrow, but I feel pretty good about it! Please keep praying hard until Thursday—I know I will!

November 13, 2007

Yahoo! Just got the call from Terry, my oncology RN, and the bone scan is clean! She said all they saw on the bone scan was bones! YES!

One down, two (brain MRI and CT scans) to go. Tomorrow is scan day, and Thursday we see Dr. Frenette for results and meet with Terry about the new drugs. Please keep praying hard, it is working!

Oh, other good news today, too! Baby Luca no longer has to wear his helmet! He looks so handsome (like a mini Joe) and has reddish hair now.

Today is the day the Lord hath made, rejoice in it!

November 15, 2007

WE GOT GREAT NEWS! THE SCANS ARE CLEAN! THANK GOD! And thank you all for all your help and prayers, they really do make a difference!

I was starting to think that my appointment today would never come. I could see the worry on Joe's face too when we met in the doctor's office lobby. The nurse led us back to our usual exam room. When we were waiting for Dr. Frenette, I noticed a calendar on the wall and went over to look at the photo because the image looked familiar. I assume it has always been there, but the previous pictures just did not draw my eye. The picture was a close-up view of none other than Grand Teton, taken from a vantage point that I had never seen before (for the new folks—I sit at the base of this mountain during my guided imagery, and reaching the summit represents to me becoming cancer free, which I will be next August when Joe and I do a four-day guided expedition to the top). I told Joe that it was definitely a good sign, and it was! The spot on the lung: gone; cysts in the liver: the same (they don't think they are cancer, and apparently 25 percent of the healthy adult population has them for some reason); brain: small but clear. Dr. F said he was 99 percent certain the rib pain was not caused by cancer. He's not sure what's causing it, "but it's not caused by cancer." WHEW!

I had been trying to distance myself from the reality of what today might hold, even though I feel like I know my expiration date now from meditation, so I was immensely relieved. The news is still sinking in slowly, though. I think my brain has shut down a bit (I've had a hard time meditating the past few days, among other things), but the joy will and is building over time. Time to seize the day again! Tomorrow, Joe and I are going to seize the lobster (a healthy seafood choice—wild-caught and antibiotic and hormone free!) at a great restaurant thanks to mom and dad. Yum!

NOVEMBER 20, 2007

Well, it has been a few days since our great news. It has finally sunk in, and what a difference it makes in each day. I finally feel like I can live instead of just going through the motions. It has taken a few days for this transformation to take place. I am not sure exactly what happened. I expected to be instantly elated. On one level I was (and unbelievably relieved), but I think my brain was so tired from all the meditation, imagery, prayers, and stress that it has taken a while for me to recover. I think I had detached from myself a bit, too, just in case we got bad news. I feel like I have been slowly recovering, like after a really big workout, and I have been easing back into life. I have been struggling a bit with my meditation/ imagery, and after talking with the instructor, I have decided to take a few days off. I am ready to get back out there and experience all the joy life has to offer.

Have a Happy Thanksgiving. I know I will.

NOVEMBER 24, 2007

Hope everyone had a happy Thanksgiving with family and friends, and found some good bargains, too! We had a wonderful day at my parents' house! It was so good to have a normal holiday, enjoying everyone's company and the good food.

Well, I had my first round of FEC (5FU, Epirubicin and Cytoxan) plus Herceptin yesterday. My appointment was not until 1:30 p.m., but due to the crowds, there was quite a wait. When they took me back to the infusion room, they brought me over to a chair in the corner right by the pharmacy. I had sat there before, and it is usually too loud to sleep. I was about to ask for the one other available seat that I saw (I'm high maintenance) when I noticed that the girl next to me looked to be about my age (on my regular day, there is no one my age), and her husband even looked like Joe but with hair. I asked them if it had been loud, and they said no. If cancer has taught me anything so far, it is to be open to possibilities, so I considered that maybe I was meant to sit next to these strangers.

We struck up a conversation shortly after I was seated and while they were poking me (three tries again, third week in a row, yuck!) to start the IV line. Turns out they are really wonderful people with such a similar story. She is three years younger than me, and they (protecting privacy) have a two-year-old son and a thirteen-week-old son. She was diagnosed with the same type of breast cancer that I have (different stage though), but she had only been breastfeeding her second son for five weeks at the time. As we talked, we found out we have quite a bit in common. It was so refreshing (and surprising and also sad) to find another local couple dealing with such a similar situation. To paraphrase that quote I mentioned in an earlier entry, "Coincidences are God's way of letting us know he is present." I think we will have a lot to offer each other as we wage similar battles against this disease. We exchanged contact information, and I am really looking forward to staying in touch!

November 25, 2007

Well, I am surprised I managed to get that much written yesterday. My mind is a bit fuzzy, and I am having to do that look-at-the-computer-sideways thing. The FEC combo seems to be quite a bit stronger than my previous Taxol. I generally felt good until around eight or nine last night when the nausea hit. I fought it off and did not get sick, but it was tough! I think it was the new drug cocktail combined with the large slice of pumpkin pie I ate. The pie tasted good and seemed so soothing at the time, and what's a holiday if you can't have pie! Hopefully I won't have any (or many) more nights sleeping with a cold washcloth on my head, the window open, saltines and water beside me, and the trashcan strategically placed on the floor. It was an eye opener. I will have to be much more careful with what I eat and do for the next week or two (or maybe for the next three rounds) until I learn what to expect from these drugs. Ahh, live and learn. At least today I have some great football to watch while I am parked on the couch.

Go Dawgs!! Go Wildcats!

November 27, 2007

*C*aution: this excerpt contains whiny material and is currently unrated by the Motion Picture Association of America (do you see what this new chemo has done to my brain?)

I'm baaack (sort of). I think I am over the worst of it now. It was an all-out mental battle not to give in to the nausea, but I won (with the ongoing help of lots of meds)! I figured it would not help my body at all to actually get sick, so I really focused on getting past the waves of nausea. I managed to sink rather than swim. This new chemo cocktail was nothing like chemo-lite (tall glass, twist of lime). It was more like a big plastic tumbler of hunch punch (same color, too), full of fruit soaked in grain alcohol. I mean, it tastes okay and will definitely get you through football season, but, damn, it packs a wallop for a few days after! I was feeling so bad that I was actually dreaming of eating something greasy from Taco Bell (must be that football season factor again—Go Dawgs!). I haven't even looked at a vitamin, fruit, or veggie since Thanksgiving. I haven't been moving much further than my bed or the couch, and that does not jive with my usual routine at all.

Rocco has noticed this. It seemed like the worse I felt, the more he wanted ONLY his mama (Luca, thank goodness, is too young to notice). I have comforted and played with him as much as I have been able, but it has been less than both of us want. I am tired of life passing me by while I lie around sick. I want to be a mother to my sons and a wife to my husband. I want to be the daughter, daughter-in-law, sister, and friend that I am supposed to be. I am tired of being on the sidelines in my own life (especially while everyone around me scrambles to pick up my slack). I want to participate. The holidays just make it more tough. There's lots of fun to be had but not too much by me. Heck, I am even sorry that I won't be out there fighting the crowds for parking spaces and gifts. What a pity party I am having—

sorry I forgot to mention what type of party it was on the invitation! I know, I know. I need to focus on long-term gains vs. short-term losses, but sometimes it is so hard to do just that.

Okay, I have whined enough (for now). I am going to get back out there and start participating in my life again, bit by bit. I'm sure the couch will be a frequent stopping point, but every journey begins with the first step.

November 27, 2007

Oh, I forgot to whine about one thing … my body is turning to mush. All the muscles are going bye-bye. This better be a temporary thing, or I am going to be really pissed. I'm already walking around with no eyebrows, eyelashes, or head hair, but I still have hair on my arms—God really has a sense of humor! The less muscular thighs might be kind of nice (I can fit much better in regular jeans now), but I want back my abs and upper body, and preferably before swimsuit season next year. I still haven't worked out the issue of how to wear a bikini with just one boob though. Lots to think about there!

November 29, 2007

Okay, today we are off to our first post-FEC meeting with Dr. Frenette. I am a bit nervous to see how he thinks I am doing. I am feeling better each day but have been having a few, odd, weak/fluttery feelings in my chest. I hope it is low blood sugar or just how this chemo plays out. I am a wee bit concerned that it is affecting my heart. I see the heart failure specialist tomorrow morning so he can monitor any changes in cardiac function, and they are going to put me on beta blockers to hopefully prevent any heart damage before it starts. I'm also going to get Dr. Frenette's latest estimate on the tumor size. Hopefully he will give me another "A" on my exam!

Next week, we are off to Duke (unless we can't get all the medical records together in time for them) to get a second surgical opinion. I'm quite happy with the surgical oncologist here, but we're just exhausting every option.

Good luck at the malls!

DECEMBER 1, 2007

ood luck everyone who is getting ready to brave the depraved masses and go holiday shopping. I envy and pity you. Godspeed, and may the Force be with you.

I have a bit of updating to do ... On Thursday we met with Dr. Frenette and thoroughly discussed all my concerns with this new, kick-ass chemo cocktail. It seems like I am on track. I asked him to measure the size of the tumor (I am a bit of a high-maintenance patient, asking millions of questions and needing a fair amount of hand holding—it doesn't matter how everyone else tells me I am doing, I need to hear directly from the mouth of my oncologist!), and he measured it at 2 x 2.5 cm! This is down from 9 x 9 cm! He also said that it is impossible (prior to doing the mastectomy and subsequent pathology) to tell how much of that remaining size is actually cancer and how much is other tumor stuff, scarring, debris ... WOW! Thank you for all your help and prayers! THEY ARE MAKING A HUGE DIFFERENCE!

On Friday we saw my other favorite, Dr. Frank. He's very bright and compassionate. He is a cardiologist that specializes in heart failure (unfortunately, he sees a lot of women who fall in this category due to receiving chemo for breast cancer, but of course, 98 or 99 percent of them are much older than me). He gave my ticker a thorough going over, and it seems like my previous Ironman level of fitness and my above-average level of fitness in general (even despite being pregnant or breastfeeding for something like twenty-two of the last twenty-eight months prior to my diagnosis) is a huge factor in my favor! My heart currently looks good, and we are going to start a beta blocker to prophylactically keep it that way, as well as do some sort of very in-depth echo. When I asked about what symptoms to look out for to know if I had the beginnings of congestive heart failure, he rattled off a few. Thank goodness they are starting me on this medicine, because all the symptoms mimic symptoms commonly experienced while on chemo. The medication should keep me from worrying myself to death.

So, all in all, we had a couple of good visits. I am looking forward to meeting the doctor at Duke on Tuesday. She is a highly recommended surgical guru, and I can't wait to ask her a million questions too.

December 5, 2007

Well, we got back from Duke late last night. I faired pretty well with the trip despite going to the doctor for a sinus infection on Monday afternoon (just what I needed—more medicine to take). We had the last appointment of the day at 4:00 p.m. and did not get seen until almost six o'clock in the evening. It was a bit reminiscent of the evening we sat waiting in the surgeon's office for about the same length of time (an eternity) to find out my initial diagnosis. It brought back some very stressful memories, but Dr. Wilke was worth the wait! It was really refreshing to me to see a female surgeon, and she had a great bedside manner. She answered my millions of questions, provided information on some other options not available here in Charlotte, and just gave me a good feeling. Basically, she reinforced what we had been told by the surgeon here. I will have to think and pray long and hard about who to use.

The only distressing news we got was about HER2/neu cancer in particular. Joe and I both know it has a greater chance of returning than the more common kind of breast cancer, but we found out it has an ability to hide in the brain. This is scary because Herceptin and chemo (like most drugs) do not cross the blood-brain barrier. They don't routinely scan for mets (metastases) to the brain because if it goes there, it is not treatable. It doesn't go there often, thank God. If it does, it is likely to happen in the first two years following treatment. I don't know if my likelihood of a recurrence is greater because I was diagnosed at such an advanced stage, or if that does not make a difference. Either way, I am nervous about facing this news (had purposefully stuck my head in the sand whenever this issue came up, but my head is out the sand now), even though I guess it is not really "news" at all. Joe and I learned this painful truth about a cancer diagnosis a long time ago.

Oh well, better go. Luca is crying to be picked up, and Rocco is running around like a maniac.

December 6, 2007

I think I miss the catharsis of the group and the one-on-one counseling I get every other week. I did not go yesterday because I was so tired from our Duke trip, and because I wanted to spend time with Rocco and my parents. I am all weepy now—can't seem to get the brain-mets possibility out of my head. I'm back to the old struggles of precognition and fear. I spent the early morning looking at oncology-journal abstracts, trying to glean more info about my prognosis. Not sure if I even want to know. Found out that there are co-morbidity factors (things you don't hear or even know about, like EGRF, unless you are a researcher or a medical oncologist) that show a more negative prognosis if present. I wonder if they are mentioned in my pathology report. Should I go dig it out of the closet?

I think this is another case of the dish running away with the spoon. That is, my brain trying to piece together data that I don't fully understand (who would without a PhD?) and creating a scary, worst-case scenario. I learned that this is called catastrophizing (try to say that three times fast), and I am quite good at it. It has been something I am working on minimizing, but, obviously, I still have some room for improvement. But the reality is, my type (lucky me) of breast cancer is more aggressive and more likely than any other kind to come back in the brain. If and when this happens, it seems you are SOL. I find the possibility of going through all this (chemo, mastectomy, radiation ...) only to succumb to brain mets in a year or two VERY scary. It leads me down that dark path where I worry so much about what would happen to Joe and the boys if I wasn't around. It is truly an awful place to go.

Acknowledging and accepting these fears is part of my recovery. I don't want to panic every time I have a headache or blurry vision during the next two years. I don't want to feel that fear, dark and sinister, lurking at the edge of my mind, or feel its presence like a chasm, threatening to swallow me whole. I will choose not to dwell on this. I just need a while to get it out of my system.

DECEMBER 10, 2007

am stressed. I have so much to do! I am so behind in everything. My body is tired, and my brain is not working all that well. I can't even seem to type correctly or find the words I want to say. To top it off, there are only two shopping days left until Christmas. Oh wait, I mean heavy chemo, which may as well be 'til Christmas. A few brave souls have graciously offered to shop for me. That is wonderful, but I don't seem to be able to figure out what to get anyone (except Rocco—he pours over the toy catalogs every night). I'm no oracle, but I don't see any bright gift ideas in my immediate future.

46 Jennifer Burnette Pagani

It is hard not to feel the holiday stresses and get caught up in the secular part of the season. I can't help but feel a bit sad about missing the hubbub: shopping, parties, baking ... I keep waiting for a moment of clarity, when I realize how silly I am being and just let go and focus on being happy to be alive and kicking and thankful to God for all he has given me.

My brain is totally fogged over. I think it is time to go.

December 11, 2007

*T*hank you, everyone, for helping me put my stress in perspective! Also, thanks for all the offers of help with shopping and baking. I will take some of you up on it. But this morning, Mom, Luca, and I went out to Kohl's and did some power shopping. Got lots checked off the list. I had a brief shopping fix and now have had enough of the holiday rush to fill my needs. All I have to do is stop watching the Food Network so I don't feel bad about all the tasty things I am not going to make this year. Last year I made three things from three different shows, and none of them tasted that good—I guess my talents lay elsewhere. Nothing like TV to make you feel inadequate, especially when under the influence of chemo!

Off to count my blessings. I hope Santa puts health, peace, and love in my stocking this year.

December 13, 2007

*W*ell, the big day has finally arrived. I am awaiting chemo with my usual mix of dread and anticipation. I still want the juice to kick some cancer ass, but I really hope they can find a vein! Apparently, I was a hard stick before all this started, and now things are much worse. The two best nurses in the place (and believe me, onco nurses are supposed to be the best) are sticking me several times and then fishing around with each stick. The actual stick is nothing, but the veins now hurt! They hurt unlike anything else and are constantly sore. It doesn't help at all that they are limited to my left forearm and hand. I have gone this far without a port, and I pray that I can make it through the next three heavy chemos without having to get a line put in. Of course, I am not looking forward to the regular feel-like-crap side effects either.

Okay, done whining. Pray for one stick, no bruising or pain while getting the IV, no infiltrating, manageable side effects and, of course, LOTS of dead cancer cells (if any are still left).

Seize your day!

DECEMBER 14, 2007

It was a bit of a long night. The nausea hit about an hour and a half after getting home. I tossed and turned all night with a wet cloth on my head, an antiemetic (a don't throw up pill) in my system, and bedside trashcan. Yuck! Definitely not feeling too hot. I also have some other side effects that are all in all making me feel pretty crappy.

The good news is they did manage to stick me only once. It took two nurses and lots of poking around while they were in there, but it was only one spot they bothered as opposed to several. We did have a bit of a concern though. It seems my labs came back with low WBCs, and the nurse had to go ask Dr. Frenette if I could get chemo or not. He said yes, and thank God, because I was a bit nervous waiting! I just have to go back today to get a shot of Neulasta (around $1,800 per single shot!), which will stimulate my big bones (think sternum, hips, and thigh bones) to go into overdrive and make new cells. The most common side effect is bone pain for a few days. It should be manageable but will naturally hit as my other symptoms are ramping up. My forecast for Sunday and Monday is a bit gloomy, but at least the weather is changing for the better—I know some of you Northern transplants don't agree! I can't wait to get over this hump!

Enjoy all the parties out there this weekend! It is prime party time. Have a drink or two for me, maybe something with vodka or Jack Daniels—I'll have the "hangover" for you! It's a win-win!

DECEMBER 16, 2007

Time has slowed down so much. Each second is stretching out to what seems like an eternity. I have doors shut, blinds down, and ticking clocks unplugged as I try to get past this unpleasantness. This is definitely the worst I have felt yet (apparently, lots of you took me up on my hangover offer!). I'm really struggling with the mental impact of the drugs too; my head is messed up. I just want time to pass. TV is no help, and I can't read. I'm just sitting around waiting to feel better and thinking about how bad I really do feel.

It's time to snap out of it, as much as I can, that is. I'm off to the basement to meditate and get my mind in a positive place. Then I'll take a bit of a rest and am going to do a "workout." I need to work these chemicals out of my body.

I was a weepy mess yesterday (poor Joe!) and noticed my tears tasted terrible. There's nothing like generating your own acid rain (so much for reducing my carbon imprint). I need to get outside and away from the sofa and bed, but I'm not sure if I can take this wind or the bright sun. I will figure something out. And I will be getting better. Maybe one more day in "the suck," and I should be crawling back out. I can hang tough. I have lots to look forward to!

December 17, 2007

Well, the past few days have been rough. The impact these drugs are having on my mental state cannot be understated. It totally changes the way I think. It warps my thoughts and keeps me dark. It is like living inside another head. And even though I know this happens each time I have heavy chemo, it is still frightening, since I don't seem to be able to stop it. It has also gotten worse, and I can't tell if it is the new drugs, the cumulative effect of all this stuff on my body, or both.

The good news, though, is that I see light on the other end of the tunnel now! My ten-mile trainer ride, mediation, and shower (I kept wondering what that smell was) had a huge impact. Joe and I actually spent some time, just the two of us, wrapping gifts last night. It was great! It took my mind off of things. And, much to my surprise (and probably Martha Stewart's dismay), it did not matter that we ran out of tissue paper, labels, and gift boxes, or that the presents were all wrapped (very imprecisely) in the same (cheap) paper. That is not the important part of Christmas anyway! I did manage, though, with Joe's close supervision, to get the right labels on the right gifts (another Christmas miracle).

Although we miss them terribly, it is a huge help to have a few nights away from the boys. I am not sure if keeping Rocco around until Sunday morning was a good idea or not. Trying to act like I felt well and play some with him pooped me out more and also got me off my healing routine (mediation, workout, shower), which right now is my saving grace. It is just so hard to be without the boys, especially when I am alone ....

Today, I don't have any appointments, and the boys won't be here until after nap time. I plan on going back to bed (I've been up since 5:30 a.m. and can really feel it!) and running through my whole healing routine again. To the grandparents, aunts/uncles, and friends who make all this possible for me, thank you! We love you so much! May God return your kindness and love a thousand times!

And I would like to thank everyone for your kind actions and loving prayers. Please pray that my echocardiogram tomorrow will go well and not show any damage from these new, heavier drugs.

DECEMBER 19, 2007

s anyone out there? Granted, it is 4:30 a.m., but still ....

The Good News: my echo was in good shape yesterday. I was worried about it a bit since I have been having some cardiac symptoms, but they seem to be chemo side effects rather than heart damage. Whew! Thanks for all the prayers!

The Bad (Not really, but the movie title already stuck) News: I am still not feeling too hot. I'm still shaky, very tired, and nauseous, and I'm having some GI problems.

The UGLY: I'm not sleeping well at all! I can't nap either. It's insanely frustrating because it is only compounding my chemo symptoms! I am using a humidifier, sound maker (waves), and a draft buster in front of the bedroom door, and I still wake up EVERY time the baby or Rocco makes a sound. I lay awake for hours trying to sleep and thinking about how bad all the not sleeping is on me, especially now. The last time I had a truly restful nap was ten days ago, which is not at all good on chemo! I can't remember the last time I had a full night's sleep. I took my usual Ativan last night and, out of desperation, an Ambien too. I slept from 10:00 p.m. to 3:00 a.m. *That sucks!* Especially when I know the baby will start his waking-up noises in another hour and fifteen minutes, and I am not even tired (well, I am completely exhausted, just not sleepy). There will be no quiet time here today, at least not the kind I seem to require to sleep lately. A nap is doubtful. Not sure what to do if this continues ... I am getting *desperate!*

December 21, 2007

Yesterday was a strange day. The oncology waiting room was a ghost town. I was expecting a pre-Christmas rush, but it was quite the opposite. I saw Dr. Frenette before chemo-lite (no lime this time, stomach has been very touch and go) and found out that he thinks I should only do one more round of chemo! I thought I was due a "bonus" (since we switched protocols after one round of AC, I'll spare you all the rest of the treatment details, it is quite complicated and boring) ninth round, but he thought otherwise. It seems all the research is done using eight rounds, and since we are quite concerned about damaging my ticker, we aren't going to boldly go where no patient has gone before (even though normally I am up for a good challenge). He seemed really surprised that I didn't argue for one last blast. I asked a few questions and then was in total agreement with him. Joe and I both feel really good about it.

After that surprise, I went to the infusion room expecting a crowd there for sure. I thought it would be packed, IV pole to IV pole, with holiday cheer, but again, it was almost totally empty. My usual RN was in a meeting, so I fully expected to get stuck forty-seven times instead of just three. The new gal (actually a seasoned veteran but new to my veins) got in on the first try without even poking around (okay, just a teeny bit)! Things were getting stranger yet.

I sent Joe back to work and settled in to some guided imagery on my iPod. A bit later, a very loud voice woke me up. It was this very strange, older couple who come every week. I noticed them a long time ago because they have no inside voices, despite being elbow to IV pole with lots of people who do not feel well. They drive in from the hills somewhere, Gaston County maybe? Picture a very short man in his seventies shaped exactly like Humpty Dumpty with a mild bald spot and very dramatic "wings" (yes, like Farah) meticulously combed and hair-sprayed at an angle up and over his ears, kind of like Paulie on the Sopranos but with salt and pepper coloring instead of skunk stripes. His wife, also short, has huge eyeglasses and a very big bouffant hairdo. She obviously does not want to be out-beautied by her husband.

So anyway, I open my eyes to see them walk toward me. This in itself was alarming because they are too loud to be anywhere near, and she actually has a ventriloquist doll dressed like Mrs. Claus on her arm, which is very creepy and even scarier when awakened from a trance-like state while receiving chemo. The doll (who was even louder than Mrs. Bouffant) wished me a Merry Christmas, and they both looked expectantly at me while I mumbled and smiled a response. I did not want to encourage a potentially long winded, deafening, and unescapable conversation. I know I had the deer-in-the-headlights look. Mrs. Bouffant's lips were moving the whole time, and I must have looked confused enough for them to move on. The husband and wife went around spreading cheer (I could tell they were disappointed by the turnout, too) and worked the room in their unbelievable loud but friendly way. Everyone else seem genuinely amused by the shenanigans. I was glad for the seasonal merriment (I had expected some) but could not get rid of the feeling that I had just seen Peggy Hill, from the *King of the Hill* cartoon, in the flesh.

Did all this actually happen? I have no witnesses to say it did. But, if I wasn't dreaming, I just got one less round of chemo for Christmas.

Merry Christmas, everyone!

Peace and health.

December 27, 2007

What a great Christmas week we've had! It was wonderful to spend so much time with family (really!), and Rocco was so much fun to watch! He was so excited about Santa and then could not believe it when he got to open gifts three different times. Luca got a third tooth and has really started to crawl. How exciting! It is fun to watch him scooting all over the floor, trying to grab all of his and his brother's new toys.

Thank you again, everyone, for all you do and have done for us! We have really come a long way from a few months ago. We offer our thanks to God every day.

December 31, 2007

Finally, 2007 is drawing to a close. What a year. My initial thoughts were *good riddance, this year sucked.* We had a house flood and five months of restoration, the death of our boxer, Tiger (my very first baby), semi-bed rest during the last few months of my pregnancy, and then of course the stage 3 breast cancer diagnosis. In some ways I am so glad it is finally over! But, the more I thought about the year, the more I realized some incredible things happened too. We now have Luca—our beautiful, wonderful, curious, and very active boy (and thank God, a great eater and sleeper!). And Rocco is doing great (despite the two-year-old antics).

And, we found out that I have cancer. I mean, thank God we found out! God has given us a chance to beat it before it could beat me. In some ways the cancer diagnosis has been great (very few things can cause such introspective and existential examination). I see with more clarity now just how important all of you, our family and friends, are to us. I am coming to understand, really KNOW, what is truly important. And I am learning from this experience all the time.

2008 is a new year. I intend on looking forward rather than back. Only one round of chemo left (this Thursday), surgery in early February, then radiation, and I am done (well, I will have Herceptin every third week through August—but that is nothing!) Let's hope and pray that I will be done FOREVER with the disease. I will, however, have the lessons it is teaching me for the rest of my life.

Make the most of your year. You all deserve it!

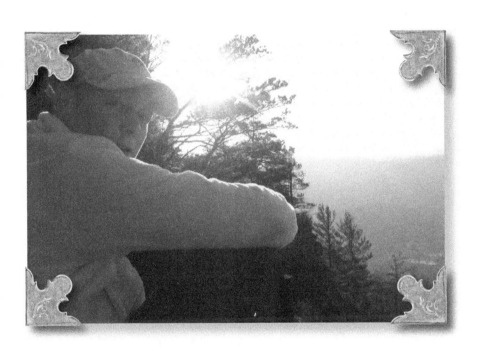

2 0 0 8

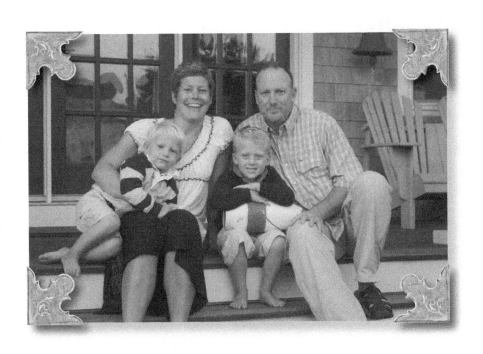

January 3, 2008

Wow! I can hardly believe today is my very last heavy chemo! What a long, strange trip it's been (and it ain't over yet). These last six months have managed to both drag out and fly by at the same time.

I am feeling a mixture of excitement, dread, and fear. The excitement part is obvious, but I am dreading the next few very dark, sleepless days ahead. And the fear, well, from what I hear from other survivors and counselors, it is a very natural part of ending this part of treatment. Right now, my fear stems from those terrible "what ifs." What if the chemo did not get all the cancer and after my mastectomy they find out that I have positive nodes? What then? What if all these headaches (and a number of other symptoms I am having) mean the cancer is in my brain? What if the cancer starts to grow again while I am awaiting surgery?

So many scary things keep creeping into my brain. I am trying to focus on the positive (there are lots of positives!), but it is tough. The really hard part is knowing that over the next few days my mental status (and physical, too, although that bothers me to a lesser degree) will be taking a nose dive. It reminds me of the lyrics to a Stone Temple Pilots (I think) song "I Fell on Black Days." That is what makes these particular drugs so hard on me—they totally screw up my thinking. And knowing that is about to start is never easy to deal with ....

Okay, enough whining! Please pray for me. I need a bit of help to get past this last blast and lots of prayers to make sure ALL the cancer is GONE! In the meantime, I am going to try and focus on Jeremiah 30:17 "For I will restore health to you ... says the Lord."

January 7, 2008

Well, I have been out of the loop since Thursday, but I got the last chemo under my belt! It was surprisingly bittersweet. There were many tears as I was leaving. I felt like I had a river to cry. I was overwhelmed by mixed emotions and a huge sense of relief tinged with some fear. Fear that maybe only others who have walked down this same path can truly appreciate. Fear that maybe some cancer is still there and knowing there is no more chemo to fight it (yes—I know I still have surgery and radiation, but they are backup defense measures, not offensive ones), fear of not seeing my medical oncologist weekly, just plain fear ....

Friday and Saturday weren't too bad, definitely not the insane rollercoaster of emotions that I was on after the seventh round. On Sunday I woke up a bit apprehensive because it is the first day after my chemo-specific anti-nausea meds wear off. I felt good, slept well, and was going to get to see the boys; the day looked promising. Things took a down-hill turn around 11:00 a.m. I experienced back pain, GI problems, and I could not get comfortable, so there was lots of hunched-over pacing. This persisted for hours. I talked with the on-call oncologist four different times. Joe was on pins and needles all day as he waited for me to decide what to do. The doc recommended I go to the ER. I really did NOT want to go, because I have no veins left to poke and cannot afford to be exposed to all the germs in the waiting room. At seven, I finally gave in. I was too exhausted and just could not take the pain anymore. We went to the ER.

I got some pain relief from a couple of IM injections (before chemo, I remember these hurt; post chemo, they feel like a sweet kiss), I had a CT scan (just what I needed: some more exposure to high doses of radiation). But they found out I have a large kidney stone, which is a huge relief! It was terrific news! The pain has nothing to do with the cancer! Thank God. I kept thinking, "God has chastened me sore, but has not given me over to death" (Psalm 118)! The stone is also low, which means my body has done most of the painful, hard work of getting it out.

I slept tons of hours. I'm still exhausted today, but there's no pain, just discomfort. I don't know if I passed the stone or not. I will find out on follow-ups with a specialist. And I figure if I can get through a kidney stone three days after my eighth round of chemo, I can probably get through anything.

January 8, 2008

I feel weak right now. My body is shaky and uncertain. I am the most tired I have been during this entire ordeal. My body and soul are worn thin. I feel like I should be starting to get stronger instead of weaker, and it is so maddening.

At therapy today, I got a call from the urologist. It seems the stone is too big to pass, and they want to do a minor surgical procedure tomorrow. I was totally stunned—I told them about my situation and my precarious white cell counts and agreed to an appointment tomorrow. I then called Dr. Frenette and my surgeon to collaborate. I cannot afford any surgery at this time and cannot risk the exposure to germs my body doesn't have the ability to fight. It is a waiting game to see what the docs say, and now I am a bit worried that I still have to deal with more of the stone's fury.

Just writing this is helping a bit. Thank you all for listening. I am so looking forward to the day when it is just good news to report. Seems I am due ....

JANUARY 9, 2008

kay, after a dozen or so phone calls to my growing team of physicians, we got some things straightened out. I will go today for a blood draw and then to the urologist. If Dr. Frenette says my labs are doable, then we will most likely schedule an outpatient procedure ASAP. There won't be any cutting; they just go up through the urethra (lovely!). I'm not worried about the procedure per se (other than it sounds rather undignified, which I guess is why they put you out) but rather the possibility of infection because it is still invasive.

After getting a more informative rundown, I decided to drag myself out for a walk. It was, for the very first time, hard to put one foot in front of the other. I was tired, shaky, and apparently hurting quite a bit more than I thought. But, I managed to go (very slowly) for about thirty-five minutes. By the time I got home, my head was clear. I felt much less dramatic, the shakes were almost gone, and I felt so much stronger!

Exercise clears my head, strengthens my body, and renews my spirit! Thank God!

JANUARY 9, 2008

a, la, la! Caution: writer under the influence. I have taken a few pain meds, and they're finally kicking in! Yeah, now I can sit and stop pacing.

Went to see the urologist, Dr. Irby (VERY nice!). Also went to the oncologist for labs, and they were relatively good. Apparently, the stone is stuck, and there is no way it will come out on its own. I also can't be shock-waved (lithotripsy) because it needs to be fixed now. He tried to send me directly to the OR, but they were too busy. He tried to admit me, but I would rather try oral pain meds and sleep at home. My kidney is hugely swollen and leaking urine out into my abdomen (it's not permanent, but it looked awful on the CT scan), and my ureter is in the same shape, which explains all the discomfort/pain/pressure in my back and also why my right leg is not doing so good walking. He asked why I was not taking lots of pain meds, and I said they make me feel like crap. After two car rides and poking and proding, I had to take enough for a horse this evening though, but now I can sit down on both butt cheeks.

So tomorrow we leave way before the crack of dawn, and if all goes well, I'll be home and feeling much better (except for some nausea) late tomorrow afternoon.

JANUARY 11, 2008

The procedure was a breeze. The tough parts were before and after: getting up at 4:00 a.m., being NPO (I usually cheat and eat a little something before surgery, but I didn't this time; I figured with my recent luck, why risk aspiration pneumonia?), and then going without any pain relief until 7:00 a.m. was brutal. The nurse did not help. Okay, she wasn't mean, but she wasn't the least bit sympathetic. Hello, did I mention that I have a big kidney stone that has grossly swollen my insides and that I just finished chemo and am still having some nausea from that? I am sorry that I had to check some "yes" boxes on the intake form, but I would have preferred some nursing care rather than a secretary with an RN badge.

In addition to the lack of sympathy, I was totally on edge for the whole IV start part. I only have two decent spots on my left arm remaining, and I needed one for Herceptin. After getting that in, finally getting every anti-nausea medicine available (really), the nurse still seemed a bit surprised that I was constantly shifting on the gurney. I would have been pacing the room again, but the IV set up limited me. Let me mention again that "I need something for pain!" Maybe she watches the Springer show and needed more drama to get motivated. I will consider this for next time: I can wail if I have to. The pain meds finally came just before they wheeled me into the OR. Unfortunately, the tears came first. I am turning into a thirty-eight-year-old blubbering baby. I tried to get it together before Joe came in but couldn't.

The operating-room guys were great. The whole operating-room part only took about forty-five minutes. I don't remember a thing (thank you, Versed!) except waking up and, with very fuzzy vision, seeing my "huge" (according to Dr. Irby) kidney stone in a jar right up in my face. It was kind of an odd way to wake up. I also remember the doc saying that my ureter was so swollen it was cork-screwing up. Normally they are straight and the width of the inside of a pen, but mine was swollen up to thumb size—I figure if you are going to get sick, why do it half-assed? But he seemed so happy it all went so well!

So that forty-five minutes was a breeze. A non-chemo person would have been out of there in another two hours (by 10:00 a.m.). As a post-chemo patient, my body apparently had other plans. I stayed until three. I got my money's worth! I had to have every anti-nausea medicine available. It seems that the last six months of attacking my healthy cells, as well as the cancer, does not seem to promote quick recovery from anesthesia. Mmmm, how surprising! The recovery-room nurses were really nice though. One of them told me to tell my upcoming mastectomy surgeon that I need every available anti-nausea med and to be aggressive with them. No problem there!

I even managed to sleep a few more hours when we got home. The pain is gone, and now just some soreness and pressure will remain until the kidney and ureter go back to normal size. I plan—I know, "Man plans, God laughs" (He has been having quite a good chuckle on my behalf lately)—to get better and stronger each day before my surgery (February sixth). I can't wait to do normal stuff again and be a regular wife and mother! Onward and upward.

January 13, 2008

*A*hh, the saga continues. I can't wait for it to end! I feel the need to rant, so consider yourself forewarned!

Well, my intention was "onward and upward," but I think I fell flat instead. I have been so weak, shaky, and uncomfortable. I can't figure out what is causing my plethora of symptoms. Dr. Frenette recommended I get a blood transfusion Friday because my red counts were a wreck, but he also suggested I talk to my urologist first. My urologist said my counts were just low due to dilution from all the surgical- and recovery-room fluids. But my labs have been trending down for the past couple of weeks; they are nowhere near normal. Dad and I left Friday a bit concerned after the oncology nurse said she really thought I needed a transfusion. What a fun way to start a weekend!

I decided to take action despite the fact that my butt has been parked on the couch with the heating pad. I have been on an aggressive nutrition plan to replace all the missing red blood cells and iron with sugar and fat. It seems to be helping! I am not shaky all the time now. Today, I even managed to walk to the end of my street and back. I was moving at a blistering thirty-min/mile pace—I can normally swim much faster than that! I am a wee bit ticked off that I managed to hold on to a few muscles during chemo only to see them wither here in the last bit.

My plan was to go into my mastectomy as a fit, healthy-looking woman who looked like she was kicking cancer's ass. Instead, I seem to be moving in the wrong direction. I look ten years older than I did in June, and I am pale, flabby, weak, and apparently quite whiney (maybe this is where Rocco gets it from). I wanted to go into surgery feeling like I looked pretty good before my body was altered forever. The likelihood of that happening now is low. How insanely frustrating!

There are a few good things to come from this whole experience though. I have been too distracted to be nervous about the mastectomy (please pray REALLY HARD that my margins will be clean and ALL nodes will be negative) or my meeting tomorrow with my heart failure specialist (let's hope the ticker is still just as strong as she was). I am, however, nervous about all the swelling in my kidney and ureter. Let's hope when I get the stent out Tuesday that Dr. Irby says there is no permanent damage and the swelling is improving!

Okay, time to hit the heating pad once again. Please send a few extra prayers my way; I need them.

JANUARY 16, 2008

The past two weeks have been the most difficult since the first days of my diagnosis. The fear of finding cancer after my mastectomy and the weariness and pain from the eight rounds of chemo, followed by the kidney stone from hell, finally overcame me. My body was weak, and my spirit was broken. My mind kept wandering down the darkest of roads.

Tonight, the dam broke. I had the house to myself, and I knew that I could no longer safely keep it all in. I finally got the catharsis that I so desperately needed. I paced, kneeled, prayed, begged, pleaded, wept, and wailed. I wanted desperately to smash things. I may not be done. I may still have more to purge, but I feel better.

Earlier, in the midst of a fervent prayer on my knees, I opened my eyes to look out the window, and much to my surprise, the heavens looked different. The color of the sky, a gray/pink blanket (it is actually supposed to snow), shifted for just a moment to a brilliant blue/purple, which is the color of the sky in several of my Grand Teton photos. I know there are several logical explanations for what I saw, but I also know it was another sign.

I pray that God answers my desperate prayers. I feel a bit different now. Again, I feel the caress of His touch. I know He has been with me all along. My most impassioned hope is that my desires match up with His plans. This hope is also the wellspring of my greatest fear. Sometimes it is terrifying to utter the phrase "God's will be done ...."

JANUARY 21, 2008

Well, today and tomorrow are big days. Today I have my mammogram, and tomorrow I have my pre-surgical appointment with Dr. White. It brings back a lot of memories of my first diagnosis way back in August ....

Being the nervous and thoroughly prepared patient I am, I have an entire page of questions for tomorrow's appointment. Most of them are of the future prognosticator type, so there are not as many about the actual demise of the boob. The thought of going around with only one ta is a strange one indeed, but as long as they get all the cancer, I think I can put up with the inconvenience. I mean, I barely filled out a bra before this all happened anyway!

Please continue to pray (I know you all are!) for clean margins and NEGATIVE nodes! Thanks!

I am just back from Dr. White's and still reeling a bit from the meeting. Overall, I think it went pretty well. We started with the exam, and he seemed pleased. Clinically, my breast and nodes are much better than before. "A marked improvement," he said.

When we reviewed the radiologist's report, it freaked me out a bit. Things sound so different in person than they look in a report. In person it sounds like, "We see calcifications, and although we can't say for sure until the pathology report comes back after surgery, this could be consistent with the death of cancer cells due to your chemo." But on paper it reads like this: "Extensive mammographically malignant calcification in the right breast, measuring ... the calcifications are much more numerous and extensive now than on the prior study on 07/30/07." Crap.

I asked in a rather pushy way (surprised?) if we could do the surgery sooner, but he was a bit hesitant, and it turns out they're booked anyway. Besides, I still need to get my kidney ultrasound to make sure it is good and happy before I go under the knife.

The surgery itself doesn't sound too bad or too long, about two to three hours. The recovery sounds doable too. The part I really don't like is that we will most likely have to wait seven to ten days to get the pathology reports back. Crap again. God is really testing my patience here! Perhaps this is what purgatory is like.

We did not discuss those dreaded "what ifs," like what if those calcifications are live cancer and not dead? What if the nodes come back positive? What if the cancer is more extensive than expected? What if we don't get clean margins? You know, those really big questions with answers that directly translate into my odds for long-term survival. As Joe points out all the time, and Dr. White pointed out today, statistics don't mean anything if you are the one who makes it! Joe is convinced that I am THE ONE, but I definitely struggle with doubts.

On a lighter note, it seems my angel followed me around today. I have a little wooden angel, I got as a gift, on my bedside table. After the appointment, when Joe and I sat down to talk, I looked up and saw the same angel, very out of place with the other décor, sitting high on a ledge above where we were seated. At that moment, I decided (I had been thinking, praying, and debating about this a lot) that Dr. White will do my surgery. As soon as I told this to Joe, I felt some weight lift off my shoulders. It is the right decision. And it is a good thing my shoulders are still strong even after all this chemo, because the "what ifs" are still VERY heavy.

Please continue to pray for a great surgical outcome—negative nodes, clean margins, and no evidence of active disease. Please pray that I live a long, healthy life with my husband and get to see my sons grow up and have kids!

I still think the voices of many are bound to be louder than just one.

JANUARY 31, 2008

Yesterday I had my kidneys looked at by ultrasound. The right kidney and ureter are back to normal size! Yeah! It is now safe to resume my nightly three-martini routine (just kidding—besides, Ativan has no calories). I also got my lymphedema sleeve yesterday. It looks like a flesh-colored arm warmer (for those cyclists out there) or one of those burn stockings. It shouldn't be too bad looking with a tan. I am still not sure how much I will have to wear it, but I will have to make a few changes in my lifestyle. Like I said when this all began, if I live a full life after all this, then this journey has been nothing more than an educational inconvenience. I still believe that! I am hoping to come out of this healthy, much wiser, and with a few more scars, which will, of course, add to my charm and character!

Today should be a good day. I get to take Rocco for his swim lesson for the first time. Fun for me, trauma for him.

FEBRUARY 2, 2008

Well, Rocco wasn't too traumatized at his swim lesson, and there were only a few tears in the beginning. They did not, however, make him put his face in yet. This is supposed to change soon, and I hope I am there the day he does it! I also got to take the big man to his very first day of school since this all began! He did great! It was wonderful to meet his teacher and see all of our old friends from CLCC! I am really looking forward to being able to do that after my surgery! I have been out doing lots of fun, normal stuff, which has been wonderful!

Yesterday afternoon was a bit tough though. I went alone to my Pre-Op check-in at CMC. I was warned the process could take between thirty minutes and two hours. I figured I would be on the quick side because, aside from a little breast cancer and a few kidneys stones, I am the picture of health. The whole affair took almost three hours! It was about two hours, one blood draw, and two tests more than I could sanely take alone. I passed the first forty-five minutes or so quite well, mediating and doing guided imagery. But then the sporadic healthcare worker or test prevented me from doing anything further than staring at the incredibly bland, sterile walls.

Naturally, my mind turned inward, and then, unfortunately, it went to those dark places again. I had been doing a really good job of not thinking too much about things until then.

I got a bit stuck in that pattern. One minute it's normal stuff, and I'm present in the moment, but then that's followed by bad thoughts and dark projections. It has been a real rollercoaster ride since yesterday morning. I decided to have my evening cocktail (Ativan) a bit early tonight to take the edge off. Joe and I had a big, crocodile-tear-filled (me not him) talk today, and that helped.

I am going to try my best to have fun during my last three days with two boobs! And I am glad, as one of my friends put it, that my boob "will soon go to boob heaven." I think it will be happy there!

-Jen, the soon-to-be Uniboober.

P.S. I guess I will have to get out my hooded sweatshirts and big aviator glasses then write my manifesto.

February 5, 2008

Well, today is my last full day on this earth with my two boobs. I feel a bit like an astronaut who has been training and working hard for many months for the big trip into space. It is currently T-minus twenty-one hours and counting until my surgery at CMC. Tomorrow at 5:00 p.m., we find out if all the hard work pays off.

Tensions at mission control have been running a bit high. Emotions all over the place. We are finally approaching the moment of truth. Was all the effort and expense (I think NASA's budget must be similar to that needed for a cancer patient) for a flight cut short? For one that ends much too quickly and crashes back to earth in a fiery ball? Or will it go as planned, with a perfect landing (obviously, I have been prepping for a ride on the space shuttle, not in a rocket) after a long, beautiful flight? We won't know for a while. Pathology results won't be back for a good week to ten days after tomorrow.

The past few days, I have been trying to come to terms with what the results and implications of my surgery might be. It has been very challenging, to say the least. I finally feel a bit more prepared for this scary trip into the great unknown. Now, if my flight is destined to be a short one, I know I will be able to smile and enjoy the fast trip back down, not fall back to Earth, crying and screaming.

Please say plenty of prayers for me and my flight team tomorrow (at least it's not rocket surgery) from two to five o'clock. AND PLEASE PRAY FOR NEGATIVE NODES, CLEAN MARGINS, AND A LONG, BEAUTIFUL FLIGHT.

FEBRUARY 6, 2008

Hi Everyone, this is Joe.

Jen's surgery is now complete, and the doctor said everything went well. It is 10:00 p.m., and she is in her hospital room. She did great! The doctor wasn't able to give us any indication about remaining live cancer cells, pathology will have to do that, but he did say that the surgery went exactly as he wanted it to go. He did seem very happy and relaxed, and it gave me a good feeling about the whole procedure. She recovered from the anesthesia in record time (no chemo influence this time), and was alert and smiling thirty minutes after the operation. It was an emotional event, as you all understand by now, but Jen handled it with the inner strength that we all know she has. I am very proud of her.

I'll let her fill you in on the details, for it is her words we have all come to look for.

I will say this: I cannot overstate the tremendous power of all of you who are praying for us, thinking of us, caring for our children, feeding our family, writing notes of inspiration, and sending those positive vibes. Without all of you, I don't know how we would make it through this. Each and every person who has been so kind and giving and thoughtful is a direct contributor to saving Jen's life, and I thank you all. We are so very blessed, and there is not one moment of one day that we forget that fact. When this is behind us, and Jen writes her book (I really hope she does), the dedication page will have to be its own chapter.

Good night, and God bless you all.

-Joe

February 8, 2008

orning everyone, Uniboober here! Boobs away! Surgery day went as well as it could have. No tears and no drama, even though we had to wait until an extra forty minutes for the actual operation to start. I did not even need any "happy juice" in my pre-op IV. I think my calm and composure was a result of a few things: having Joe and my parents in the pre-op room, having a caring pre-op healthcare team, and of course, all your prayers on my behalf. I was also fortunate enough to have a CMC chaplain, Sara, do guided imagery with me both pre-op and during surgery. She led me through a specific imagery session tailored just for me while we waited to go to the OR and, thanks to an open-minded surgery and anesthesia staff, for the first two hours of surgery. She was even able to touch my head and say prayers over me! I came out of anesthesia smiling and joking, was only in the recovery room for thirty minutes, and was not nauseous!

I'll spare you details, but it sounds as if surgery went as well as it could have. They did not see cancer in any surprising areas, and Dr. White said he got all the tissue he wanted to get. However, much to my dismay, no one would comment as to whether the additional calcifications were active cancer or not, nor would anyone venture a guess as to whether or not the lymph nodes removed were positive or not. We will still have to wait a long seven to ten days for the pathology results to get these answers. Dr. White again told me I wasn't a statistic and that radiation would hopefully get any cells that might have been left behind. Again, please pray for negative nodes, clean margins, and a long, happy, healthy life!

Anyway, me and my remaining, healthy boob got home from the hospital around 4:00 p.m. yesterday. Dr. White gave me the option of staying another night, but I figured if I had any hope sleeping that I better get the heck out of there. For some reason, I feel a bit more rested when I am able to sleep in a solid block of time rather than getting thirty short naps. I finally fussed at my nurse around 2:00 a.m., after the fifteenth or sixteenth visit from hospital staff, and she said no one would bother us again until 4:00 a.m., and no one did, but, of course, I had to get up to pee at 3:30 a.m., which is a little bit of a production on wobbly legs, with a sore wing, and lots of IV tubes. The constant stream of medical personnel started up again around 4:15 a.m. They make those poor first-year residents, the ones who don't have any answers and seem a bit awkward, do rounds at the worst hours! By 7:30 a.m., I had seen another six or so doctors and was feeling a bit like an interesting lab specimen (one with crusty eyes and only one boob—not really a good look for me).

Last night, all the unanswered questions got to me a bit. I did shed a few tears. But after a good night's sleep, I feel like I am back in a positive space again. I think I will need some serious distractions and lots more prayers between now and next Thursday to keep my mind off of the pathology.

-Jen, the no longer crusty-eyed, Uniboober

February 11, 2008

WARNING: THIS LACKS HUMOR AND CHEER AND IS DOWNRIGHT PITIFUL!

I cannot think straight. I am not sure if this is due to my general state of mind or the fact that I desperately need a nap and took a Lortab two hours ago, thinking I could get some rest (and relieve some discomfort). While I am stuck here in the doldrums, waiting to hear pathology results, it has been so hard to deal with the both the chaos and the mundane of daily existence. The struggle to be able to accept pathology news that is most likely far from best-case scenario has been compounded by the toll the past few months have taken on my body and mind, the current physical restrictions due to the surgery, and the challenges of life with a teething baby (who has a double ear infection) and a precocious two-and-a-half-year-old. Luca is by all accounts an easy baby, and Rocco is typical for a boy his age. But as I am trying to fight for my life, it has frequently been, over the past few months and despite all the help, extraordinarily difficult to deal with the task of raising two small (even though they are wonderful) children.

Yesterday, a darkness settled on me that I am having trouble shaking. This morning, I awoke to the light, but, alas, darkness has settled again. I am finally near my breaking point and, thanks to surgery, have no way to escape. I recognize my symptoms as those of depression, and I hope they don't take root before I can beat them back on my own.

This is really so discouraging. Where is the personal growth that I have fought so hard to achieve? How am I going to find the joy and determination to live, especially if my remaining time on earth is only a few years, when I am so tired and worn thin? How can I beat the odds and survive when I feel like this? My immune system needs to be working at its very best to beat the odds I am facing, and right now I am a f***ing mess. From the start, my docs and Joe have stressed that my previous accomplishments (Ironman) have put me in a survival category that defies odds and statistics. Okay, I have always accepted this, but on some level, I knew there was something not right about that too. Today, I finally realized that the body and mind that did fine for a couple of Ironman races is the very same one that allowed cancer to grow in the first place. Granted, I did have lots of stressors early last year, but what about the stress load now? THIS is stress. I think I will give myself a few more days to try and beat this on my own before I seek some medical help.

-One sad boob, Jen

FEBRUARY 12, 2008

*T*hank you all for such an incredible and immediate response to my last entry! Your love, prayers, and words of hope and determination are helping.

Joe (my incredible husband) called the doctor right after reading my entry. Both my surgeon and medical oncologist discussed my situation and got back with us right away. It seems this is not all that uncommon (which makes me feel a ton better) to have these feelings at this point in my recovery. Apparently, the waiting for results can cause even the toughest to crack. I am now taking Ativan (at the doc's suggestion) around the clock until the appointment on Thursday. Hopefully then we will have the pathology results back, and the wait will at least be over.

The Ativan, trying to stay distracted and not talk about the situation at all, and the help from you (family, friends, and my medical team at CMC) is making a difference! I am still teetering a bit, but now I know help is just a short call or email away.

Thanks, from the somewhat tired but still moving forward, Uniboober.

February 14, 2008

Well, the results are finally in. Some of our prayers have been answered. Dr. White was able to get clean margins, and some good-sized ones at that! The mass that showed up on my mammogram that had me so worried was in fact cancer, but now it is gone! Fourteen lymph nodes were also removed. Unfortunately, eight of these were positive for cancer. This is quite concerning, because cancer presence in lymph, especially after chemo, means the disease is either still out there somewhere in my body or is more likely to go somewhere other than my breast. This is, quite frankly, worse than I was expecting. My first thought upon hearing this was that I am a dead woman, that this will kill me.

Dr. White told us that statistics are of no use to us. I can still win, but I will need to access my inner competitor to beat this. It is potentially still curable, but I am really going to have to fight. Monday, we will be meeting with Dr. Frenette, and we will also talk with Dr. Marcum, my medical oncologist at Duke, to discuss the possibility of more chemo. There is no data on giving chemo at this point (Dr. White says it is currently being hotly debated), so we will have to weigh the pros and cons and make a somewhat blind decision. I imagine there will be some discussion as to whether or not it is worth it to fight an unquantifiable disease or wait until it metastasizes and then treat it then. We are still on tap to meet the radiation oncologist tomorrow morning, so that is still in the mix.

The shock is starting to wear off a bit, and it has given way to tears (despite the Ativan). Hopefully, after they pass, it will give way to an unstoppable will that ignores all the odds and negatives, and fights like my life depends on it, because it does!

On a positive note, we are in an uptown hotel, thanks to some very good and generous friends, and we will get to process this for a few days on our own. I really must gather my inner resources and steel my nerves and prepare for battle before I see my sons again.

Please continue to pray for us. Pray for successful radiation, and whatever other measures, to work and to give me a long, happy, healthy life with my husband and sons, the rest of our families, and our friends!

February 15, 2008

Don't read this if you are looking for encouragement. You won't find any here.

Last night was a long, sad night. I was and am stuck at a crossroads, and I am not sure I have the strength right now to choose the right path. Joe practically had to drag me out of bed this morning to go see Dr. Fraser, the radiation oncologist. It is an effort to even move. The only reason I went was the glimmer of hope that we might get some good news, some incentive to fight some more, some indication that I might have a real future, not just a short one filled with treatments and a decreasing quality of life until I die. That really holds no appeal and does not motivate me to move forward.

And, apparently, I will have to wait longer to hear any good news, if there is any. They said they had our appointment down for 10:00 a.m. this coming Monday. Well, at least I got to see the office. It is small, depressing, and smells like a hot ashtray. I guess there must be a few smokers in there getting zapped for lung cancer, and they figure, "What the hell, I am already dying, why quit now?" It was far from encouraging.

I have been staring out the window of the hotel, through the overcast skies. I have been watching the cranes and the men walking up on the girders, way up in the sky. It looks like freedom and like they are really sucking the marrow out of life up there. One misstep and it is curtains, the line between life and death so certain. This seems so very refreshing to me. I feel like, if I could climb to the top of a crane, walk way out to the end and just sit for a while, I could really think clearly and figure things out. The rush of cool air whistling in my ears and caressing my skin, the total quiet, the long look down ... I know these things would give me the moment of clarity to see into my future and determine my present. I would know, looking down to a certain, sudden death if I had the will to fight in these very uncertain circumstances.

Right now, though, without the benefit of walking in the sky, I am still unsure as to whether I have the strength or the will to move on. My future is not that beautiful black and white. I may opt to fight only to find that it gave me a few more miserable years of half living while still dying and suffering until the end.

I will thank you for your concern in advance. I am already medicated and under the care of doctors. This is just my honest assessment of what my future currently looks like to me. Maybe Monday we will get some good news, but I am not holding my breath.

February 17, 2008

I am slowly starting to come out of the spell I have been under. Thursday, I just wanted to lie down and die and get it over with. I have been trying very hard to find my will to fight, and each day is getting a bit better. I still have not reached that helpful point of anger to fuel my desire to fight, but I can finally feel it building.

I will say that your emails and guestbook entries have been absolutely invaluable. I cannot overstate how important they are to me! They are a visible reminder to have hope.

I am trying very hard to find a balance between reality, faith in God's plan, and indescribable sadness. I am trying to figure out how to find joy in what is most likely a short, fiery trip back down to Earth. How do I acknowledge the reality of horrible odds while still hoping for a miracle? How can I steel my nerves and stop the negative messages from my subconscious and conscious brain? How can I forget, relax, and enjoy my time with my family and friends when images of my funeral and my husband and sons in years to come, without me, keep popping in my head? I desperately want these struggles to end, but how do I get them to?

I am also questioning all the efforts I have taken to ensure my recovery. Is it all just a bunch of crap? And are the prayers falling on deaf ears?

We will meet with Dr. Frenette (probably) tomorrow. This is highly unusual and a last-ditch effort. Usually, when you have chemo and then surgery, it is off to radiation, and there's no more chemo unless you get mets, and then they try to buy you a little more time with more chemo. This both totally freaks me out and gives me a bit of hope at the same time. My medical team does think I am the one who can beat impossible odds. We will see what they say … In the meantime, I am not dead yet ….

-Uniboob

FEBRUARY 18, 2008

Well, the saga continues. Before I do the doctor recap, let me tell you all that your incredible messages are VERY important in healing my body, mind, and spirit. I gather strength daily from you all for this fight, the fight for my life. I can't thank you enough!

We met with the radiation oncologist, Dr. Fraser, today. He had already reviewed all my information and spoken to Dr. White and Dr. Frenette about my situation. Basically, he said chemo did not do what we wanted. I believe he used the term "failed." BUT WE HAVE NO REASON TO GIVE UP HOPE. We will do some more scans to see if the cancer spread anywhere else in my body, but more than likely we will do six-and-a-half weeks of daily radiation followed by more chemo. Thank goodness I have a "beautifully shaped head." It looks like bald, uniboobed, and beautiful is what's on the horizon for late-spring fashion.

This week will be full of appointments and some more scary time waiting for results. I am still a mishmash of emotions but am gathering strength, determination, and JOY. I have been praying for JOY. I feel pretty good at the moment, although fear and worry about the future also shift and blow around me (and my family) like the wind. I want to just get as much joy as I can with what time I have left, whether I die old and gray, or (somewhat) young and bald.

-Jen, the temporarily-haired Uniboober

FEBRUARY 19, 2008 4:43 P.M.

This just in! Spring fashion headlines all wrong: bald women with "beautifully shaped heads" everywhere are depressed. It seems hair is back in!

Per our meeting with the chemo doctor this morning, we will start with radiation next week, after I get my other drain out, and then do weekly chemo. The drug that has been selected by my CMC docs, the doc at Duke, and to be reviewed by Sloan Kettering next week, does not cause hair loss. Immediately, Joe and I were suspicious; I mean, what do you lose if your hair stays in? It seems there are some perks to getting more chemo ... The duration is to be determined.

I will be scanned again this Friday from head to toe. I won't know anything until next week, of course. KEEP THOSE PRAYERS COMIN'!

February 22, 2008 8:14 a.m.

Well, today is the big day: scan day. I will have five altogether. By five o'clock tonight, I will be covered in black marker, have a few blue tattoos, and will probably be visible by satellite. We will have to wait until next week for results. Of course, I begged Dr. F for quicker results, but that was a no-go, because we need accuracy not speed for results. It is a bit scary, and it's another long wait. But no matter what they find, I am prepared to fight for a long time. I AM THE ONE. I CAN DO THIS. GO JEN GO!

February 23, 2008

Well, I thought I would look a bit like a lightning bug when the sun set yesterday, but I think most of the radiation was already gone! I got scanned, molded, marked, and three very small tattoos. It went as well as it could have, but I am glad it is over.

Everyone at CMC and Mercy Hospital was very nice. They all remembered me (not sure if this is a good or bad thing) and seemed extra sweet. Dad did waiting room/distraction duty. God bless him: it's not an easy job on a day like yesterday! Did not even get so much as a "no comment" from brain/chest/abdomen/pelvis scan peeps. But the bone scan guy's wife was a breast cancer survivor, and he told me my bones looked "lovely!" Great news! And, just think, if I never got cancer, I would never have known about my beautiful head or lovely bones!

Two friends also visited for a couple of hours when we got home yesterday. It was really enjoyable and helped pass the time in a good way. We are going to run with this idea and have a full weekend planned. No talking about the scans or cancer stuff!

FEBRUARY 24, 2008

MY SCANS ARE CLEAN! MY SCANS ARE CLEAN! We just found out a short time ago. Out of the blue (at 2:14 p.m. to be precise. I will remember this call until the day I die), our phone rang, and it was Dr. Frenette. I did not even recognize his voice, and I was not at all expecting the call. In one quick breath he said, "It is Dr. Frenette, your scans are CLEAN." He must have said it that fast to prevent the heart attack that I would have had if he had paused.

Joe and I were totally stunned. We thought we had to wait at least until tomorrow morning (an eternity), and Dr. Frenette did not say he was going to call today. We laughed and cried (for a long time, still doing it a bit) and hugged. I dropped to my knees to THANK GOD. Please thank God! He is listening! We still can hardly believe it! It will take a while to sink in, a while for the burden of this tremendous weight to fully lift. But we are so thankful. Thankful for our merciful, wondrous, healing God and thankful for all of your prayers!

Now I can go to radiation and chemo with JOY and rediscovered purpose. My will to battle has been renewed! Please keep those prayers comin', there is such strength in them. GO JEN GO!

-Jen, the girl who couldn't be happier with just one boob!

FEBRUARY 26, 2008

Wow! Waking up the past two mornings with clean scans has been so incredible! We are still reveling in the awesome news, and hope to be for the rest of our long, healthy lives! I have been walking around with a silly grin now for quite a while, the darkness from last week already starting to fade ... God is soooo good!

Despite the euphoria, it has been a bit odd in these days following our clean scan report. I liken it to an emotional tsunami. We had been swept along in this wave of fear, worry, and extreme stress for so long that hearing the news, even THE MOST FANTASTIC NEWS EVER, left us emotionally and physically drained. Lying around the living room Sunday night following THE CALL, Mom, Joe and I all looked like we had just weathered an awful storm (I know there were storm victims all over that evening). We were elated but wrung out. Now, thanks to the incredible news, each of us, in our own way and time, is gathering strength and floating along with buoyant hearts and souls.

We'll all float okay ... Uniboob

FEBRUARY 27, 2008

While all of you have been sharing in our fantastic, clean scans news, a few of you have said, "Jen, that is truly a gift from God and is so incredibly wonderful, but what the heck does that mean?" I have been getting that "it's all Greek to me" bewildered look or tone from some of you. Not to worry, because BC (before cancer, in case you forgot) I had no idea what the implications of "clean scans" were either, or why they would even scan in the first place.

Basically, the clean scans are an indication that the cancer has not spread to my brain, lungs, bones, or liver. If breast cancer goes to one of these spots, it is still breast cancer and must continue to be treated as such. Those are the places breast cancer likes to go once it is able to leave the breast/lymph areas. Long-term prognosis changes if the disease is able to metastasize to these spots ....

Does that mean I am done with treatment? No. I will start six-and-a-half weeks of daily (just Monday through Friday—they give the machines the weekends off) radiation as soon as my remaining drain is out. After radiation, I will start weekly, heavy chemo (the hair-sparing kind—I need to show off all my grays) for an unspecified period of time. It's just a wait and see kind of thing. Herceptin (chemo lite) treatments have already started back up and will most likely continue until August.

Why will I still do all these treatments? Because even though cancer was not detectable on the scans, there is still the possibility that there are some cancer cells out there floating around and looking to give me some major trouble again.

Blah, blah, blah ... I am ready to get on with my next round of treatments and kick breast cancer's ass (does breast cancer even have an ass?) once and for all.

-Uniboob outta here

MARCH 11, 2008

*F*orgot to post this from yesterday. Suffering from severe toddler interruption syndrome!

Ding-dong, the witch is dead! The drain is out. Thank God! It is a bit of a shock, this newly found freedom. I finally got to drive (I guess it's like riding a bike, you never forget how to do it) and run an errand all by myself, just like a big girl. The best, though, was picking up Luca and Rocco for the first time in five weeks! Okay, maybe I fudged and sort of picked up Rocco a few times in the last few days and was scolded: "Mommy! You're not allowed to pick me up!"

All of the inaction—I guess it was also a healing period—had grown extraordinarily difficult! I was a bit desperate (on the inside only, I looked normal on the outside) by the time the appointment rolled around. I told Dr. White that I had been exercising the utmost restraint (drain was in four weeks and five days) but had almost cracked and taken it out myself on more than one occasion. Dr. White was his usual compassionate, charming self. I just love this man! He actually let me (with his guidance of course!!) remove the drain during the appointment. Apparently, this was an office first. It was so much easier than just lying there and letting him do it like the last time. I have some serious control issues to work on!

So, thank you all for the prayers! If all continues to go swimmingly, I will have a great radiation appointment today and then start therapy Wednesday (at best) or Thursday. I am so ready to let the zapping begin!

Oh, some other prayers were answered too: Rocco spent his very first two nights in his "big boy bed" and stayed put all night long! It's a Festivus miracle.

Soooo happy to be free again, Uniboob

March 12, 2008

Today was the first day of radiation therapy (RT). It was a piece of cake, and the actual zapping went by very quickly. They make you lay (lie? I hear a former English teacher screaming somewhere in the distance) down for it, so how hard can it be?

Before RT was a bit odd though. I arrived early (I was fortunate enough to drop off Rocco at school today! I love to do the normal stuff!), popped on my iPod, and wandered around the hospital. I had a strange, slightly nervous feeling and needed to roam. It was a bit surreal. I felt like I was in a movie, an actor playing a role in a story about someone else's life. It was a Talking Heads *Once in a Lifetime* moment that left me asking if this life was really mine. Thoughts of "this is not my (semi) bald head" and "this is not my chest full of scars" were in my head. I also wondered what the others roaming the halls thought of me as I passed. I always notice the lingering glances. I can see them wondering if I am in treatment for something or if I was just under duress at the hairstylist. The experience left me reeling a bit and feeling like maybe the earth had shifted slightly on its axis, but I was the only one who noticed. It was similar to a dream that ends just before you wake up. It influences your mood and sometimes your whole being, but you can't quite make out why you feel the way you do, you just know you feel different.

Aside from my "I'm not a cancer patient, but I play one on TV" experience this morning, I am having a little bit of a tough time. There are twin barbarians at the gate: fear and fatigue. While I was patiently (hah!) waiting for the final drain to come out, some red spots popped up around my scar. The consensus from Dr. White (my surgical oncologist) and Dr. Frazer (my radiation oncologist) was that there is no need to do a skin biopsy to see whether or not they are cancerous, because our course of treatment would not change. Dr. White actually asked me if I was looking for something new to worry about when we discussed it. I wasn't sure whether to hit him or laugh when he said this. I have enough worries, but still I find these blemishes quite concerning. Perhaps this worry is contributing to my lack of sleep and the off-and-on icky feeling I have had for the past few days.

All of this is being compounded by, or perhaps is a result of, my current level of fatigue. The RT fatigue won't set in until around the three-week mark, but I am flat-out pooped even though I still have peppy, or at least normal, moments each day. I am just about to the point where I am running on fumes. My heart feels fluttery in my chest, and my body feels weary. I am not sleeping well at night and have only managed two or three naps in the past two-and-a-half weeks. I seem to be getting more jittery when I should be getting sleepy instead.

Okay, I'm complaining. I have made plans so that this will hopefully change soon. Let's hope I settle into some quality Zzzz time and things even back out.

-Uniboob

MARCH 15, 2008

My surreal, inner space odyssey this week continues. RT itself is quite quick and painless, and in my heart, I know I do not fear the process. But when I leave the house and drive to the hospital, I begin to feel wired (an odd nervous energy akin to pre-race jitters.) Perhaps I am mentally putting on my "game face." I crank up the music on the way there and get lost in the songs. Joe burned me some incredible new stuff: Amy Winehouse, The White Stripes, Fiest, Kate Nash, MIA, Arcade Fire, and the Kaiser Chiefs, to name a few. I park in the same spot in the same lot every time (yesterday, someone actually had the nerve to park in MY spot!). Then I put on my iPod and turn to the exact same tune I had going in the car. I literally don't miss a beat. I flip my sunglasses down and start walking (or maybe pacing). It is far from a leisurely stroll: it is a very determined walk. I have my head up, and I can feel the look on my face. It's not quite the thousand-yard stare (it is not hardened and beyond help), but it is determined and at the same time detached. Perhaps it mirrors my mind. It reflects the dichotomy of my thoughts: a fearless ready-to-fight attitude combined with angst about the spots and what they might portend. I do a convoluted loop through the grounds and several buildings before heading to the chapel. I get some quality time in with God, and then the pacing continues ... I have it timed perfectly to arrive just in time to check in, change, and get nuked. They should have a beep from a microwave-timer ring when you are done.

Speaking of deadlines, Holy Week starts tomorrow. Go hurry up and drink some green beer or maybe just a stiff shot of something Irish.

-Uniboob

MARCH 16, 2008

*E*rin Go Braugh! The luck of the Irish was with me. I found just what I was looking for.

I had been looking forward to Mass for days. I was going come Hell or high water. Well, high water definitely came, but I went anyway. The pounding rains seemed to be what I needed to cleanse my mind and soul. The thunder and lightning were the perfect accompaniment for the catharsis I was seeking. The sun shone brilliantly through the black clouds as Mass ended—it was the perfect meteorological backdrop for the "rebirth" I was seeking.

The Palm Sunday Mass was beautiful. I felt touched by the hand of God. I asked to feel His light flow in me, through me, and back out again. And it is. I can feel it. And in my mind's eye, I now have the most beautiful picture. It gives me strength, inspiration, and peace at the same time. I can't wait to go back.

I was under strict doctor's orders to have a bourbon this weekend. Actually, I think Dr. Frenette said to "curl up with a bourbon and a good book." Surely, he meant a good bourbon and a book—life is too short to drink cheap liquor! I got the best half of that prescription right!

The night out with friends was fantastic. The only thing lacking was Joe's presence. I am so thankful that my friend included me and a few others to party with his family, the Federal Clan. And party we did. A private tent, a fantastic band, and a few hundred drunken Irishmen make for a very lively evening! The Federal Clan knows how to celebrate! Next year maybe I can get myself invited to participate in the float, private bar, and party bus. I have one year to get my liver ready. Never have I been more excited to be half Irish.

God is good. Have a beautiful Holy Week.

-Uniboob

MARCH 18, 2008

*T*hank you, everyone, for the many kindnesses you continue to do for our family. They are each appreciated. Every gesture, no matter how big or how small, is noticed.

We are so grateful for the prayers. Please keep them coming. We have come so very far but still have a long way to go. Please pray that my family finds comfort and peace. Please pray that I have the courage and stamina to move forward with five more weeks of radiation and then what will most likely be four more months of chemo. I will get the heavy stuff weekly this time. I know it is a blessing to receive and that it will hopefully knock any remaining cells into oblivion, but I am a bit nervous about my ability to handle more chemo after all my body has gone and is going through.

When I started on the heavy stuff last time, I was fresh out of the gate, but now I am fatigued and growing a bit wearier with each day. These past two days, I have been quite pooped, tired even, when I get out of bed. The fatigue is ironically settling in my thighs, the thighs that never really got tired when doing the Ironman. I can't tell if it is the radiation fatigue setting in already (I thought I would have another week or two before that hit), the fact that I am on medication for a sinus infection, post-St. Patrick's Day stress disorder, or a combination of all three. This fatigue scares me a bit. Although I must say it is a different fatigue than the kind I experienced while doing chemo, it still, for lack of a more eloquent word, sucks (I gave up cancer, not cursing, for Lent).

So, with all that being said, please pray for me to find strength, stamina, and perhaps my Thesaurus. Thanks, Uniboob

March 25, 2008

I am woefully behind in all things correspondence. I have missed being able to sit and write. It is so hard sometimes to be quiet and reflect when I am in the midst of life and all its joys and challenges. And, of course, I am still suffering from T.I.S. (Toddler Interruption Syndrome).

It was a beautiful Easter Weekend. It was so great to relax and enjoy both boys and some family fun. We even managed to do two church services—a Pagani Family first. Easter Day was lovely, and we had fun at Gammy and Papa's with family and friends too. Dinner was dee-lish, the kids went on a lakeside Easter Egg hunt, and then we went out for a boat ride. The weekend was almost perfect.

In the midst of all the beautiful moments with family and friends, I still found (and find) myself struggling with fear and worry for what the future might hold. The mirror was and is a powerful reminder of the demons I still face, demons that haunt me at the most inopportune times. They have no respect for the sweet times I spend with my sons or the quiet times in the evenings when I am alone with Joe. They follow me into and out of the shower and all around the house. I can see their handiwork right there on my chest. It is not the scar, the stickers, the marker lines, or tattoos. No, I have red spots where their devilish hands caressed my skin, marks of the disease their embrace left behind. I pray fervently that radiation stops them. It is my most solemn prayer that the chemo banishes them from my body and into Hell forever.

-Uniboob

March 26, 2008

I re-read my previous journal entry, and the last line seemed, well, a bit dramatic. I definitely do have some very intense feelings about my skin situation, but I am usually not so histrionic (or at least I was not b.c.). Anyway, my rant is already out in cyberspace, so there it is.

On a much lighter note, spring has sprung. The trees and bushes are all blooming or getting ready to burst forth in color, and the wildlife is all a twitter. Our backyard is bustling with activity. It is so beautiful to witness. And love is in the air, literally. We have been listening to the owls in our backyard for a couple of weeks now. I wonder how long their mating season lasts? All of this life and energy is good for my soul. I love the impact nature has on me.

As I mentioned in my last entry, I am a bit behind in journaling. It is tough to find quiet time to sit and write. This week alone, I have five radiation treatments, one ultrasound (the tech told me I was in really great shape, which I thought was a very nice thing to say to a woman who has recently had two babies and only has one boob), and appointments to see two different doctors. I am starting to feel like CMC is my home away from home. Not sure how I feel about that ... At least I am out and about, because I am already dreading the upcoming four months of chemo-induced seclusion.

Joe and I did manage to get out to the Charlotte Track and Tri Club meeting on Monday night, though. It was really great to see some old friends and make some new ones. I found the whole evening quite inspiring and fun. Of course, it is hard not to have fun if you are drinking really good tequila.

Get off of your computer and out to enjoy this day. If you happen to go by a Cantina 1511, have a margarita for me.

-Uniboob

April 1, 2008

It is a sad day at the Pagani house. I am out of Dove dark chocolate. I made a mental note last night, when I ate the last of it, to pick some up when I was out for RT today. I remembered the Desitin, but I forgot the chocolate. I must be a good Mommy—Luca's butt really is more important than my daily cocoa cravings. Of course, it is easy to say that now, but later in the day when I am really tired and desperate, I might think otherwise.

Perhaps I can cope without the chocolate after all. I went yesterday morning to get my head shrunk again. It helped. My mental state has been rather precarious lately (I know this comes as a surprise to a few of you). I'm struggling with lots of "what ifs" and negative thoughts again. I'm contemplating an antidepressant, and I might still go that route, but today I feel like I am on more solid ground. Let's hope that continues.

-Uniboob

April 2, 2008

MVA-L- This segment is intended for mature viewing audiences only, language.

Oh shit. I met with Dr. Frazer after I got zapped today. The spots have changed and not for the better. We are bumping up radiation from once a day to twice a day starting tomorrow. The thought is that the extra radiation and more aggressive timing will impact the "rapidly growing cells." As he told me all this, my first thought was "this is going to kill me." I thought it clearly and without emotion. I could actually see the words float through my mind. It was a clear headed, dispassionate moment. It was not laden with fear or loss. I did not panic or breakdown until a bit later when I began wondering if this was fear or precognition, when I began to think about Joe and the boys and all the incredible, normal things I would miss. Unfortunately, it seemed like it might be a bit more like precognition, because I felt truly detached.

A friend, a doctor at CMC, came by to visit while I was in radiation (okay, so you know you are at CMC a bit too much when friends stop by to visit you there). I paged her after my appointment, and we went to a private place to hang out and chat. I filled her in on the latest news and then shed a few tears. She is a great listener as well as quite inspiring. And I love the fact that she is an MD (not in oncology though). I showed her my chest (or where by chest used to be—I flash more (un)boob than a drunk girl at Mardi Gras). We decided the spots look a bit like ringworm, just not in rings. Boy, wouldn't that be wonderful! I'll just go out and buy some anti-fungal spray, and then I'll be sure to live to see my boys go off to college. Shit! The worries are creeping back in again.

I am doing all I can to get better. I just need to leave it to my doctors and to God, and if I die soon (hopefully, I will have at least a couple of years left), then that is just going to be the way it goes. I do plan to go down swinging. I do hope to stop crying about it. I hope the tears stop sometime soon.

Soon to be visible once again from space,
-Uniboob

April 4, 2008

It has been a whirlwind of appointments this week I am ty-erd. They should really think about changing the way they spell that, it could be tyerd or tyyerd, depending on where you're from. Anyway, I have lots to tell.

Joe and I met with Dr. Frenette and discussed the state of things. It looks like the skin is not the big concern right now. Hopefully, my "hyperfractionated" (two-a-days in laymen's terms) RT will work. The bigger concern is the possibility of a systemic spread of the disease (breast cancer cells moving somewhere other than my chest).

The possibility, however slim, still exists that I may not have any cancer cells anywhere. Because this is not too likely, we will start chemo the day after I get my port. So, I will finish RT on April 18 or 21, go to Duke on the 22nd, get my port on the 23rd, and then start chemo on the 24th. That should be a fun week.

I will get re-scanned the week following chemo, an even more exciting week.

As Dr. Frenette has mentioned several times, we are entering un-chartered waters with chemo at this point. There is no data out there on what to do in a situation like mine. So, after consulting colleagues at Duke and Sloan Kettering, we have selected a course of therapy for me. It will most likely be Navelbine, unless the scans show something ....

To sum it all up, in a few weeks we are somewhat blindly (but with a consensus) starting a chemo drug that we have no way to measure whether it is working, but we can only measure if it is not (i.e., I get distant metastases and become a stage 4 (there is no stage 5), which would show up on a scan). So, my job, aside from continuing to do all I can do to find a cure, is to stop projecting and start finding joy in the here and now. To paraphrase a quote, "Worrying does not change tomorrow, it only robs today." Hopefully, I am up to the task. There is still lots of fun to be had.

-Uniboob

April 13, 2008

I spent a good part of last week at appointments, fifteen in all (fourteen this coming week). By Friday, my soul was worn thin. I was spent. It wasn't the fatigue so much as the constant flirtation with the issue of my mortality that wiped me out. It silenced my muse and made me quite sulky and surly. But yesterday was rejuvenating. It was a day spent with Rocco and Joe (we missed Luca a ton: he was with JuJu) doing normal stuff. Hopefully, we will have many, many more such days.

Please pray that my radiation therapy is working to kill any and all local cancer cells and that my upcoming (end of the month, dates not yet set) scans will be CLEAN.

APRIL 15, 2008

Tomorrow, I am getting a biopsy of my axila (armpit). It is a bit swollen and tender again in what feels like the lymph node that started this whole process. It could be from the lymph edema that is starting. I should get the results back later tomorrow. Please pray the biopsy shows no cancer.

Dr. Frenette also wants to re-scan me prior to starting the Navelbine next week. His nurse is setting up my scan appointments for this Thursday or Friday. Please pray that all my scans come back negative and that there is no evidence of disease.

We need these prayers! I believe many voices are louder than just one. I know in my heart God answered all the prayers and gave me clean scans the last time. We need divine intervention again (and always!). It would be incredible to start the Navelbine (four more long months of chemo) with clean scans and lots of hope for a long future! Please ask God to let me grow old with my husband and see my boys off to college!

Thanks for all your help,
-Uniboob

APRIL 17, 2008

The results are in, and they are not good. The lump in my armpit is cancerous. I just found out a bit ago. We have tons of questions and won't know a lot of answers until after the results of my scans tomorrow are in and we meet again with all my various docs.

Please pray that my scans are clean (meaning the cancer has not spread to any other organs) and that the cancer is confined to my armpit and will be wiped out. If my scans show it has spread, it is a different ball game, and the discussion moves to prolonging life, not curing the disease. But it ain't over 'til it's over.

APRIL 18, 2008

FULL SCAN RESULTS ARE IN. THEY ARE ALL CLEAN!!!!!!!!!!!!!!! This is Joe taking over Jen's site for one minute to let you rejoice with us today. Jen is COMPLETELY exhausted, both physically and emotionally, and can't come to the computer right now. When she has some strength back, she will give you all the details. We still have that spot of cancer to deal with, and this doesn't mean we will never have any metastases, but for now Jen is NOT a stage 4!

Thank you all for your LOUD and effective prayers!!! And Thank You, Lord, for watching over us.

April 20, 2008

Thank you all for your prayers and inspiring words. THEY WORKED! My scans are CLEAN (just wanted to say that again)! God has given me yet another chance! I have to be on my fourth or fifth life by now. I must be part feline, nine lives and all that. It's kind of funny, I always considered myself a dog person. Go figure.

We did manage to get out and do some celebratory things. We went to the range with Rocco and Uncle Jeff, had dinner with good friends, and did a playdate with a good friend and her daughter this weekend, all the while trying to rest from the insane ups and downs and catch our breath before the whirlwind starts again. And it starts again bright and early tomorrow.

I see Dr. Frazer in the morning, and then I have a meeting of the minds with Dr. Frazer, Dr. Frenette, and Dr. White to review the next line of attack. I am still going to Duke on Tuesday, and they will discuss their opinions with us and the Charlotte team. At this particular moment, it looks like the plan will be surgery to remove the mass in my axilla, more radiation, and chemo. Details will follow after we know more.

Thank you again for all the prayers, and thanks to God for restoring our hope. Still lots of fight left in this dog, I mean cat.

-Uniboob

April 21, 2008

What's life for this cancer patient without a little drama? Went in (early) for my radiation and appointment with Dr. Fraser this morning to talk about our plan of attack for the armpit spot. We got a preliminary game plan from them both. I mentioned that I had a sore spot on my neck that was swollen. I figured it was probably due to pollen, but this was examined and not taken lightly.

Three needle biopsies to the neck later, we are waiting to hear results. Preliminary (must be my word of the day) results show atypical cells. This is NOT good news. I have heard this twice before, and both times the results were cancer. The location is quite perplexing. We are still hopeful that it is not metastasis. We should know results later today or tomorrow at the latest. Please get on those knees again and say some more prayers for us!

-Thanks, Uniboob

April 23, 2008

For those of you anxiously awaiting my neck biopsy results from Monday, we still have not heard the official news. However, based on our exam yesterday, we will only be surprised if the results come back negative for cancer.

We arrived home from our marathon trip to Duke last night. We were scheduled to see both Dr. Marcum and the surgeon, Dr. Wilke. We ended up only seeing Marcum. It turns out that surgery is no longer a good option, so no removing the lump in the armpit today, or ever. Also, I don't need a port at this point either. So, strangely enough, I currently have nothing scheduled for today. This might change as I have been battling some sort of virus or bacteria or whatever, and today I have a fever and feel like I have been beaten with a baseball bat.

The meeting with Marcum was a mix of good, bad, and ugly. The good: there is a trial starting next week (a miracle?) for my particular situation. With what we know now, we still have some treatment options. Bad: he said, basically, I have distant metastases (although, thank God, not in any organs or bones that were just scanned), which puts me in the stage 4 category. Dr. Frenette will order a PET scan and a brain MRI. Please pray that these additional scans do not show any more mets, especially anything widespread on the PET or anything at all in the brain, which would mean I am SOL and would have two years at best. The fact that the cancer has spread outside of the breast, hence the stage 4 diagnosis, means I will get treated forever. Please pray that forever for me is a lot of years! I want lots more time with my family! I want to see my beautiful boys hit all the milestones .... The Ugly: how long might I have? We won't really know until the study ends. If we don't get promising results soon, then my end of days will be sooner rather than later. Hopefully and prayerfully, they will find something that works and buy lots of time.

Thanks for your help and prayers!
-Uniboob

April 23, 2008

YAHOO! My neck biopsy came back negative! We are quite stunned, and so are my docs. Apparently, the pathologist kept doing different stains on my slides because we all expected it to come back positive for cancer, given the rest of my situation.

We are most thankful (thanks, Big Guy) and quite encouraged. The rest of the deal is still the same: I'll get my PET scan and brain CT tomorrow, followed by a visit to Dr. Frenette. We will take copies of these tests when we go to Duke next week to start the trial.

-One happy, one boobed lady!

April 25, 2008

YAHOO, NUMBER TWO!! My PET scan and brain CT are CLEAN! Thank you, God!!! Thank you, Team Go Jen Go, for all your help!

All of the excitement during the last week and a half (or maybe over the last nine months) has really tuckered me out. I seem to have a bit of a virus and a sinus infection. I can't wait to feel a bit better and celebrate! Currently, I am in convalescing mode (how extraordinarily boring and frustrating, but I suppose necessary) and trying to use this time to get back to feeling like my regular old self. I will keep you posted as soon as we learn about my treatment plan.

-Uniboob

MAY 1, 2008

*O*ur little life raft has made it through the doldrums and caught a mighty wind; our wait for a treatment plan has finally ended! No longer will we wash about, adrift at sea, wondering if we might get rescued. Today, we put our feet down on solid ground. Tomorrow, we start attacking my little cellular foes once again.

Duke finally called this morning to give us the details on the GSK clinical trial and to let us know if I even qualified for the new drug. It was insanely frustrating to hold off treatment for a study that I might not even meet the criteria for. After lots of info gathering and more question provoking discussion with Duke, we went to see Dr. Frenette and his nurse armed with our new info. After graciously working us into the schedule on a moment's notice, we discussed all my treatments options, both here and in Durham, at length.

Blah, blah, blah … both doctors agree we have three good options to choose from—two here, one at Duke. Boring medical details and lots of shades of gray later, Joe and I were initially quite stressed because we thought, after the prolonged wait/drama for the Duke info, that I was not even going to qualify for their trial. I did qualify, and thus we had to choose. After more discussion, a lengthy pros/cons list, and prayers, it came down to a gut decision. As Dr. Frennete put it, "There is no way to make a wrong decision with the information that we have." Our guts led the way, and we are going with an option available here in Charlotte.

I start an oral chemo, Tykerb, ASAP, and will be on it indefinitely. As of right now, I will also be starting the weekly IV drug, Navlebine (navy bean), next Tuesday. I will unfortunately have to get a port. Oh well. Let's pray Dr. White works me into his schedule right away!

We are so excited to get going in the right direction again and continue in our fight to Kick Cancer's Ass! I already feel like a different person, one back amongst the living and not wandering aimlessly about in purgatory. Although I have VERY much enjoyed the last few days with my family (Rocco and I have had an especially great time playing spiderwebs), I have been in a bit of a fog as I tried not to focus on not getting treated. Well, the fog has lifted, and I am back! Let's go, chemo!

MAY 5, 2008

What a great weekend! I hope everyone enjoyed the beautiful weather as much as we did. We did a very low-key celebration of Luca's first birthday. Hard to believe a year has gone by .... He is such a big boy now and was just a little squirt back when I was diagnosed. He is so much fun. He has a great, smiley little personality, until one of the trucks he is playing with tips over (then we see a glimpse of his little Italian temper), or until his brother tries to grab something out of his hands. Sharing is not a concept Rocco gets just yet.

Please keep those positive vibes comin' our way. I start on IV Navelbine (pre-port) tomorrow. I will get it three weeks out of every four for the next four to six months, as well as the oral chemo, Tykerb, which I will be on indefinitely.

-Uniboob

MAY 10, 2008

I have missed my peeps, and you guys are my peeps. I have been offline for a few days for system maintenance, and now I am back. Welcome to the new and improved Jen, version 2.1, if you will. I can now offer instant IV access 24/7! My transformation into the Bionic Woman is now almost complete.

Can you tell I am still under the influence of some drugs? I still feel a bit odd but much better than yesterday. Yesterday, I woke up feeling like I'd had a fifth of tequila, which would have been fine if I'd had the good times to go with it. But all I managed to get was the bitchin', head-splitting headache, exhaustion, and very fuzzy thinking.

We had another marathon visit at CMC on Thursday. The catheter went in fine. I was awake and chatting during the whole procedure. I am sure I said nothing the least bit stupid and that I was my normal, witty self. The cath placement was not too bad (they would not let me watch though), but the tugging and pushing on my left shoulder really put a hurtin' on me afterwards. I had this very persistent, deep joint ache that I used to get pre-shoulder redo. So, I had pain meds and anti-nausea meds several times over, hence the major hangover and post-UGA football game flashbacks.

Anywho, I am feeling much more like my normal self. My biggest concerns (okay, not really my biggest) right now are: will the catheter be in the way of my bikini top? And will I be able to sleep on my left side again without discomfort? These types of problems I can deal with! Happy Mother's Day!

-Jen 2.1

May 12, 2008

We had a great Mother's Day weekend. We had a family gathering at the lake Saturday, and yesterday was a normal (don't have too many of those anymore) day with my three boys. It doesn't get much better than that.

Tomorrow, I am due for Navelbine again. Even though time seemed to really drag its feet last week, I can't believe it is time for IV chemo again. This one-week schedule (as opposed to my former three) will take some getting used to. I know I shouldn't end a sentence in a preposition, but today I am throwing caution to the wind. I still haven't sorted out what exactly is causing my current bevy of symptoms. I can't tell if it is the oral drug (Tykerb), the IV Navelbine, the after effects/drugs of the port placement, the stress of the last nine months, or a combo of all of the above (wah, wah, wah) .... I do know that I seem to be under some sort of sleeping spell. I can hardly stay awake. Thank goodness it is mainly weakness and sleepiness, and not tiredness.

I am a bit anxious to try out the new port. Hopefully, it will go without a hitch. I can't take the navy bean in another peripheral vein. My arm still throbs and burns all the way up from last week (man, am I whiney today—and I am holding back—don't get me started!).

Better go before the violins start playing.
-Uniboob

May 16, 2008

Well, the port passed inspection with Dr. White on Tuesday! He asked about the post-surgical pain in my shoulder (apparently, most people who get ports haven't had their shoulders re-done), and I told him it was a still a bother but not nearly as bad as it was following surgery. I went from White to my chemo appointment la-la-la-ing, happy to get the go-ahead to swim and looking forward to not getting my arm maimed.

Chemo in the port was a breeze. The RN was a bit apologetic that I still had to get one needle stick, but she did not seem to realize that the skin piercing the needle is nothing more than a small annoyance—the pain comes from the screaming veins that like to collapse, spasm, roll, or blow. I'm so glad there is no more of that! The navy bean is not too bad. It is still chemo, but most of the side effects seem quite manageable so far. The most challenging side effect at this point is a crazy amount of fatigue, which is a blessing when compared to some of the side effects from my previous treatments.

It is like I am under a sleeping spell from some strange potion. I am only good and awake for a few hours at a time, followed by a couple hours of napping. I am even managing eight to ten hours of shut eye at night. A few days of this probably sounds fantastic to some of you, but I am worried about this lasting for the duration of this treatment. Frequently, I am too tired and unmotivated to do even basic things (except in spurts). This "rest" would be fine if I wasn't a wife, mother, daughter, sister, friend .... I don't want life to pass me totally by these next few months. I am supposed to be seizing the day!

I have lots left to say, but I am too tired to write right now.

Nap time ....
-Jen

May 23, 2008

I have been absent from this site and life in general the past few days. This round of navy bean has hit a bit harder than the last two. I have been primarily off the grid, shuffling back and forth from porch to den, in the quiet. My brain is slightly askew. I am in a strange state. I feel tired and wobbly, dreamy, and maybe a bit like I am slowly coming off of some weird party drug and have yet to get my bearings. Maybe now would be a good time to pick up a copy of *Fear and Loathing in Las Vegas*.

All this weirdness aside, we are actually leaving for the beach tomorrow. This is the trip that was originally planned for last year, but then I got diagnosed, so we postponed it until now because we thought I would be done with treatment. OMG! I am excited and worried at the same time—so much to pack and organize, so little brain and body power to do it with. Just getting myself out the door would be a feat right now, let alone the boys too. I am sure we will forget tons of stuff (anything but my drugs we can live without for a week), but we'll manage.

The sun, surf, and sand will be so therapeutic! We haven't been to the ocean in so long. I am sure it will be rejuvenating and life affirming. And, hopefully, lots of fun to boot!

See ya in a week.
-Jen

June 1, 2008

Well we made it to Oak Island, along with most everything we needed (a Memorial Day miracle!) in a mere six hours (including an hour-plus stop at a fast-food play-place to burn off a little baby/toddler energy). It had been a long two years since we last had a beach vacation. It was wonderful, soothing, invigorating, and good for the soul. It was rejuvenating to be away and concentrate on just enjoying rather than on treatment. We all had such a good time. It was so fun to see Rocco so busy playing in the sand (he's still a bit iffy when it comes to the waves), and Luca loved every part of the beach, water included. Watching them experience the ocean, with its myriad of delights and with the joy only children can exhibit, was beautiful. And even though I spent each afternoon quietly tucked away inside, napping to regain my energy, I have never felt more grateful and privileged to spend time with my family. Each moment with them was truly precious, a little gift from God, and one of the blessings of this diagnosis.

-Uniboob

P.S. I didn't look too bad in the bikini tops, despite the obvious, and now I finally have a little color, too. Gotta run, TIS.

June 11, 2008

I finally gave up on more sleep, but I am fairly happy with five hours of good rest and no icky Homer Simpson/Wonka side effect. I lay in bed and mediated for a while. My mind went directly to summiting Grand Teton (I hadn't been there in a while). My meditation began with most of the long climb behind me. I had almost finished the difficult struggle that I frequently picture occurring after a sliding fall near the top. I reached the summit, arms outstretched, Joe standing a few feet below me. As I looked around, I noticed the skies were ominous, low, and pregnant with dark thunderheads. Lightning flashed all around. The breeze was still, however; and I stepped off the ledge and flew out into the valley, taking my usual form of a great hawk or eagle. The valley was beautiful and vast below me, and as I flew, lightning began to strike all around. I did not fear this; I only woke and wondered what, if anything, it meant.

June 27, 2008

This week has been such a blessing. Boy, I love my chemo "off" weeks. Rocco has been out of school and around for most of the week. It has been so wonderful getting to do normal stuff with him and Luca! Luca is totally incredible, walking around everywhere and babbling up a storm. It is so beautiful to see him grow and change almost daily. And speaking of growing, I had the pleasure of taking Rocco to see his first big-boy movie this week, *Kung Fu Panda*. He did great. We were able to watch most of the movie, with the exception of a few run-around-out-in-the-hall breaks, which was way more than I had expected. The movie had a good message and a few good quotes. Two of which, following in the style of the Kung Fu movies of old, had great messages and really got me thinking: "Yesterday is history, tomorrow is a mystery, and today is a gift, that is why they call it a present" (could this be any more true following a cancer diagnosis?), and "Our destiny is often found on the very path we take to avoid it." Hmmm, Shifu is one smart, red panda.

Get out and enjoy!

July 2, 2008

*M*y brief sojourn to the land of normal living was great! Lots of good time spent with the boys doing regular, fun summer stuff: a movie, trips to the grocery store, painting a few pieces of backyard furniture, a trip to Discovery Place, and lots of giggling. But alas, I'm back to the weekly grind. It seemed way too pretty out to have to go and sit through several hours of chemo today. But all went well. I saw Dr. Frenette too, and he addressed some concerning symptoms I have had of late. He thinks most are post-radiation therapy related, especially considering my aggressive treatment, but he suggested a follow up with Dr. Fraser and a CT scan in three weeks to more convincingly rule out concerns.

July 9, 2008

I have been largely off the grid for this past week. Let me say though that we had a nice Fourth of July. It was a bit low-key, but fun nonetheless. And, huge bonus, we took Rocco to see his first fireworks display over at Carmel. It was fantastic! He was such a big boy, especially considering we sat close enough to need sunscreen rather than bug spray. We got there just before it started, and I was wondering why we got such a great seat. I love fireworks! What a fantastic, visceral link to the joyous summers of my youth, made all the more real when feeling the vibrations of each shot reverberate in my chest. It was a perfect evening made even better because I got to share it with my son (hopefully, with both sons next year; Luca was at JuJu's and is way too small not to be terrified, especially when we sit in the "fall" zone), my husband, and neighbors.

-Uniboob

July 16, 2008

I hit a milestone yesterday. I completed the halfway treatment for my IV navybean. Whew! Let's pray the next three months will be it for the IV chemo, so I can get on with things.

Speaking of praying, please put in some words with the Big Guy for me about my upcoming scans. I am having a few symptoms Dr. Frenette would like to check up on, so Monday I am having a head/chest/abdomen/pelvis CT scan. I will see Dr. Frenette next Thursday to get results.

Please pray that there is no new cancer and that my existing lump is shrinking away to nothing! I am nervous about this and the fact that I will be getting results just before Rocco's third birthday party and the anniversary of my one-year diagnosis. I'm stressed and concerned and need some major prayer help! I really want to hit the one-year mark feeling positive.

Thanks, Uniboob

July 24, 2008

The verdict is in: CLEAN SCANS ONCE AGAIN!!! Thank you, God! Thank you, everyone, for all your kind words and prayers—they worked! I wanted to get out the news right away. I have a bit more to tell (none bad), but now I am going to unplug the phone and nap until Rocco gets up. I am pooped!

One happy, one-boobed lady!

July 25, 2008

Thanks, everyone, for writing in and calling! Now that we've rested (Whew, scan week is exhausting!) and had some time to let things sink in a bit, we are ready to get on with life.

Tomorrow is Rocco's Spiderman-themed third-birthday party. I am so excited and really looking forward to celebrating his big day with high spirits! The only downside is we are also giving up the pacifier this weekend too. Big boys don't need paceys. We'll see who this is harder on, Rocco or Joe and me. Who knows, maybe the trauma of not having a pacey will snap him out of his super-clingy phase? I can dream, can't I?

Have a good weekend, everyone!

July 29, 2008

Whew! All the excitement of the past few days has pooped me out a bit, but it is a damn good tired. It all began with a great celebratory meal Friday night. The tremendous bar bill (I even managed to have a cocktail!) reflected the magnitude of our good news. And I must say, the Pagani boys (the big ones, not my sons) can really rally after a night of heavy drinking. I expect my sons will be able to do the same in a few years.

The big-boy birthday party was great, too! It was everything I had hoped for and, most importantly, I think it exceeded even Rocco's expectations. The kids (and more than a few adults) went nuts on the bouncy things, and the surprise visit by Spiderman was a HUGE hit! What a fabulous day! I felt so good and was so thankful to be able to truly celebrate. I said several prayers throughout the day, thanking God for my clean scans and giving us the great weekend. I had so much fun. I haven't had fun like that in a long, long time. What a gift!

And, huge bonus! I hope I am not jinxing us, but Rocco has slept through the night both nights since giving up his pacifier. He is a big boy now, and I hope this continues, especially since it is back to the weekly grind in a few hours.

Off to see the wizard ....
-Jen

July 30, 2008

Let me start by saying this is long—sorry in advance, and due to my drug rattled brain, it is not nearly as eloquent as I had imagined it would be.

Tomorrow is a significant day for me. A day that, prior to last week's scan results, filled me with more fear and dread than joy. It is the one-year anniversary of my cancer diagnosis, a noteworthy day in the life of any cancer patient. I have over the past several weeks relived the shock and horror of that fateful day. I can remember it in such vivid detail. It provokes the darkest of feelings. It has dredged up images of the past year that I would largely like to forget—so much suffering, so much fear.

Although I am sure that some of these thoughts and emotions will come unbidden to me tomorrow, I have for the most part moved past this. In light of the clean scans (the armpit thing is still there but is getting very hard to see), the great birthday weekend, and Joe's positive influence, I am more able to focus on the great strides we have made since that awful day. I now have a year of treatment under my belt. Think of all the cancer ass I have kicked in that time!

Despite the negatives, the diagnosis has been a blessing in so many ways. Joe and I have both grown in our relationships with God, I can now see the good in people first instead of the bad, I now appreciate and see the beauty in the smallest of things and strangest of places, and I have learned over and over again of the kindness of strangers, acquaintances, friends and family alike.

I have also come to understand that nothing should be taken for granted. But while this is true, I cannot spend my time in fear of what may or may not come to pass. To quote Aristotle speaking to Dante in *The Divine Comedy*, "The way out is the way through," and I am hopefully and prayerfully almost all the way out.

August 6, 2008

J need to whine about the weather. It is too damn hot. It has been making me feel like kee-rap. I have some (previously unmentioned to you guys) treatment-related, not disease-related, swelling in my right lung, which is making my breathing a bit of a challenge of late, since it has been humid and a million degrees out. Wah, wah, wah. Done bitchin' for now; my usual DAC (Day After Chemo) rant is over.

I have been way more tired of late, but I have really enjoyed the boys. Rocco is such a card. He actually makes really funny jokes and has us in stitches at least once a day. Of course, I had lots of funny stories and quotes to share, but chemo-brain strikes again. Luca has been a scream lately, literally. He is so cute, fast, independent, and loves to be chased around, especially if he has something he knows he shouldn't or thinks you are going to tickle him. But he has only two forms of oral communication: babbling or screaming. Lately, screaming has been his MO. I used to call Rocco "Mr. Squeakers" because of all the cute sounds he made at that age. Lately, I have taken to calling Luca "Mr. Shriekers."

Lastly, let me say that yesterday I really did NOT want to go to chemo. I was dreading it, feeling a bit pitiful, and did not want to leave the house even for a swim (I have been swimming for exercise, my very most favorite thing!). It totally poops me out but does wonders for my body, mind, and spirit. While in the pool, my thoughts ran to the negative. In the midst of struggling mightily (again, not a pool usual for me, even during chemo), I tried to gain control of my mind and spirit. Finally, I managed to do so. I realized that chemo is a gift, and all I had to do was to go and receive it. Wow! My circumstances did not change—only my perspective—and that might be the most important thing.

So let me leave you with one thought: find what out what your gift is today, and go receive it willingly.

August 13, 2008

Okay, thanks to the steroids, I got my usual post-chemo four-hour nighttime nap. But I am pretty proud, and relieved, to now be officially done with another four months of chemo (next week is my off week). Hopefully, just two more months to go. That's only six more treatments, one little surgery to pluck out that spot under my arm, and a wee bit of radiation left. I CAN DO THIS!

When I am so tired it is hard to even walk down the stairs; it is so incredible to get up at this hour and turn on the Olympics. Could anything be more inspiring than the most beautiful spectacle in sport? A triumph and celebration of the potential of the human body and spirit. It is a combination of grace, discipline, and determination unparalleled anywhere else on Earth; an event to unite all the world in competition. How fantastic! I watch the athletes (especially those in the Water Cube—Phelps and Torres are my very most favorites) and gather strength from their achievements, and determination from their presence and their performances. That they have all overcome great odds and worked tirelessly is not lost on me. I revel in it.

And, in my own way, and due to labs that have gone from sucks to shitty (it doesn't count as cursing between the hours of three and six in the morning), I will soon be joining the ranks of some unscrupulous Olympians (and Tour de Francers). Pending approval of my insurance company, I will be blood doping (starting shots to boost my body's manufacture of red blood cells; the four I have left don't seem to be hauling their weight) in a day or two. I hope they won't start testing the Olympic spectators too, because I will be really pissed if they don't let me watch the games.

One Huge Phelps Phan!

-Jen

AUGUST 19, 2008

PG-13 (Whiny Content, Language)

I have been struggling mightily lately and decided not to write in. My mom always said, "If you don't have anything nice to say, it is better to not say anything at all," thus the silence on my end. I was all psyched-up last Tuesday (thank you, Team USA swimming!), but oh, how things change. Since early last week, I have been feeling lousy: ridiculously tired (the blood-doping shot to boost my red blood cell production takes weeks to produce really noticeable results), terribly cranky, comically achy, and sometimes downright pissed off.

Nothing happened to spur on my anger. It just came out of the blue. Apparently, some part of my brain is quite ticked that life has gone merrily by for most folks, while I (I speak for my family here too) have been dealing life and death on a daily basis for what seems like forever now. A few oblivious comments that normally would have rolled off my back have infuriated and depressed me, and made me feel very isolated. I know how incredibly lucky I am to have so much support from so many people, and that is why the anger surprised me a bit.

AUGUST 22, 2008

We (just Joe and I) are off to the mountains today, thanks to Gammy and Papa, who practically had to throw us out. This will be our first weekend alone (and to vacation) in a very, very long time. We are excited!

I think it will also be good for my lung, which is starting to be a real pain in the patootie. For the first time ever, since the beginning of chemo, I have been told to withhold my drugs (Tykerb only) to give my body a chance to recover from side effects. I will get re-scanned next week to check that this is a side effect of lung swelling and not cancer. Hopefully this little break will be just what my body needs to get back in the swing of things.

Enjoy the cooler weather,
-Jen

August 27, 2008

We took the scenic route to Beech Mountain on Friday. It took me most of the day to feel better and settle into vacation mode. A relaxing dinner at a rustic, outdoor café in the cool mountain air helped me shift gears and shed most of my aches, pains, and worries. We stocked up on supplies at Fred's General Mercantile, took in the soft colors of the Blue Ridge, met a very cute but camera-shy groundhog, and spent the night tucked away in a log cabin on the side of the mountain. Ahhh. Saturday was even better. I woke up leisurely to the sound of birds, sipped on some coffee, read on the big porch, and had the luxurious pleasure of snuggling in long pants and a fleece. The crisp cool air was fantastic, invigorating, and much easier on my lungs. I really should live somewhere cool and preferably high; it is the perfect fit for my soul. Our first adventure was a trip over to the original Mast General Store in Valle Crusis. It is so beautiful there, and I love that store! It is always on our mountain itinerary. Oh my gosh, am I writing a novel? Cut to the chase—our getaway was great! And it was a huge bonus not to wipe anyone's butt but my own!

Quick re-cap of visit with Dr. Frenette yesterday. My lungs are improving. I will stay off oral chemo until I am 80-90 percent side-effect-free, and then I will resume it at a lower dose. My red blood cell counts are a bit better, but they could be much better, so I might get the blood-doping shot again. My white blood cell counts are so-so. And I only have five more Navelbine rounds to go!!!

-Jen, the girl who is tired of political coverage and ready for UGA football to begin. GO DAWGS!!

September 3, 2008

Caution: this might be hard to follow. I'm tired and am suffering from T.I.S.

It seemed like a great idea at the time to show Mr. Shriekers how cute Thomas was on the computer, but now I am starting to realize I may have to hide in a closet to successfully use the computer when he is around.

As per usual, lately, I have been off the computer for a few days. There is lots of craziness going on, and a new school-year stomach bug is already at our house. We like to be on the cutting edge.

Yesterday, I went in for a little swim (picture lots of hanging onto the walls and frequent stopping and starting) before chemo yesterday and ran into a small problem. My left arm (port side. Oh great, now I sound like a freaking boat) was swollen, looked reddish purple, and it felt like it was being strangled. It seemed rather important not to go home but stick around the hospital area. I tried to use my cell phone about twenty times to call Dr. Frenette's office but kept getting a "No Network Available" message. Naturally, I was fantasizing about doing some nasty stuff to the phone company people or, at the very least, ripping my flip phone in half (even in my chemo-weakened state, I think that was a viable option). But it occurred to me that Rocco and Luca were playing with my phone just the day before and maybe this had something to do with them. It did.

In the meantime, I went to a good friend's house that is just around the corner from the hospital. She fed me and let me play with her daughter and use her phone. Thanks to her, it worked out well. I got worked in at CMC for an ultrasound (by the time I was seen, my symptoms were declining and the impending arm-explosion feeling was mainly gone). I then went to see Gary, and then went on to the imaging center for a chest X-ray. I was too tired by the time (four-ish?) I saw Gary to even think clearly but it seems I have a small blood clot that partially obstructed flow in my arm. So, for the first time ever in ten-plus months of treatment, I am not on any chemo. Yikes! I started Coumadin for the clot and should start back with the navy bean next week. I'm waiting on X-ray results which I should have by this afternoon, to see if I can restart the Tykerb. I'm a bit nervous about the lung X-rays. I seem to get nervous whenever they take my "picture" now.

Waiting for the phone to ring, Jen

September 10, 2008

I had a fantastic day yesterday. I had a leisurely (okay, that may be an exaggeration: fun and rambunctious is more accurate) morning with both boys, and it was nice to feel good and not have to rush them off anywhere. It was so incredible just to do regular mom stuff! I was able to take Rocco to his Sports Camp Class. Both he and I hate that I miss so many of his activities, so it was great to see him in action and to hang out with his buddies' moms. These are the gals who have done so much for us over the past year, and it was my first real chance to sit and talk with them probably all year. What a gift! I actually came home afterwards and wept tears of joy at how fantastic it was to feel good and get to do some of the things I usually miss out on.

I am most happy to report that I got my navy bean. Whew! Hopefully, my lungs will be okay enough to restart my Tykerb next week. I did not see Gary, so I have no updates on the malignancy under my arm, but I am feeling like, at least with some chemo in me, I am moving in the right direction. I'm ready to get that damn thing taken out (scheduled for October 29th). They also doubled my Warfarin (blood-clot med) after testing my blood. I am a bit relieved by this because my arm was still looking pretty scary every evening, and I figured that probably wasn't a good thing.

Thanks again to those of you have joined the team, take the boys for playdates, and even still bring us dinner. You inspire me to continue this fight!

-Jen, the almost 'normal' mom

September 15, 2008

I had a busy, fun-filled weekend! I love the normal stuff! On Saturday, we went to the Serve for the Cure tournament again. It was so wonderful to see everyone from last year and meet some new folks too. What a positive, empowering experience for the girls involved. Celebrating female athletic achievement and at the same time raising money for charity is a combo that is hard to beat. Many thanks to those who worked so hard to raise over $35,000 for Komen.

I have a chest X-ray later today to see if my lungs are ready to restart Tykerb. Please pray that this is the case! Also, I meet with Gary tomorrow to discuss the malignant tumor in my armpit (sounds so undignified). Please pray our discussion goes well and they find everything this time!!! I am SOOO ready to be a doting mom and wife (I have already been warned that next year is the Year of Joe), and I have lots of people I want to help.

-Uniboob

P.S. Rocco and Luca can both do the Go Dawgs war cry. I think that is why we squeaked out that win over Spurrier.

SEPTEMBER 18, 2008

OMG! What unbelievable weather! I feel like a new woman! The season of air-conditioned isolation is finally over!

It was so pleasant yesterday, I was even able to walk outside without feeling like I might croak. I was so giddy and light-headed from the low humidity (not from blood clot problems), I even wanted to run a bit. I did not; sanity prevailed at the last possible moment.

I did, however, get the okey-dokey to restart my Tykerb. I'm very psyched about this. You know your life has radically changed when you get excited about restarting chemo! My last chest X-ray showed no change in my lungs, but my symptoms had improved, so Gary gave me the go-ahead to start back. I am on a slightly decreased dosage and hope to be able to take it until a few days before my surgery. Kickin' some cancer ass! Go Dawgs!

-Uniboob

SEPTEMBER 22, 2008

What a great weekend: we had perfect weather (okay, I prefer it even cooler), I did fun stuff with my boys, we got to see some friends, and the Dawgs won (sic 'em!). Ahhh, life is good ....

Today I played America's Top One-Boobed Super Model. Thanks to a good friend's recommendation, I was selected to be the Asana Sportwear's Hero of the Month for October. Today, I had some pictures taken in various outfits, doing workout stuff. I am NOT a natural in front of the camera, but after a while I loosened up a bit. It was fun and for a good cause. My photo and bio will be up in various spots for October (Breast Cancer Awareness Month); more on this later ....

Thanks again to everyone who has signed up and raised money for our Komen team, and all of you who continue to do so, so many things for our family! We thank God for you every night!

-Jen

SEPTEMBER 24, 2008

Hello, fellow insomniacs and insanely early risers (I'm looking at you, triathletes and workaholics). I'm just getting up after my usual four-hour or so post-chemo nightly nap and thought I might say hello. I woke up thankful for treatment and for all the blessings bestowed on our family this past year by all of you. It is definitely not a bad way to shake out the mental cobwebs. And, I must say, it is worth the loss of sleep to be out on the porch with the windows thrown open, the cool air rushing in, and the owls hooting in the woods. Fall is delightful!

It is really hard to believe, but I only have two navy beans left! Just the thought of ending chemo, having another surgery, and then another blast of radiation fills me with both joy and trepidation. We are praying fervently (and hope you are too!) that my results will be much better this time, that we kicked cancer's ass for good, and that it is time for us to get back to the business of being a normal, healthy family—a family that has a new and improved perspective on the value of life and the innate goodness of people in it; a family that is filled with love and gives back to others. I pray frequently that God will guide me to follow that path in the right way. I am really looking forward to making a positive impact in the lives of others (survivors and supporters), and I plan to be doing it for many, many years to come!

-Uniboob

P.S. Go Dawgs! Roll right over 'Bama's Crimson Tide!

OCTOBER 6, 2008

The Komen Race weekend was fantastic, incredible, amazing! I am still reeling from the emotional impact of it all. What a testament to the generosity, compassion, love, and enthusiasm of the members of Team Go Jen Go and of all the thousands of other people who came out to support and do the race. It truly was a celebration of life, and you made it possible! Joe and I are deeply and profoundly touched. It was a powerful demonstration of the goodness of the human spirit and a gift that perhaps only a life-threatening illness can bestow. Thank you, Team Go Jen Go members and everyone who has provided us with so much support during this long journey. You have made us better people. Oh, and by the way, we all looked great in the new shirts and we really kicked some fundraising ass!

-A very humbled but empowered, Jen

October 7, 2008

TODAY IS MY VERY LAST IV NAVELBINE! Good riddance, goodbye, farewell! Time to get Joe a T-shirt that says: "My wife went to the oncologist 237 times, and all I got was this lousy T-shirt!" I'm trying to feel the JOY, but I am feeling a bit more of the cautious optimism currently ….

Please pray for clean scans on October 13th and 14th, and a 100 percent successful operation on the 29th!!! Then the joy will really sink in!

-Jen

October 10, 2008

Well, the navy bean isn't going down without a fight. My head is pounding, I'm achy all over, tired as you know what, I have more zits than a limo full of kids on the way to the junior prom, and I'm deathly pale (and apparently very whiny). It's not really a good look for me, but at least Halloween is right around the corner. I am just going to pretend I dressed up early this year.

Please pray extra hard for me this Monday and Tuesday! On Monday, I have my CT scans and an echo with my heart failure doc. On Tuesday, I have my bone scan. Pray for CLEAN SCANS and a good echo. I will start pestering Dr. Frenette and the gang for results as soon as the scans are done. I hope to have them by Wednesday-ish.

Thanks again for your prayers and all your incredible support!

-Go Dawgs! Jen

October 14, 2008

*T*he barium shakes were delicious yesterday! The new Creamy Vanilla (it sounded so promising that I fell for it) is so yummy that I only gagged once or twice. I would much rather have those than a large cup of steaming hot, very caffeinated coffee and my usual breakfast.

Okay, so I am a bit sassy this morning. CT scans are waiting to be read, and the results should be in sometime tomorrow. I will be sure to call Dr. Frenette's office nonstop until I hear what they have to say. My echo and appointment with Dr. Frank, the heart failure specialist, went well. Apparently, my heart can take a licking and keep on ticking. That was great news! One less thing to worry about. And he and his RN are just great, caring people!

I have the bone scan today. I'm not sure when these results will be in. This is the one that has me the most nervous this go-around. My right ribs (mastectomy side) are very sore, which has been an ongoing concern for most of my treatment. Hopefully and prayerfully, this is just a non-specific muscular problem and not a serious, metastatic one. It does seem to get aggravated when I play, tackle, and swing the boys around.

I'm off to consume and get injected with more radioactive isotopes. I will be glowing like a jack-o-lantern just in time for the holiday.

October 15, 2008

I got one great phone call already! My CT scans look good!!! The spot in my right axilla (armpit) is still there. We were expecting this because I can still feel it, but it has not increased in size! They are hoping and we are praying that at least some or even all of it is necrotic (dead tissue—basically a scar). We will find this out when we get surgical results following the procedure to remove it (on October 29th). Also, the swelling in my right lung from radiation and Tykerb has decreased in size.

All around, this is fantastic news and the answer to many prayers! Thank you!! I should hear the results of the bone scan test later today. So, please, please keep those prayers coming!

OCTOBER 15, 2008

*T*HE BONE SCAN IS CLEAN TOO! WHEW! THANK YOU, GOD!!!!! THANK YOU, EVERYONE, FOR ALL YOUR INCREDIBLE PRAYERS!

We are elated (to put it mildly) and exhausted too. We are one very important step closer to our plan of being cancer FREE!

Kickin' some major cancer butt,
-Uniboob

OCTOBER 20, 2008

*O*MG, I am pooped! We had a great but busy weekend, and today was a marathon of pre-surgical appointments. The visit with Dr. White was a bit nerve wracking. Please continue to pray for us. Please pray for great surgical results on October 29th. Hopefully, this will be a simple procedure for a small spot that is at least partially just dead tissue. This is still a rather significant hurdle to jump.

On a lighter note, Joe and I leave for a "mommy and daddy" vacation tomorrow, immediately following a first-thing visit to Dr. Frenette. I'm so ready for a vacation! You know you are desperate to get out of town when you leave your oncologist's office and go directly to the airport, and then have surgery within twelve or so hours after getting home. Southern Utah, here we come!

OCTOBER 30, 2008

*J*oe and I had a great time on our vacation. There's nothing like the majesty of Southern Utah's scenery to melt away all (well, almost all) fear, stress, and worry. It was a true getaway!

We arrived back in Charlotte late Tuesday night and went straight in for surgery first thing Wednesday morning. Dr. White was able to get margins, and he said there were no surprises. Good news! I go in for my post-surgical visit on Tuesday, and hopefully, we will get more good news then too. I'm a bit nervous about this visit because last time the news was far from encouraging. So please pray for a confirmation of good news. I am ready to be officially cancer free!!!!!

I am a bit slow and sore, but I'm looking forward to the weekend festivities. Happy Halloween, everyone! Go Dawgs, kick some Gator butt!

November 5, 2008

First of all, I am so glad I managed to drag my butt off the couch (the small surgery wiped me out much more than I anticipated, or was that my vacation?) on Friday for all the Halloween festivities. We had a great time with the boys! Luca was too cute and kept trying to give candy back at every door. Rocco was a very serious but polite Superman. It was also great to see so many neighbors. Thank you all for your prayers! It really makes my heart sing when people come up to me and say they follow my story and pray for us all the time! That is a precious gift and one of the blessings bestowed by this disease.

Down to brass tacks. We got the news about my surgical pathology results yesterday afternoon. It was not quite as clear-cut as I had anticipated, and thus I have been struggling mightily with what to write. I am conflicted about the results. Basically, they saw evidence that the chemo worked (good) but there was still an 8 mm or so cancerous tumor present in my axilla. We expected this but hoped otherwise. As per Dr. White's expectation, the tumor was encapsulated—think of it in a hard, self-contained shell, which is what we hoped for—but there were cancerous cells present in the perinodal lymphatics. These are the channels leading into and out of all lymph nodes. I had no idea about these channels until yesterday, although their presence makes total sense. I went to the appointment thinking "encapsulated" meant cancer was surrounded by a hard shell, making it unlikely to spread anywhere, and that would be really good news (the best-short of no evidence of cancer at all). I figured I'd have radiation and get on with my life!!!

But, although the doctors understood what an encapsulated node meant, I am still trying to adjust to this news that the cancerous node was more like an old potato with eyes on it rather than the walnut I had pictured. Crap! There is also the matter of margins (non-cancerous area around the tumor). The margins are great on one side, good on another, and close to non-existent on the third side. Crap again! I wanted nice margins all around. Of course, this is what radiation is for. So basically, I am trying to get my head around this uncertain news. Where is my written guarantee? Why couldn't I get a nice "no evidence of cancerous cells" report? Insert frustrated scream noise here!

So, as one of my good friends pointed out last night, it is time to get on with life and get past the not knowing. No one knows what the future holds. IF (NOT WHEN) I have to cross the cancer bridge again, I will do so. My job for now is to enjoy my life and savor every precious moment (even if Rocco is being very, very bad) with my family and friends. My job is to seize the day and to get myself back into the best shape possible to be a lean, mean cancer-fighting machine.

November 8, 2008

Yikes! I finally managed to get back on the computer. I still can't do it with Luca around because he immediately and constantly screams "choo-choo!" for the Thomas site. I am so soothed and buoyed by what you all have written in response to my pathology results. I also reread my last journal entry and decided that I am so long winded that my parents really should have named me Wendy. Thank you for your comforting and encouraging words! They move me and soothe me. I think I am managing to seize the day and get back to my old self most of the time. I am, however, getting seized by fear a bit too.

The fear is creeping in because I have a bit of fluid under the incision that I think needs draining again. Dr. White drained some on Monday when I got the pathology results and stitches out. This is potentially problematic because it can interfere with radiation. It effects the calculations or distorts the beam or something. Can you believe I have never, ever taken a physics class? Please pray for the radiation to start on time (by November 19) and for it completely wipe out every last cancerous cell!

-Jen (Wendy?)

November 12, 2008

J have way too much to say but will try to limit it a bit. I haven't been on the computer for a few days due to TIS. It's probably a good thing that I couldn't find the time on Monday. The entry would have been too dark. It was a long, emotionally difficult day. I had a mini breakdown or two. I had four doctor appointments, asked lots of stressful questions, developed new concerns, and I waited a bunch. A packed oncology office waiting room is really a great place to pass the time—not!

I wanted some answers to questions about the chances of distant mets (cancer that spreads to my organs), local recurrence, and the effectiveness of all these treatments. I got the standard "you are such a unique case, and there is no data out there" answer. Dealing with the probabilities vs. possibilities is so very difficult. I will just have to continue to defy the odds, whatever they are!

Ironically, it was and continues to be the very challenges (and of course, all the good stuff that goes along with the parent thing) of child care that got me out of my funk. Monday evening's dinner chaos and poop explosion made me forget all about my fears. Even though I still get frustrated and overwhelmed sometimes (and am tired all the time), I have real appreciation for every single moment I get to spend with all my boys. What an incredible blessing, and one I would have not received (I was a previously an easily frustrated, self-centered person) if it weren't for our current situation.

A quick story: I tried my first nap while the boys were home. Luca was napping too. I kiddie-proofed everything, locked up the house, and put a very sleepy Rocco on the couch with a movie of his choosing. I was so happy and confident that he would sleep, and I felt like my mommy ears would alert me to anything out of the ordinary; but I woke up later to the door bell ringing and the dog barking. Rocco was outside ringing it. He was playing with a squirt gun and had run out of water and needed to come back in. He had managed to get the gun off the top of the fridge (the Halloween candy was up there because I thought it was secure!) and fill it up in the sink all by himself. I realized how very impressive this was—check out the brain on Rocco!—while I was in the middle of scolding him. I told him this was quite a feat. He found the squirt gun (Joe and I had forgotten it was up there) after he rewarded himself with some candy for "peeing in the potty." Judging by the discarded wrappers, he thought about two pounds of candy was an appropriate reward. Aside from a tummy ache, we were quite lucky with the outcome!

November 14, 2008

So far, no more "Pagani prison breaks," which is a very good thing. And now my neighbors know if they see the boys outside without a parent, they need to come over and wake my butt up right away.

Yesterday, I went to see Dr. White for more post-surgical tending to. That went fine. We will, however, be postponing my radiation (after total assurance that it won't effect outcome) for a week to ten days, until we get this fluid thing under control.

But (there is almost always a but lately) he wanted to do a skin biopsy on a rash just above my radiation area on the right side of my chest. I have been worried about this. Why would an itchy rash appear adjacent to my surgical/radiation area and nowhere else? I don't believe in coincidences anymore, and I don't think Dr. White ever did. So they did a skin biopsy, and I had an emotional breakdown right there in the office. I'm not scared of the procedures; I'm scared of the potential results. One of the nurses (a short, big-bosomed African American woman who reminded me of the nurse in *Ferris Bueller's Day Off* who came to tell Sloan that her grandmother had passed) gave me a big hug, and I just cried right there on her shoulder and chest. Those big breasts really do provide comfort. I know most men think they are just for entertainment purposes ("motor boating" and all that), but they really are multi-talented. Everyone was very, very sweet and patient with me. They certainly helped calm me down.

So, if you aren't burnt out on asking the Big Man (or Woman!) for help on my behalf, please pray that my biopsy is negative, my radiation is 100 percent effective, and the cancer stays gone long enough for me to see Rocco and Luca graduate from high school!

Thank you!
-Jen—Mrs. ifs, ands, and of course, buts

November 19, 2008

Good morning, everyone! Great morning, actually. Joe here. The biopsy results are in, and they are negative! Jen is now truly NED! (No Evidence of Disease). We wanted to get this posted as soon as possible to thank all of you out there (our family, our friends, and the huge teams of Prayer Warriors) from the bottom of our hearts. We are truly grateful to have so many caring and compassionate people praying for Jen's continued health; and those loud prayers continue to work.

I know Jen will want to tell you more soon, but I wanted to share this wonderful news with everyone in the hopes that it will lift up your spirit as it has mine. My family will never lessen in our thanks for your love and support.

-Joe

November 21, 2008

I have wanted sit and write for so many days now, but I have been a mommy on the go, which has been completely fantastic.

Thank you all for supporting us and for celebrating with us too! I am so completely shocked by these great results that I haven't seemed to make the adjustment to the good news just yet. Seems that most everyone else has (thank goodness). I am indescribably relieved but seem to be a bit gun shy and afraid to totally give myself over to joy, only to be potentially devastated again at some later date. I think feeling the aches, seeing the scars, taking all the pills, and going to get manipulated (got to love those sexy radiation stickers) and laser beamed for the start of my radiation is leaving me with a slightly different take on the matter.

Don't want to look a gift horse in the mouth (and this is some horse!) and all that, but I am still a bit caught up on what the phrase No Evidence of Disease means. Does it mean that I am certifiably cancer free, like most everyone seems to think? No. It means that I have no cancer that can be detected on scans. Microscopic disease (the kind that has the potential to become a big problem later) is still around. Hopefully and prayerfully, it is limited to the area to be radiated!

I don't mean to be a party pooper; I'm just trying to come to terms with it all. I do start radiation today and am pretty psyched about that!

NOVEMBER 24, 2008

Can you believe I have already gotten three trips to the bug zapper (radiation) under my belt? I am so excited to be done before Christmas! I will need my energy to elbow folks out of my way at the sales racks; I've got to have those bargains this year. I am also lucky to have gotten an appointment time that lets me drop the kids off at school in the morning and get to CMC in time to visit with a friend or drop by the chapel. I spent some quality knee, time in there this morning—despite the very random and somewhat startling construction noises—asking God to make the treatment 100 percent effective and to continue to bless me with clean scans.

Thank you all for your prayers and inspirations! Please keep them coming, and also ask God's help for everyone suffering with illness this Thanksgiving.

NOVEMBER 30, 2008

We had a wonderful day at Gammy and Papa's. We all have a lot to be thankful for this year! I am still getting my head around the fact that treatment will be done soon. It's a very scary proposition for a person who has been actively fighting cancer for a year and a half. I am currently trying to get my body and mind back in that kick-cancer's-ass mode. I know that daily exercise, eating lots of organic fruits and veggies, prayer and meditation, plenty of sleep/naps, and enjoying every second of my family are now the ways I can keep this disease at bay. It sounds like an easy plan, but it is a bit hard to manage it all. I am working on it.

The boys are also proving to be a wonderful affirmation of life, and a distraction too. Luca is finally making that shift away from Mr. Shriekers (after a lot of instruction on how to say "no" instead of shrieking and shaking until he is red in the face). Last night, while we were out to dinner, he was shrieking at a very high volume, and I told him to stop and start using his words, to which he responded, "NO!" It was good for a chuckle.

And, to paraphrase a line from *The Departed* (The Depahted), I leave you with this parting thought: we are all on our way out, so act accordingly.

December 5, 2008

We finally saw Gary (Dr. Frenette) yesterday, the first visit since my armpit surgery (sounds so glamorous). It was a great appointment. After a brief exam, I actually changed out of my gown and sat in one of the regular office chairs to talk with him about my status, instead of remaining on the exam table. I felt like a big kid who just made the leap to the "adult table." It took me a year and a half, but I finally made it!

I had my usual question list. He answered them all. And now I have finally heard what I have waited a long time to OFFICIALLY hear: I am now considered NED (No Evidence of Disease). Remission is the laymen's term! How absolutely, indescribably fantastic!!!! What a beautiful answer to so many prayers and so much suffering!

We were so overcome with the joy that we were taken completely by surprise (at least I was) by his next statement: "This coming year will be the most difficult." WHAT? When he quickly explained that he meant emotionally, I knew then what he meant. The prospect of getting no treatment, everyone basically thinking you are cured (I'm still far from officially out of the woods, but every day I am a step closer), and the near constant fear of recurrence is tough to handle. I am already struggling a bit with these things, and I haven't even finished radiation yet (I will on Tuesday though). Why put off worrying tomorrow when you can worry today?

So for now, Gary (isn't that the name of the Sponge Bob's pet snail that meows?) recommends getting scans every three months. He also said he would not be surprised if we have to do another biopsy or two in the upcoming year to keep on top of things. He also recommended going to therapy and getting back to living like a normal person as much as possible. He said the rest is in God's hands for now. Let's hope that God and I have similar plans for my future. That "Man plans, God laughs" quote always haunts me whenever I start to ponder this.

So, getting back in good shape, getting plenty of rest, and eating well are also going to have to be priorities for me. I kicked cancer's ass once, and I plan on staying on my toes if it comes back for a second visit. All this should be easy with two wide-open, Italian-tempered (how did they manage to get just the temper and not the beautiful dark skin?) little boys, right?

December 9, 2008

This morning I had my last radiation treatment. My dear friend Susan came with me for the occasion. I brought some sweet treats and heartfelt thank yous for the staff. We took photos, and they gave me a Certificate of Achievement. Apparently, I am Outstanding in the Field of Excellence. I don't think I received a certificate the first go around, so I figure this must be a really good omen. This is what I have wanted for eighteen months now, a written certificate saying I BEAT THE DISEASE. Breast cancer can't come back because I have it in writing, and I will sue big for breach of contract.

A few of you have asked, "How does it feel to be done?" Believe it or not, I have not been overcome with joy just yet. Today was my LAST DAY OF CANCER TREATMENT, and I feel mainly just exhausted, flat. Honestly, it was a bit anticlimactic. The world did not stop to celebrate, my kids are still sick (at least Luca is getting tubes in his ears this Monday), the market still stinks, more people are losing their jobs and homes, and everyone is off in their own holiday-induced frenzies. I feel a bit alone and like most everyone is going to expect me to pick right up where I left off b.c. But the reality is I have a long way to go until I am up to speed (on so many levels), and now I have to deal with a world that seems like it's on a bit of a downward spiral. That and every ache, pain, and itch I have scared the crap out of me.

But on the upside, this evening when I got a brief moment alone (in the bathroom when the kids where in bed), I realized what I need to start to get my head on straight and get out there and enJOY. I need some time alone (sleeping time doesn't count). I need catharsis, and until I get it, everything else (but the boys) will just have to wait, whether I want it to or not.

December 11, 2008

Since Tuesday, I have been celebrating my new-found health swamped in various colored goo from my two boys. Fluids seem to be leaking or flying out of every orifice. Last night, after Gammy left and before Joe got home (that lucky duck got to work late), I was chuckling to myself that the only bodily fluid I escaped getting covered in was vomit. Naturally, Rocco woke up projectile vomiting, like that scary chick in *The Exorcist* about thirty minutes later. Poor guy. At first I thought, "poor mommy," because he ruined a favorite shirt, but then I remembered that this was exactly the kind of stuff that I signed up for: normal, everyday life with its multitude of ups and downs (or, in this case, ins and outs). And if I get the flu or the plague or whatever it is that has infected our household, it will still beat getting chemo; or on an even more positive note, maybe the vomiting will be just the catharsis that I need.

DECEMBER 16, 2008

Whew! What a week. I can't believe it has only been seven days since my treatment ended. I've definitely hit the ground running, but I am running way too slow. All things but essential mommy and Santa duties have fallen completely by the wayside. Laundry qualifies for essential duties, but apparently, grocery shopping and healthy-meal prep don't. I just don't see that improving much anytime soon. At least we've managed to conquer most of the bugs that plagued us last week. Luca's tube surgery was successful yesterday. They warned us that most children come out of the anesthesia very grumpy, but that term really didn't do justice to his post-op fury. But now that all the screaming has subsided, he is so happy and feels so good. The operation already has made a difference. Dad had his back surgery today, too, and it sounds like that also went well. Hopefully, his recovery will go just as well (and more quietly) than his grandson's. So, now that is all behind us, we have a lot to do (or not do) before Christmas. But no matter how tired or behind we might be, we are still so very, very thankful.

P.S. Look for my new book *How to Ineffectively Parent* for next year's Christmas rush.

DECEMBER 29, 2008

I have wanted to write so many times, but it just did not happen. I was either too busy, too tired, or trying too hard to think clearly while Luca smashed his golf clubs against the wall and Rocco did kick flips while screaming and jumping on the couch. I was going to try to sum up the holiday in a clever tribute to "The Twelve Days of Christmas," but I couldn't figure out numbers five and eight. You get the picture. I have lots to say, but I can only manage the quick version.

We've had a fantastic holiday. It has been blessedly normal (I have been on my knees thanking the Big Man quite a bit) and hectic (and not just because I have two wild boys). We managed one school Christmas program (Rocco smiled but did not sing, and Luca had to be held by one of his teachers because he was screaming like a banshee), one sports camp party, three separate and terrific family Christmas celebrations, and quite a few gatherings with friends. It was all good! I wish it could go on and on ....

It has been incredible to focus on celebrating life rather than just clinging to it. It is such an incredible gift to be healthy! I pray so often and so fervently that I stay this way. I go back to see Dr. Fraser tomorrow for a follow up. Let's hope all is still well!

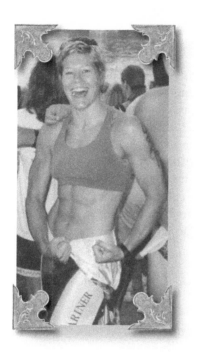

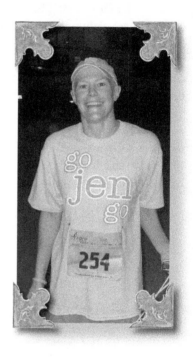

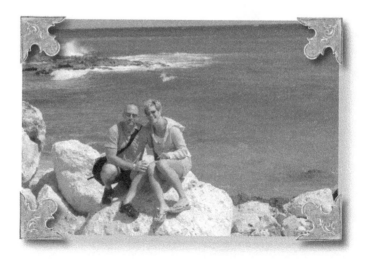

2009

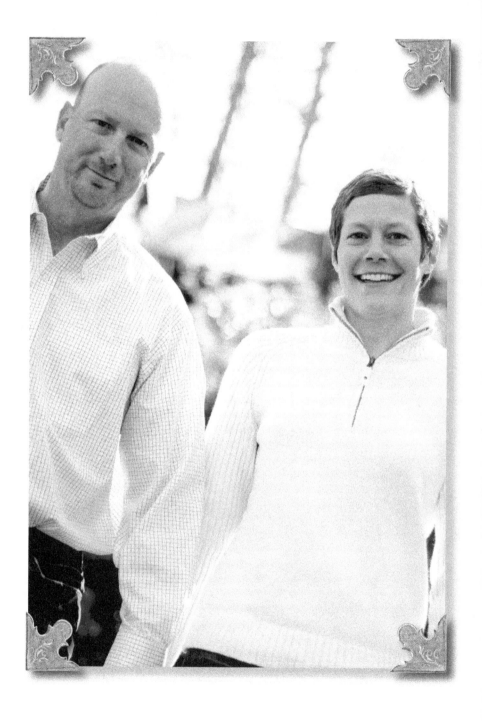

January 1, 2009

2009 is finally here. We celebrated with a quiet home; well, relatively quiet—JuJu brought over cupcakes for the boys, and the resulting sugar rush was long lasted and loud but great. I managed to get a hangover, which is quite a feat for someone who hasn't imbibed in months. In the post-sugar mayhem, I forgot, for the first time ever, to take my bedtime Ativan. So, I kicked off my New Year with a series of twenty- to forty-minute naps last night. I thought the spicy chili I ate for dinner was wreaking havoc on my whole body when, at 3:00 a.m., I realized that I may have missed my nightly chill pill. I confirmed that guess first thing this morning. Hmm, I guess you can't take an anti-anxiety pill every night, eighteen months in a row, and then expect a blissful night's sleep when you miss. You live and learn! At least I won't have to permanently give up chili!

The holiday has caused me, like most everyone else, to reflect on the past year and wonder what lies ahead. The fact that I now have an appointment with my oncology surgeon, Dr. White, on Monday for a couple of spots that are "cause for concern," makes this a difficult thing to do right now. It is easy to get caught up in the uncertainty of my situation, but that Emerson quote keeps popping in my head, and I remember that it is not what lies behind or before me, but what lies within me that counts. That is very good advice to heed this year.

January 6, 2009
Rated G (for Grumpy)

I now have more holes than a pound of Swiss cheese. I saw Dr. White yesterday and am now sporting some new stitches and two new biopsy sites. He was inclined to only do one, but I insisted both spots be looked at. Dr. White's impression is that they will be negative, meaning no cancer, like the last spot. Let's hope and pray he is right. I should get results on Thursday or Friday and stitches out in two weeks. I can't shower until tomorrow, which ordinarily wouldn't be a problem for me in the middle of winter, but did I mention that it is sixty-five degrees out, icky humid, I am having hot flashes (I think the chemo has kicked me into what I hope is a temporary menopause), and I have a monster headache? Apparently, I am a wee bit grumpy too. Steer clear (not just 'cause I need a shower) if you see me coming.

January 6, 2009
Rated S (for Shocked)

Shortly after I posted earlier, I received a very unexpected call. The boys were screaming, and as soon I as walked into another room to hear better, I knew immediately that the news would be bad. Dr. White had called to say that both biopsy spots were positive for cancer. The overwhelming flood of dark, intense, hot emotion rushed over me and made it very difficult for me to get any of what he was saying. But basically, I think he has consulted with my other doctors, and they are putting their heads together to come up with a plan, which will most likely be more chemo—surgery probably won't solve the problem long term. Tomorrow, I will get rescanned head to toe, so they can re-stage me. I'm not feeling too positive about this at all. Thursday we will see Gary and talk about a game plan. Please pray for us, all of us, for the strength and determination to keep fighting, for good scan results, and for an effective therapy regimen.

Thanks, Jen and her boys

January 7, 2009

The family gathered at our house last night to weep and deal with the shock. It was hard to keep our minds from wandering to the multitude of what ifs and even harder to digest the fact that the normalcy we had a taste of (and desperately needed) over the holidays is quite possibly gone for good. It is such a jagged little pill to swallow. I have decided to pull an Amy Winehouse and medicate some of my stress away; don't worry, I am not pulling lines of coke out of my hair or stumbling around just yet, but the Ativan is mostly definitely making this a bit more tolerable.

The scans are done, and now I am just waiting for the other shoe to drop. We see Gary tomorrow at 11:45 a.m. for the news. I will pre-medicate for that too—I think I am probably supposed to die from cancer and not a massive, stress-induced heart attack, but who knows? We also have two appointments at Duke and will be enthusiastically researching our options over the new few days. Please pray hard for us.

JANUARY 8, 2009

*A*ll five scans are CLEAN!!! I can't even believe that I am writing those words. This is Joe; Jen is in an Ativan-induced coma (nap) right now, and she wanted me to get the word out. The doctors are thrilled and completely surprised by those results. Her two spots on her chest are still very much a cause for concern, and we need to attack right away to stay on the offensive. But there is no other evidence of distant cancer right now. So, Jen will start a new regimen of chemotherapy right away (in one week) with some new drugs and some old. This will be weekly for six months to a year; we're not sure exactly because we are, again, flying off the grid. We will get a second opinion at Duke in one week, but Dr. Frenette has, once again, proactively contacted Dr. Marcum at Duke, and they concur. Gary has also spoken to two other respected breast-cancer experts, and they are in agreement as well.

We have our dear friend Mindy in Houston connecting Dr. Frenette and Dr. Massimo Cristofanilli, a well-known expert in inflammatory breast cancer at MD Anderson, so that they can confer on this choice of therapy also.

All that being said, I can only believe that the loud and heartfelt prayers of all you Go Jen Go supporters out there have brought us this unexpected chance at a cure. I could never describe to you the overwhelming fear and heartache of the drive to Gary's office today. Maybe Jen can, but the thought of the positive biopsies and "this is often the tip of the iceberg" screamed in my head all morning. I had lost almost all hope for clean results. But upon hearing Gary say, "All your scans look great," I could only think of everybody out there praying for us. I don't want to call this a miracle, because that would be forgetting that we have a very long struggle ahead of us. But to have the chance to fight ahead of this monster is SO great. And I know my wife is up for that fight now. She just needed this little bit of God's grace to push her back into fight mode.

Thank you all again for your prayers. Know that they are working and continue to have a very real and positive effect on our family. Keep them coming, as this year is going to be another tough one for my girl.

-Joe

January 11, 2009

Thank you, everyone, for praying so hard for my good news! God must have really been listening. I really do believe the voices of many are louder than the voice of just one. How else can you explain clean scans when all evidence and expectations pointed to the contrary? To say we dodged a bullet would be an understatement of huge proportions. To say I am not stressed about the current situation would be the same.

I am still totally reeling from both sets of news. I can hardly eat (stomach is a wreck but getting better), can't think straight (Joe thinks this was a pre-existing condition), and randomly get super-anxious (forget giving up the Ativan for a while). I am guessing that any week that you seriously think you are going to have a heart attack, not once but twice, will take a bit of time to get over.

Please send us some more good vibes and prayers. I want more than anything to see my sons grow up, to be there for the tender and tough moments, and to see them turn into men. I need a lot more time with my husband. And I need effective treatment and a decent quality of life to do so. Off to my nap and hopefully some sweet dreams.

P.S. I think God had his phone off the hook during the Panthers game.

January 14, 2009

I am going to try a quick entry while Luca sits beside me and repeatedly asks for "choo-choo." Maybe some soda, a snack, and a video will buy me some time? This nifty trick will appear in my book *How to Ineffectively Parent*. A multitude of thanks to everyone, again, for all their prayers, well wishes, and help; they sustain us.

Lots of you have questions. Since there are a lot of questions about what is going on, I'll list a few relevant answers regarding the current state of things:

- This is considered a local recurrence of my breast cancer that has occurred in the skin, on my chest and in the area that was initially radiated. It is called *chest wall recurrence*.
- Even though it is in the skin, it is still breast cancer and thus must be treated very differently than skin cancer would be.
- The best course of treatment is currently systemic therapy. We can't surgically remove it, because historically, they have poor results with this and can't get it all.
- I will get treated weekly, on Thursdays, for the next six to twelve months. I will get two drugs at the chemo center via my port. My side effects should be much more tolerable than previously.
- I am incredibly fortunate that it has not spread to distant organs (usually brain, liver, lungs, or bone), especially given that it has been resistant to all my previous treatment.
- Generally speaking with cancer, the longer you go before you have a recurrence, if you have one, the better your long-term survival chances. A recurrence this soon, to put it bluntly, sucks.

Hopefully, this will work. If not, we still have an option or two. Please pray this will finally kick the cancer's ass, or at least stop it in its tracks.

P.S. Off to Duke early on Friday. Hope to get back to "normal" soon. We need it!

JANUARY 18, 2009

A lot has gone on since my last entry. Treatment Thursday wasn't too bad, just long (six hours or so), and it left me with an icky, hungover feeling. They should have water or juice in party cups with umbrellas or something there so at least you can pretend you are working on your hangover the old-fashioned way. I have a bitchin' headache. Oh, and I found out I only have to go every other week, which is a huge bonus!

On Friday, we left before dawn to go to the Breast Clinic at Duke. I'm sure the name sounds intriguing to some of you, but it's not the party you might be picturing. They told us right away that they had been in contact several times with Gary discussing my case, and after a thorough evaluation, they confirmed everything he said. I managed to ask a few tough questions (the kind that make you break into a sweat and prompt your guts to clench), ones I hadn't asked before at Duke. Because they see more women with case histories like mine (remember, lucky me, I'm special), I wanted to know if they had seen anyone with a disease presentation similar to mine be cured. No. We suspected this, but it's a little harder to hear out loud.

Then I asked the really tough question: does he think I will be able to stay in front of the disease, meaning, nothing has killed it so far, so will it just keep spreading and grossly shorten my time on this planet? Dr. Marcum said it "is reasonable to think" that is possible. Most likely, and he has yet to see an exception, it will eventually spread through the rest of my body, and I'll be pushing up daisies at some point. When that is depends on how effective this treatment is, whether or not I can tolerate it (I guess they prefer you die of the disease rather than the side effects these days), how I respond to other currently available options (there are about four), and whether or not they develop new drugs before the progression is too far along.

We did eat lunch at a great place, and it was nice to spend the day with Joe, but damn, Durham stresses me WAY out. I managed to keep it together all the way home until we got in the drive way, then pity party, party of one, started. I partied for a good hour and a half or so and then pulled it together just before Joe returned from JuJu's with the boys. The catharsis was good, and I'm sure I'll need to do it again and again, but for now, I am trying my best to stay healthy and get back to living. To quote 50 Cent (yes, that's right, the rapper), "I got a lot of livin' to do and ain't got time to waste."

January 21, 2009

Rated HC (for Heavy Content)

The news from Duke finally came spewing out from the deep recesses of our souls. Neither of us could stop sobbing and shaking for a long time. I felt like my heart was ripping in half, and Joe, the love of my life, my soul mate, seemed to be suffering even more than I was (and am). We are both still trying to choose (we CAN control, to a certain extent, what we think) to focus on what we have now and find the joy in daily life, rather than look ahead to a future neither one of us cares to contemplate. We did have a great day sledding, making snow balls, and sipping cocoa with the boys! To say it is difficult to focus on the good things is a huge understatement, but we have to for the boys.

Thank you for sharing this journey with us. I know it must frequently be difficult to read my site and perhaps even more difficult to figure out what to say (I'm not sure I would know either), but thank you for your entries and prayers. We are sustained and can continue to find the will(s) to go on. Please pray for a miracle; we need it.

January 22, 2009

We find such strength from your words and prayers! They help us refocus and concentrate on living in the now, and last night we did just that. Joe had an invite to the opening of a new pizza restaurant at the Epicenter, and I managed to get the boys ready and meet him uptown after work (a somewhat incredible feat considering evenings are high fatigue and stress times). It was a wonderful distraction! Luca was fascinated by all the lights, towers, construction equipment, and escalators. He screamed, "SCHOOL BUS!" at the top of his lungs every time a CATS transit bus went by, and that happened often because we were very close to the depot. He did his happy side-to-side big boy swagger and took it all in with the joy only a child can experience. It uplifted our souls to see it! But when did he turn into a restaurant screamer? Oh God, let it be a one-time thing fueled by excitement and twelve ounces of a sugary drink! Rocco (he's been uptown at night before, so he tried to act cool and point out things to his little brother) kept talking about how these were the kind of buildings that Spiderman swings from, which is a rave review in his book. They both were even deputized by a very nice policeman we met. Rocco had to promise to eat his vegetables to get his badge sticker.

All in all, a great, but very tiring, normal night—just the kind we want and need.

Please pray for peace, strength, courage, determination, health, and joy in the Pagani House.

JANUARY 22, 2009

I flipped a bit this afternoon. I have rage and frustration inside me that desperately needs an outlet. I can't lift until I hurt or run until I drop, I can't beat my kids or my husband (just joking, I beat them all the time—they deserve it), I can't get drunk, I can't even shoot my shotgun anymore …. It seems that my Burnette sensibility or the need to protect my fragile health always prevails, even when my soul is crying out for some relief. Sometimes being levelheaded just sucks. Screaming only helps for a second, and if I break stuff, I know I'll just have to clean it up (so much for smashing the windows or throwing some glasses). So, what's a gal to do?

In true feminine fashion, my catharsis came in the form of a somewhat passive-aggressive self-done new hairdo. After an hour and a half of hacking, I decided, "What the hell? Screw you, cancer! Take my hair!" Every hair in the sink was one less tear to cry, one less minute to focus on dying (which I have been doing very regularly lately; I've almost accepted it as a forgone conclusion) rather than on living. Despite feeling a bit crazed, and like I should have a cigarette barely hanging out of my lips and an empty bottle of Jack on the bathroom floor, I was feeling better, more empowered; I felt less cancer-victim and more cancer-warrior.

What started out as a somewhat aggressive trim became an eyes-closed, haphazard, hack fest. But somehow, despite all this misguided attention, my hair didn't look too bad. I was shocked. Then, in for a penny, in for a pound, I decided it was time to learn how to use Joe's clippers. And, despite a somewhat tentative learning period, I am now sporting a number-seven, self done, buzz cut. It's not my best look (Sorry, January, Howie, and JuJu), but it's what's on the inside that counts, and now my insides feel a whole lot better.

-GI Jen, cancer Warrior

JANUARY 29, 2009

The hair didn't quite do the trick for the transformation I had hoped for. These last weeks have been tough, perhaps the most difficult since this journey began. I feel like I've been walking on a very narrow, winding path. The path is rocky in some spots, easy and comforting (snuggling on the couch with my boys) like a country lane in others. Mostly though, I'm aware of the dangerous drop-offs to either side. I keep finding myself slipping off the edge in places. It is so easy to do. Once I fall off, I have to scrabble and claw my way back for fear of falling down into oblivion. I am bruised, battered, bleeding, and weary. I have to dig so, so, very deep just to fight my way back up to an uncertain, bumpy road. It is so hard to muster the strength to continue such a difficult, unknown journey, but slowly I seem to be finding more and more. But it is taking what seems to be a long damn time, and I can't seem to hurry along despite an intense desire to do so.

So please forgive me if I have not returned phone calls, emails, smiles or even conversation lately. Just about all of my energy is focused on staying on the path and forging ahead, no matter where the road leads.

-J, gotta go: major TIS

February 4, 2009

Snow Day! We have at least three-quarters of an inch on the ground, so we could not possibly drive safely to school or to Harris Teeter (yes, people from out of town, that is the actual name of a grocery-store chain here). Good thing we have plenty of milk, bread, and brownie mix to tough it out. Unfortunately, though, Joe is going to have to "brave" the roads and try to "make us some money," as Luca puts it. But all kidding aside, this is a special day to play with the boys, and I'm going to make the most of it.

Thanks for all the prayers and encouraging words these past few weeks! Mentally, spiritually, and emotionally, I have been getting stronger since my treatment on Thursday of last week. Hall-lay-loo-ya! Its so much better to live in the moment and focus on kicking some cancer ass rather than the other way around.

Better run. Batcave to play with, brownies to make, and superheroes to chase.

February 12, 2009

This is at least the fourth time this evening I have tried to write; my intestines are currently suffering the effects of the "perfect storm" from today's treatment and a concurrent round of antibiotics (I must have picked up some cooties earlier in the week somewhere). Luca is screaming in his crib, and Rocco is wide awake and in and out of bed for various, inventive reasons.

So, in a nutshell, I had a good visit with Gary. He thinks my chest looks less red and is definitely not getting worse. I do have high blood pressure now from one of the treatment meds (Avastin) and will start some BP medicine for it (goody, more pills to pop) tomorrow. I can't risk anything new on the stomach tonight.

Hopefully, I will have a chance to blog a bit more tomorrow when all the "excitement" around here dies down.

February 16, 2009

We are dropping like flies around here, victims of various icky germs, luckily, none of it contagious. We have pharyngitis, an ear infection, and two sinus infections between the four of us. Hell, even the computer is having hard-drive problems. Just what we need: some feeling-bad crankiness to add to our high levels of stress. Perfect.

All of this (on top of everything else) has caused me to be in quite a funk that I just can't seem to get out of. Don't worry, it's not the "jumping out of a plane without a parachute" kind of funk—it's more like the "blah, I don't feel like talking" kind of funk. I am sick of sickness and feel like I am currently being consumed by it. I need to find and perhaps redefine myself, and I need some time away from the computer. What I really need is some extended time alone, but that is not realistic. So please forgive me for all the correspondence I am going to miss and the phone calls I will miss too. I'm not sure how long this will last. Thanks for your support, patience, meals, playdates, and prayers in the meantime.

FEBRUARY 23, 2009

I don't believe in coincidence, so last Thursday when I was driving to The Well of Mercy, a spiritual retreat in Northern Iredell farm country, I was pondering if larger forces were at work. From the time I heard about The Well on Wednesday and called to see if they had any availability (they had a cancellation earlier that morning), about a million things came to together to make my trip a reality. I went with no expectations (I really didn't have any time to form them)—just the most sincere hope I might recover some of the "me" that I seemed to have lost in the midst of this disease and treatment. Of course, I had no idea how to go about doing that, just an intense desire that it might happen.

What I found in that beautiful, peaceful place was more than I would have thought possible. The profound quiet, the striking beauty of the land, the ability to explore 110 acres by myself with no agenda gave my mind and spirit time to open up and expand. The first afternoon I bushwacked for a couple of hours (I'm a path less taken kinda girl) and then found myself at the labyrinth. I contemplated it a bit; after all, it seemed like it might be a bit silly just to walk back and forth to arrive at the center of a circle, but I decided it was metaphorical and started it with an open mind. I started slowly walking, letting my mind breathe, and noticed I was saying, "Let God direct your path" to the beat of my foot steps. Things seemed to just flow after that.

Shortly after, I had an appointment with Peg, the spiritual director. I walked in without really knowing just what she did or what I hoped to discover during the appointment. I began with nervous rambling, and thanks to her tender, thoughtful guidance, I gained profound insight on the root of some rather intense feelings I had been experiencing. She also helped me put a few very important things in perspective.

Later that night, after dinner, I followed everyone to the chapel, again, with no expectations. As soon as I set foot inside, I knew that God dwelled there. That was unusual for me because I usually find him outside. During the service, I felt like God, through Sister Donna, was speaking directly to me. Emotions and tears flowed out of me; they were unstoppable. I wailed, and I did not hold back. I finally had catharsis. And right there beside me, holding me and soothing me, was Sister Donna. I am not sure how to even describe her and her presence, other than to say I think she might be an actual angel.

The rest of my time there (did I mention they had yet another cancellation, this time for two nights?!), I had more revelations and more catharsis, but unless I plan on writing a novel, I will have to wrap this up. With each hour that passed, my soul rid itself of fear, guilt, and anger, and it filled itself with light, love, and life. I have drunk the water of The Well and found it to be beautiful and nourishing indeed. If you, too, need a drink, please check The Well of Mercy. It might just be the best thing you can do for yourself.

-The Old Jen

March 10, 2009

Names have been changed to protect the innocent.

We had recovered pretty quickly from all of our ailments at the Pagano house, had a great visit with our friends, and were winding down from a lovely weekend when the shit hit the fan—although, ironically, the fan was about the only thing in this story that was spared—Sunday evening. Daddy was upstairs, finally getting a much-needed shower, and Mommy was in the den watching her two sweet sons, Jocko and Lucas, play quietly and separately with their toys. Mommy decided to go put some clean clothes away (good mommies multi-task) and take advantage of the boys' good behavior. It was to be a quick trip down to the laundry room, but the quiet play enticed mommy to throw a load in the wash while she was in there. What a proud moment she had, and she smiled to herself and thought it was so wonderful that she was able to catch up on some long overdue chores because her boys were playing so well. There were, after all, no screams or thuds coming from above.

Mommy was gone at most five minutes and had her "mommy ears" on the whole time, so she was quite surprised when she came upstairs with an armful of laundry and did not see Jocko playing in the den where she left him. The quick sigh of relief when she spotted him in the playroom with his brother was quickly replaced with some very, very choice words. You see, Jocko and Lucas had found and opened a brand-new sixteen-ounce bottle of wood-glue that Daddy used to fix the train table (finally). Apparently, Daddy, also reveling in his completion of a long overdue chore, accidentally left the brand-new bottle within reach. Oops! Jocko and Lucas somehow managed not only to get the bottle open but to dump gobs of it on the train table, over several trains, two wooden chairs, one French door, one coffee table, the rug, their hair, their hands, and all over their clothes. The fan, as stated earlier, was spared.

Well, this was just a bit too much for Mommy to take. She said several words she hopes are not repeated, raised her voice, and actually slammed a door shut. Despite what you think, this Mommy does not lose her cool too often. All of this excitement left the boys with shocked, contrite (okay, not Lucas) looks on their faces and made Daddy come running. Daddy agreed with Mommy's sentiments exactly and said as much. Ah, but this story does have a happy ending. After two and a half hours of cleaning, two baths for each boy, whacked-off hair for Lucas, a brand-new clipper-cut for Jocko, and a very late bedtime for all involved, all the Paganos went to bed learning something important. The boys learned that there are things called "consequences" (What are they called again, Mom?) that happen as a result of certain actions, and that they should think about what kind of consequences their decisions might have. And Mommy and Daddy learned to count their blessings. After all, it was wood-glue, which is apparently water-soluble. And somehow, neither boy managed to get any in their eyes, so a trip to the emergency room was not needed. But more importantly, the parents learned that if their relationship can survive a challenging disease, a terrible economy, and two small boys, it can probably survive just about anything.

-Mommy Pagano

MARCH 20, 2009, 9:18 P.M.

In keeping with my minimalistic computer-time goal, I have been offline for a while now.

I am happy to say that we have had no more glue incidents (or string-cheese incidents, for that matter) since my last update. We have had the usual bumps and bruises and several terrifying (for Rocco) sightings of carpenter bees, though. Apparently, our redwood swingset is carpenter-bee Nirvana. But basically, life's been good, and we are reveling in the vibrant colors and warm weather of a Carolina spring. Of course, for every action (blooming flowers) there have been equal and opposite reactions (green, snotty noses). Trying to explain pollen to a four-year-old—even one that a doctor just this week said was "one of the most intelligent children she has ever met" (had to work that in my blog somewhere!)—is not easy, but at least Rocco now knows that bees do serve a higher purpose than just scaring the kee-rap out of him. Luca's too focused on swinging to be bothered by some noisy insects or mommy's semi-helpful ramblings.

All this enjoying life has been wonderful, incredible, and joyous! I have been focused on living not worrying (I stopped watching the news too, which helps tremendously), and I hope and pray it continues. I have recently noticed (just two days ago) a new spot on my chest and am a bit worried. I really don't want this magic to end. My quality of life is good right now, and I don't want to change at all, unless God grants me the miracle of a total cure!

Please pray that my cancer is being cured and that it is not spreading anywhere! Pray that the Avastan and Herceptin are working, and that I can stay on them for a very long time.

Thanks.

APRIL 6, 2009

So much has happened since I was last able to write, and as usual, I have a bit too much to say and two little boys who aren't going to let me say much at all. Currently though, I am not suffering from TIS because one is in his crib and the other is firmly planted in front of a Scooby Doo movie. We did, however, suffer mightily from PIP (Poop in Progress) this weekend because it is so hard for Rocco to tear himself from playing to run, in a timely fashion, to the john. And who can blame him? We did five "practice" Easter Egg hunts yesterday alone.

Gary (Dr. Frenette) wants to be "better safe than sorry" and check out the changes in my chest. Life, despite the disease-related challenges, has been quite good of late, and we desperately want it to stay that way. "Scanxiety" and stress about tomorrow's test is peaking. Scans are at 3:45 p.m. tomorrow, and I probably won't have results until Thurs. I am afraid. Please pray the scan reveals the disease has not spread. Unfortunately, the scans are incapable of showing us this in the skin. Please pray my current drug regimen is working to kill the disease we know is already there. The inability to distinguish the effects of the treatment from the symptoms of the disease is an unusual, deeply frustrating, and truly terrifying challenge with my "special" type of breast cancer. Please also pray that my current therapy, one that gives me a good quality of life, is working and that it will not be necessary to change it up for an even more toxic (but stronger) chemo.

Thank you all for all your prayers. Thanks for the dinners and playdates—they help us maintain a fairly normal life. Thanks for your listening ears and open hearts and for giving us the strength to go on when we are tired and scared.

-Jen and boys (who are now beating each other over the head with a plastic toy container)

April 7, 2009

The scan is done, and the image is just a ghost in the machine now. The stress is at times manageable and at times not. Whether my stress is managed well depends a lot on how well behaved my boys are and how much stress I can feel radiating from those dear ones who wait, terrified, with me. How dramatic does that sound?

Most likely, it will be Thursday afternoon (at my appointment with Gary) when we will find out results. I will have Joe post something when we find out, because I also get treated then, and it will be a long day. Please keep those good vibes coming. And forgive me if I haven't returned an email/phone call ... I tend to let things pile up when I am worried.

April 8, 2009

I ran off some anxiety this morning. The pollen burning my lungs and face was a great distraction from the stress of waiting. I dropped the boys off at school, but when I came home, the dark worry hit all over again. It is so very heavy and hard to carry, and ironically, I only really have the strength to shoulder the burden when I get a good, tiring workout in. It tires my body but rejuevates my mind and soul (which then, in turn, physically gives me a boost). So when the phone rang and it was CMC, I was too afraid to pick up at first. Does a call this soon mean good news or very bad news?

But the news was good! MY SCAN IS CLEAN! No spread from the skin to my more vital pieces and parts. WHEW! Thank you, prayer warriors and good-vibe senders! Now, we just need to see what Gary thinks of the skin changes. Hopefully, he is still pleased with the way things look, we can stay on the current regimen, and I can keep on truckin'. I want to keep this good quality of life!

Now, I can hop on over to the boys' school Easter parties today with a real smile on my face! I can savor the fun rather than worry too much about tomorrow! Happy Easter!

April 9, 2009

Well, in this roller-coaster battle, we continue to slide into a trough after the crest. After seeing Gary today, before Jen's chemo treatment, he thought the redness in her skin could be a progression of the inflammatory cancer. He had Jen get a punch biopsy, just like the ones she had earlier this year. She went to Dr. White, and he performed it this afternoon. We will likely not hear the results for several days because of the holiday work schedules. Please continue your loud and effective prayers for the results to be negative. Should they come back positive, we will have to face an ugly choice of different, more aggressive, and more "toxic" chemo drugs along with other therapies. We have had such a wonderful quality of life over the past few months that the thought of going back to some more taxing chemo is depressing.

We had a nice day celebrating the chest scan. I just wish it could have been a longer celebration. We'll be sure to let everyone know the results just as soon as we hear, but that may not be for a while. In the meantime, hug all your children and your parents and your spouses.

And keep my sweet bride in your hearts and prayers.

-Joe

April 13, 2009

Rated R for Language and Adult (not the fun kind) Content

I wouldn't really recommend an unscheduled biopsy the evening before a major holiday. Dr. White put a rush on it, but he said it will only matter if someone is in the pathology lab to see the label. Life has been rather hellish. I have had some fun, normal, revel-in-the-egg-hunts family moments, but that's all they've been: moments.

I keep staring into the abyss. The Waiting is just horrendous, especially to confirm what I think I already know—that the cancer is progressing in my skin and marching across my chest. I die a little bit each time the phone rings because I still feel unprepared for the moment of truth, but most likely, it won't come until tomorrow. I go from normal to completely freaking out (I guess I am having some anxiety attacks) in sixty seconds or less. It makes me a real joy to be around. My behavior is fine until it isn't, and then I can't tolerate anything, anything at all. I have to move, exercise, do something exhausting and quieting. I have to be away from everyone. What bizarre behavior. I feel the need to be away from the people that love me the most. It is one of the very, very worst things about all of this: the people that I love, need, and care about the most suffer so horribly as this disease progresses. They try to hide it from me as much as they can, but it is forever there, unspoken and dreadful. It is the fucking worst thing in the world. To continue to give those I love so much more and more bad news is such a horribly, bitter, jagged pill.

So most likely, we will know tomorrow. I will see Dr. Frasier and Dr. Frenette over the next two days to discuss results. We will most likely schedule more scans, and there is also the possibility of starting a month or two of photo-dynamic therapy, which is only done at ECU in Greenville, NC (four hours away).

Please pray for our peace, strength, and a miracle cure. I feel like I'm due and that my husband, boys, parents, and rest of my family deserve it.

April 14, 2009

Still waiting ... J

April 14, 2009 4:11 p.m.

Jen and I met with the radiation oncologist and got the bad news. The biopsy came back positive for cancer. It is still spreading in her skin on her chest. Jen was pretty sure it would be positive, so we weren't shocked at the news. But it is still a punch in the gut. The radiation oncologist said he had spoken to the director of the experimental program at ECU, and they are going to see if Jen will qualify for that treatment. It is still in the experimental stage, so they are very selective about who they accept. It was designed more for skin cancer, but there have been more applications lately, including inflammatory breast cancer in the skin. We will know if Jen qualifies by tomorrow at three (Oh good, more waiting.) She will hopefully be able to tell you all about it tomorrow.

Thank you all for your endless prayers and support. I know it seems to us that we ask and ask and ask. You all have never tired from giving, and I thank you from the bottom of my heart.

-Joe

April 16, 2009

Well, we've had some good news! ECU thinks I will be a good candidate for the photodynamic therapy (PDT). Now we just wait to hear from them to get the ball rolling. This is still considered experimental, so there will be hoops to jump through for insurance (if they agree to pay at all). I hope all this gets taken care of quickly, because Dr. Fraser indicated it should get taken care of soon. Waiting more sucks, but thank God we have had some hope restored.

As for now, I am crazy, borderline exhausted, and I hope to get some rest over the next few days. I feel like I need about a week to lie around and do nothing just to get back up to speed. The past week or two has really depleted me, but at least now I can be pooped with a smile on my face!

Thanks for all your prayers, food, help with the kids, and love! They make the difference. Please keep 'em coming. Please pray that insurance will approve this therapy, and do it quickly, and I will be able to start it in the next week or so! I'm most nervous about this part, because I don't have time to wait, and the insurance company seems to have all the time in the world. Also, please pray that this is the miracle cure we've been waiting on.

APRIL 17, 2009

This will be quick (TIS). I have a major prayer request for this weekend: please, please pray that the very nice nurse manager at ECU can squeeze us into the treatment schedule VERY SOON. Currently, the next opening is June 22, and that is most likely too long to wait. Please also pray that this laser stuff works and totally eradicates any and all disease!!!!! Thanks!

APRIL 22, 2009

Very quick, until I get some more time and can compose myself a bit ... mountains were moved on our behalf, many helped, lots prayed, and I am now on to start treatment at ECU on Monday, May 4 Thank you!!!!!

APRIL 23, 2009

This is Joe. I just wanted to let everyone know some details from yesterday until Jen has a chance to write. It started out very early as Rocco had a small procedure at CMC that required him to be put under for a couple of hours, which freaks me out pretty badly. He was a champ throughout the entire thing, and he woke up from the anesthesia like a happy-drunk frat boy.

That stress combined with the waiting to hear from ECU was taxing, to say the least. We finally heard that they could not see us until June. This sent Jen down hard. I spent the next several hours contacting everyone I could think of to influence the director of the program there to change something and get us in. Key players were on vacation or at conferences, so it was very frustrating. One caring radiation oncologist, subbing for our usual doctor who was on the West coast, asked Jen to come in for an exam so that he could plead our case personally with first-hand knowledge. It was during this exam that he noticed the fast spread of the disease and told us that there was no way Jen could wait for six weeks. That hit her very hard, and right then and there, she lost a lot of fight and faith. We stayed in the exam room alone for about an hour crying our eyes out. The pain spread to everyone who checked in on us during that hour, including that doctor.

When we got home, I frantically searched for other hospitals that do this procedure, only to find out that ECU was the only place in the country. It has not been approved by the FDA for inflammatory breast cancer yet, and ECU is pioneering the way. Even MD Anderson and Slone Kettering send their candidates to Greenville. I was devastated. I don't think that I have seen Jen this lost since the first diagnosis.

Around 4:30 p.m., Jen's cell rang as I was in the backyard with the boys. I had both of our cells, as Jen was napping, and it was the ECU scheduling nurse. She said we are on the books for May 4. I was running around the backyard with the cell phone to my ear, trying to speak and listen while my whole body was jumping for joy. Gammy knew what was going on from that crazy dance, but the boys didn't. Rocco looked at me like I was insane, and Luca just chased me around like it was part of a game. Minutes later, Jen opened the back window of the room where she was napping, and I gave her the news with a shout.

From deep, dark despair to bright, shining hope in less that three hours. It is a damn tough ride; I don't recommend it to anyone. But I am certainly glad we're holding on with both hands.

-Joe

April 24, 2009

Where to begin? So, so much has happened in the last two weeks that I feel like I'm aging in dog years. Joe gave you the nutshell version, which will, for the most part, have to do. Otherwise, I'll be at this computer the rest of the day telling Our Tale. But I will say that by Wednesday afternoon of this week, all the waiting had pretty much done me in. I was pretty much out of hope and ready to throw in the towel. I felt, for maybe the very first time since all this started, that it just wasn't worth getting out of bed after my nap. It took every fiber of my being to drag myself up and walk from the bed to the window to look out down below on the boys, Joe, and Gammy. I did it for them. I did it because I still had the tiniest hope that mountains would be moved and I would get in at ECU on May 4. I never, ever thought it could be so exhausting and take the efforts of, so many impassioned people to get me treatment that I needed to save my life, but it did.

So, I threw open the window and saw Joe on the cell. He hollered (this is the South) up that we got in on the date we needed! He had just heard. Coincidence? I don't believe in them. Greater forces were at work. I was dumbfounded, awestruck, speechless, numb. Gammy and Joe thought I didn't really hear what was said. Oh, but I did, my soul just needed a moment to back away from the abyss. Once you look in—really look in—through the inky darkness, you can see things that draw you in and make it hard to turn away. I went from the window to fall on my knees, to sob, and finally, to thank God for this miracle.

Yesterday, I had the opportunity to thank in person and hug all the folks who worked so fervently, passionately, and with incredible determination on the CMC end to help make this happen. Their dedication to helping others is nothing short of extraordinary and cannot be fully expressed here. And at ECU, many people moved mountains to get us in so quickly. I owe them so much and am so unbelievable grateful, and yet we have never even met. Wow!

Thanks to so many. We will leave for a one-week stay in Greenville, NC, where I will receive this new therapy. We leave on May 3, and treatment starts on the 4th, which is Luca's second birthday. This is the most amazing present to Luca and us all.

-Peace, Jen

April 26, 2009

We had a great, normal weekend! And I can't wait to start at ECU! I have been given a new opportunity at life and am so indescribably grateful and ready to get the ball rolling! Let me tell you a bit about the treatment I will be getting. It's called Photodynamic Therapy (PDT). The use for breast cancer, chest-wall recurrence specifically, is experimental. It entails injecting (via my port) a drug called Photofrin on Monday, May 4. This drug is a photosensitizing agent, not a photosynthesizing agent (which seems to jump out of my mouth initially every time I go to talk about it). Think of it in terms of this: they are going to make all my cells, in particular the cancer cells, very sensitive to light. Or, dumbing it down a bit further (this analogy helps me and seems rather romantically amusing), they are going to turn me into something like a vampire, rather than a tree.

Remember photosynthesis from ninth-grade biology? Normal cells excrete the Photofrin by forty-eight hours, but cancer cells don't. So, on Wed the 6th, they stick me under a laser and zap the still glowing (I am picturing the cancer cells lighting up like a glowworm) bad cells, three millimeters at a time, with laser-tube things. The laser treatment should take about five or so hours and is done in increments of fifteen minutes (don't know why). On the following two days, Thursday and Friday, they check to see if I need to be re-treated and see how I am doing … I should go home Friday afternoon. It will take about four to six months to heal.

There are the usual, potential side effects: pain, possible infection, and healing problems, but one is a bit unusual. After I get injected with the Photofrin on Monday, I will have to stay out of direct sunlight for four to six weeks. I initially figured, no big deal; I mean, I could really use a tan, and what could be the harm in a little sun? Well, it turns out that I have to be covered from head to toe (meaning, every inch of skin and with sunglasses on) and shouldn't be out during daylight other than for moments at a time, or I will get second- and third-degree burns! Hmmm, not the "little bit of color" I had hoped for, hence the vampire comment above. Trees thrive in the sun light, but I, on the other hand, will apparently burst into flames if I am exposed to the rays of the sun for more than a minute. I can't help but picture Vampire Bill (yes, that is the character's real name, and he is a hottie, especially for a guy with no pulse) from my very most favorite trashy show on Showtime, *True Blood*. I picture him bursting into flames as each ray of the sun hits his body, and he is forced out into the light of day to save his lover, Sookie. God, I can't wait for next season to start!

This will take some serious getting used to, but is so, so, so worth it!!!!! I am kind of, in a very weird way, looking forward to this very odd shake-up. I mean, could there be a more fashionable time to be a vampire? Who knows what fun this little adventure will hold? I will be a night owl for the first time ever. It will, however, be a challenge to Rocco and Luca who, this time of year, want to be outside every second and, I am sure, will not understand or accept (despite repeated attempts) that Mommy just can't do it. I am hoping for lots of outside playdates, or Mommy (and probably the boys, too) will go nuts, and I am sure our house will get totally trashed by all that pent-up kiddie testosterone.

Better go get some sun while I still can.

May 4, 2009

This last week has been wonderful! We managed to do lots of fun, normal stuff and tons of outdoor play with the boys. It was heaven! We even had an incredible family get-together at Tommy and Judy's (thank you for hosting, again!) for Luca's second birthday. The party was perfect. Luca totally enjoyed himself, and so did Rocco—he got lots of gifts and cake too. Luca didn't notice at all when we all got really excited while watching the Derby. I still don't know how we didn't win a little something; the boys and I had money on six horses ....

We made it to Greenville. It's cute. Yesterday afternoon, after we arrived, I made Joe walk for over an hour in the heat and humidity, all around campus and through downtown. My last few hours of sun were not wasted. We even sat outside at a Mexican restaurant, and, of course, wistfully stared at other people's kids. I enjoyed a margarita, and Joe had a few beers. The drinks were, of course, medicinal—we were both a bit stressed.

Blah! (the vampire kind, not the humdrum kind). Our meeting and my injection went ab-fab this morning. It was great to meet Teresa and Dr. Allison, two folks I can't wait to be indebted to forever for saving my life. They were positive about my prospects, and we are relieved to be starting the show. So now, we have a day and a half to go to work on my un-tan before the laser part of treatment on Wednesday morning. I am already chomping at the bit to get outside. I will take another walk (lucky Joe) after the sun sets.

Better go, time for din-din (real food, not vamp fare),
-Jen

May 5, 2009

This vampire thing is much tougher than it looks onscreen. It has only been a little over twenty-four hours since my injection, and I am already starting to go stir crazy. Plus, I am under advice from my doctor not to exercise. I know, I know. It sounds like the answer to quite a few people's prayers, but not mine! No exercise makes the dark confinement all that more challenging for this motion addict.

We did do an after-dark trip to WalMart last night. It was very exciting and interesting at the same time. Let's just say that they apparently don't see a lot of women-folk in these parts with shaved heads. Now I want a T-shirt that says "Go ahead and stare." We bought the boys each an ECU sports outfit, but despite our new allegiance to the Pirates (don't worry, I'm still a Dawg fan, too), I just could not manage to buy myself a purple and gold T-shirt. Were pirates color blind? Are they still?

We did, however, get accosted by an overly chatty man in the very slow checkout line. He informed us he's had four heart attacks (as he was stacking tons of frozen potpies up on the checkout thingy), he is not yet forty, he can't get disability, and he is currently being charged with child abuse. Maybe we will fare better at the CLT Walmart late at night? Or maybe we won't.

Anywho, time for me to lay (lie? still don't know, haven't bothered checking and probably won't at this point in my life) down in my un-tanning bed and get a nap. All this sitting around in the dark is exhausting.

Please send some extra prayers for us tomorrow. Pray the laser kills ALL the cancer cells on my chest, and that they will not (and have not!) spread elsewhere in my body!

Also, we are in good spirits! I will be in even better spirits tomorrow due to pain meds (which start first thing). I'm so ready to kick some more cancer ass! God doesn't mind if I cuss occasionally; I asked Him.

-J and J

MAY 6, 2009

Hi Everyone,
    Joe here, in Greenville. We just now completed the laser procedure, and Jen is back in our room recuperating. She was the perfect patient: no complaining, fidgeting, moaning, or screaming, even though they were slowly burning half of her torso over a six-hour session. Everything went according to plan, and the doctors were pleased. The burns on her chest are extensive and may take months to heal. Jen is on some pain meds now and hopefully will get some rest.

We both wanted to thank everyone for the outpouring of tender wishes, prayers, and thoughts over this trying time (the past two weeks or the past two years, you pick.) The amazing and moving basket of gifts and cards that came along with us for the ride were inspirational, to say the least. A scrapbook of notes and artwork from our extended Go Jen Go family gave Jen the extra boost she needed to get back into attack mode. It was lovingly done and no small task, I am sure.

Judging from the past two days of no sunlight, the next six weeks will be very challenging for Jen. She has always thrived outdoors; she feels her best after a long run, bike, or swim. She will still be able to exercise, thank goodness, but being away from the sun is going to weigh on her mental state. Please keep the guestbook notes, emails, and cards coming. They mean so much to us, and they give Jen an unbelievable amount of support to her spirit.

Sometimes, it is difficult for her to return all of her emails and other correspondence, but please know that everything is read and everyone is felt. Reading all of those notes from caring people all over—from close neighbors to far off relatives, from long lost friends to people we have yet to meet—fills us with hope and happiness, and I thank you deeply for it.

One more set of thanks goes to JuJu, Gammy, Papa, and all of the other caring hands that are taking such good care of our boys. We miss them dearly, and we can't wait to hold them tight.

Quietly typing with all the blinds drawn.

-Joe

May 7, 2009

*B*lah! I am vaiting for the sun to go down. A little burn isn't going to keep me in for too long. Actually, yesterday's treatment wasn't too bad (thank you, pain pills and Ativan). Initially, it was just going to be the prescribed, pre-administered pain pill, but when I got in there and realized it was going to be me, two "fizz-eh-cysts," an RN, and the doctor, and that I needed to keep perfectly still for five or so hours while the lasers made bacon-sizzling noises from the skin on my chest (not really, but it would have been very appropriate), I opted for an Ativan too. It was a smart move, and it kept the nausea at bay. They asked a few times about my pain tolerance level and remarked on what a great job I was doing keeping still. They thought it was me, but I knew it was my old friend Ativan.

Well, about three-fourths of my chest is now burned—it's not like the grill marks on a hot dog, which is what I had anticipated in my rather active imagination. It's more like a boiled, spotty lobster. Parts of my chest feel like a bad sunburn and other parts are much more "ouchy." But there is an upside, due to the swelling, my left breast looks fantastic! It's too bad it will only last two or three weeks. It's also too bad it is only temporary and not really in the mood to play—God really does have a sense of humor. Sorry, Joe.

I might be rattling a bit, oh well. We did go in for a checkup with Teresa and Dr. Allison this morning. Dr. Allison felt that it looked good and did not want to re-treat this morning. We will do another checkup tomorrow and then it is back to the Queen City, vampire style. Joe used foam board to cover the back windows of the car, so I'll run out to the car dressed like some crazed, post plastic-surgery starlet with really bad fashion sense.

Picture this: me in a big floppy Columbia hat; wide, summer-colored scarf wrapped totally around my head, neck and face; big Armani Exchange sunglasses that look like cataract glasses but are masquerading as the latest in fashion; whatever long sleeve and long pants I decide to throw on; white socks; purple Keen sandals; and of course, my black Carolina Panther gloves with the claws on the palm and fingers they gave out at a game like five years ago. Then I can slowly, cautiously unwrap parts of my outfit after I determine there are no rays of sun peeping into the car that would cause me to burst into flames. Joe then has this great habit of pointing out sights and asking where we are because he can't read the road signs. He keeps forgetting to bring his driving glasses when we go out. I'll very sweetly remind him that I can't see shit and to bring his damn glasses next time.

Better go. Dark clouds are brewing, and I am chomping at the bit to take a slow walk around outside.

May 12, 2009

We made it home in one piece, no arguments (Joe wore his glasses). I just chilled (get it?) in the back of the car with some ice packs and a pain pill.

Our Mother's Day was fantastic! I was totally pampered and showered in homemade cards and gifts, which could not be more precious at these ages. We "celebrated" in the morning with a trip out to Harris Teeter to get some much-needed groceries and to see how I faired in non-blackout car conditions. We learned three important things:

- I can't drive or manage to get the boys in/out of the car safely while the sun is up.
- Covering myself from head-to-toe (in this part of town) makes me more recognizable, not less. I ran into a somewhat confused neighbor on the way into the store who asked, "Jen, is that you?"
- Lots and lots of folks do very last-minute Mother's Day shopping.

It is funny how exciting a trip to the grocery store can be despite the fact that I kept going from feeling quite icky to okay over and over again—it was a big deal to go out so soon. I picked out all the things I like to eat, and we ended up having a great, impromptu cookout at our house with the family. It was tons of fun. Everybody pitched in (even me, 'cause I wanted to), and the mood was festive. And nobody cared that I had to partially cover myself in ice packs (it helps to cool the burns and decrease the swelling) and take it easy on the couch in the relative darkness of the porch. No worries.

I will have to wrap it up soon. I keep thinking my time to get lots done will start any second. So far, I have found it is hard to do stuff while covered in ice, and my motivation seems to be lacking just now. So, the 140 DIY projects I have been inspired to do by HGTV will just have to keep piling up.

But let me just say we can't thank you enough for your continued prayers! The cards, dinners, playdates, and the amazing gift basket with the scrapbook have been immensely appreciated! THANK YOU!

MAY 18, 2009

Apparently, I am the laziest active person around. My laptop died rather unexpectedly on Wednesday (a fix doesn't look too promising either—power problem), and I just have not been able to make it all the way downstairs to use the desktop. It doesn't matter that I'm down there fifty times a day anyway, it's the thought of having to walk all the way down here to type when I used to be able to do it in my kitchen. I guess it is similar to what I like to call "mall parking syndrome" (or Harris YMCA parking), when you cruise the lot looking for a primo spot before you go inside to walk or workout. You get the idea ….

So, we saw Gary this past Thursday for my first post PDT appointment. He was pleased with the news from ECU and with the way my chest looked. We decided to start the Tykerb (the oral chemo I was on for four months last year) to make sure we kill any stray cancer cells that might be out there. Last time we stopped the drug because of swelling in one of my lungs. Hopefully, that won't happen this go around, and I can stay on it for quite a while, at least long enough to ensure Total Cancer Ass Kicking (however long that is). The side effects aren't as bad as the IV chemos, but I can already feel some nausea, extra fatigue, and backaches. The lovely zits I had last time will most likely be coming too (damn it). Can't they put some cancer research money into finding cures that cause fat loss, muscle gain, younger-looking skin, and a healthy glow?

But kidding aside, thank you for all your help! We are eating well, the kids are happy, and I have already survived two weeks of "darkness."

May 22, 2009

I hit a rough patch earlier this week when the effects of starting back on Tykerb, the daily oral chemo, coincided with the end of my steroid buzz (think restlessness and poor sleep). Go Jen Go ground to a halt. It was more like Stop Jen Stop. Can't you just picture the little bird holding up the red stop sign to the dogs in cars in the Suess book? I barely spent any time out of bed on Tuesday, and Wednesday was a wash. The past two days have been much better, though I am now reeling a bit mentally and still have more than my usual amount of fatigue. I can feel the tug of the "what ifs"at the edge of my consciousness. They're threatening to pull my mind back toward the darkness, and I don't want to go there again. I'm sick of the dark. Some vampire I've turned out to be.

But instead of using my time productively outside of spending as much time with the boys as I can, I've had my nose stuck in a book. I'm currently reading *Twilight*, which, despite being written on a sixth-grade level, still provides an interesting escape. I have thank-you emails, correspondence, piles of "stuff," and lots of household and home projects (thank you, HGTV) to do, but I seem to be not doing much of anything at all. Sure, I need time to rest and heal. Sure, I need a little time to indulge and feel better. But now I think I need a good kick in the pants to get out of my rut. I'm frustrated and a bit worried that this is what the Tykerb is doing to me this time around. I hope not. I pray not, especially because I am on it indefinitely.

So please forgive my manners and my whining. And in the meantime, I'll work on digging myself out of this hole. Blah!

MAY 28, 2009

I am totally coming around. We had a really fun weekend with lots of visits from family and friends, and we got a few errands done too. I love the normal stuff! And I have managed to get a few things done, which seems to be helping my mental/emotional state. I even drove (covered up very well) a bit and did not burst into flames. It was awesome to do a regular mommy thing! Doing mommy things are the best yet for my outlook, and of course, being outside wasn't too shabby either.

I must say, I am totally loving this rainy weather that everybody is complaining about. For all you *Twilight* fans, I feel like we live in Forks; and that feeling, paired with my current situation and complete enthusiasm for the start of the new season of *True Blood,* have me really feeling the vamp thing. Plus, I don't have to obsess over watching the weather channel ten times a day now, and I don't care that the humidity level is 88 percent every day. And now, everybody in Charlotte is stuck inside with me.

Our yard also looks so lush, more like this wooded, mature neighborhood looked when we first moved in years ago. What a treat to gaze upon. The green really gives off some amazingly good, healing vibes. The vibes are so good, in fact, I decided to get off my ass and bring the outside in. In one of my brilliant-idea moments, I decided that the best time to paint my workout room would be now, while extra fatigued, restarting chemo, and with a hurt chest and arms that don't stretch much at all without a loud protest. But stupidity has never slowed me down before. Why let it now? So, to recapture the feeling of nature, I have wisely chosen to paint the walls the same vibrant green (my entire house is neutral, slightly masculine tones) as the bush I see from my kitchen window. Let's just say, after some perusing and purchasing and painting, paint always looks different on the wall, and they don't make that color. I was shooting for inspirational and soothing. I think I hit closer to manic. Gammy called it chartreuse. I don't know if that's accurate, but I know that's supposed to be a very ugly color. Anyway, it has grown on me. I'm all in. And to top it off, literally, I am painting the ceiling sky blue. I have clearly watched too much "Color Splash" on HGTV. I'm not usually into a lot of color, despite this story, but I love that hottie show host. I think Joe is going to cut me off from HGTV before I do something really radical to our 1960s bathrooms.

Yikes, I better shut up now. I could go on and on (the boys are at their cousins' house). Have a good one.

-Elvira

June 1, 2009

Hi Everyone, Joe here. Jen is having full scans today, so I wanted to send a message to ask for prayers on her behalf that all will be clear and clean. We probably won't have the results until Wednesday or Thursday, so these next few days will be ones of great mental strain. We've been here before, and it doesn't get one bit easier.

With that in mind, Jen and I would like to help the many other women out there who are there stricken with this disease but without the army of support that we are blessed with. Over the next few months, a group of us will be gathering to form a new charitable foundation called Go Jen Go. The main goals will be to provide a network of support to those who do not have that key component to fight breast cancer and to raise funds for the important and effective groups already working toward a cure.

I will keep you all posted on our progress. We will take it slow and steady to make sure we create something that will endure and support women in need for many years to come. Our first goal will include having the largest team ever entered in the upcoming Komen Race in October. So put October third in your calendar.

Thanks again for all your support and PRAYERS!

-Joe

JUNE 2, 2009

I had a check-up with Dr. White this morning. I found out my scans are clean! WHEW! Prayers answered once again! More later ... I have some snuggling, snoozing, and celebrating to do!

JUNE 7, 2009

Well, it was an ab-fab week! It did take my usual break of a few days to get my head around the great news, but we managed some dinner celebrations, a trip to drop the kids off at their day care (I hadn't been since I was injected with the photofrin), and a wrap-up of the cheap makeover for my workout room. Thank God that one is over: my chest can't take any more stretching to paint! But the paint actually looks quite good, especially with the Matisse prints I put up.

Gary was pleased as punch with my scan news too! He joked that he was going to call Dr. White to give him a little hell for stealing his thunder about the news of the clean scans. He is also pleased with the way my chest is healing and said we'll continue to keep lots of eyeballs (four doctors get weekly photos) on it to make sure it continues to heal properly and doesn't show any signs of recurrence. He does want to continue the Tykerb indefinitely to stay ahead of the game, and we will continue to scan frequently to keep tabs on the rest of my body as well.

And we got even more great news! On Friday, after talking to Teresa, the nurse at ECU, I found out my vampire days are over! I do still have about 200 pages to go in the last of the *Twilight* series though! I am officially out of the dark and into the sun, humidity, and mosquitoes! The only thing holding me back from full-blown summer fun are the wounds that are still healing on my chest and in my armpit. I can't get them wet because of the possibility of a serious infection. It's a bit of a buzzkill for Rocco (and myself) who is all psyched for some major pool time. But since I can't manage a bra yet (let alone a bikini top), because my burn pain has gone way up (thank you, healing skin and nerves), it's probably a good idea to stay away from the pool or lake, anyway. Who wants to sit around tanning in bathing suit bottoms and a T-shirt? And God knows, after weeks of consoling myself in the darkness with handfuls of chocolate and nuts, my bottom half is not the part I want to unveil at this particular moment. Diet starts tomorrow!

June 10, 2009

*C*urses! I just lost a huge blog entry. To recap, we've had a big week. Rocco had emergency splinter "surgery," which was successful mainly due to the administration of some heavy-duty anesthesia (Starbursts and Tootsie Pops). Rocco made some "bombs" with partially filled water bottles and toothpaste during some suspicious quiet time yesterday. Thank God they didn't go off. And he made the transition from night time pull-ups to underpants without incident! Luca came down with a virus and is cutting his two-year molars. His normally sunny, laid back disposition has been stormy and high maintenance. It was perfect timing for mommy, who had the major yucks yesterday. I had nausea and malaise big time, but I guess some icky days are to be expected with daily Tykerb. It was bad enough that I did not even take a pain pill until ten at night, and that effort left me shaky and crankier than normal. My skin has been through-the-roof sensitive and painful (mainly late in the afternoon or at night after a day full of moving and doing mommy stuff). There are two chargrilled areas, one on my chest and another in my armpit, that are so sensitive I can barely stand to wear anything but two of the softest T-shirts in the house (both are very, very old one's of Joe's). Ironically, the pain has been getting worse as they heal. But as long as the cancer's ass was kicked, who cares?

Oh, and while I'm whining, what happened to the cool weather? I am finally okay (from the Photofrin) to go outside, but I can't take the heat or humidity. Sure, it has always made me cranky and long to live somewhere well north of the Mason-Dixon, but now I feel cranky and terrible within about two minutes of being outside. It's from the chemo, and it sucks (wah, wah, wah). All would be well for this mommy of little ones who want to be outside rompin' or splashin' around if I could get in the pool or lake with them. But no, I must wait until my wounds heal or I face the probability of infection, which could be rather serious. Super duper—cue the violins. I might as well be a vampire again (and I will be this Sunday night when season two of *True Blood* premiers).

Better go before I whine some more. I must say, I am doing this whining with a smile on my face, though, because despite the challenges of living with cancer, I am living!

JUNE 16, 2009

he boys and I went on a mini, three-day lakation (lake vacation) to Gammy and Papa's house this weekend. It was just what the doctor ordered. We had some rest, sun, a few cruises on the boat, and plenty of good food. We wrapped it up with a nice Italian meal at JuJu's house Sunday night with the Pagani boys. Yum. I was suspiciously comfortable and even needed a hoodie to stay warm as we ate out on the porch. That was my first clue (okay, second clue, but I'll spare you the TMI details) that all was not to be well.

On Sunday night, I spiked a fever and slept under piles of blankets but still couldn't get warm. Yada, yada, yada … I had to go see Gary to get two bags of fluid yesterday afternoon, but by 11:30 last night, I had a fever of 103.3 and felt horrible. After eleven hours of sleep, I am feeling much better, still not well, but much better.

I have also broken out in some very unusual spots on my chest and abdomen. We sent pictures to my doctors, and Dr. Fraser wanted to see me today at ECU's request, but I postponed until Thursday morning because I am not up to going anywhere today. We are praying (and suspect) at this point that they are related to whatever weird bug I have or the PDTI got at ECU. Please say a prayer or two that this is the case.

Time to go back to bed.

JUNE 18, 2009

ast night, I hit that sorry trifecta (sickness, self-pity, anger, and frustration—I guess I meant quatrafecta). I felt bad, was stressed about getting the spots checked out by Dr. Fraser, and was very ticked off that it is always something in the expenditure department. I'm already a money pit, we don't need the house to be too. We have just discovered water coming from our inside A/C unit that has seeped through the walls and warped floor boards in the basement. I was in a foul mood to say the least. I kept trying to shake myself out of it and adopt the Navy Seal "so what?" motto, but it just wouldn't take. I was a seething, not-feeling-well ball of anger.

But today was a new day. And even though it started an hour earlier than I expected it to (thank you, Rocco), I felt better all around. Dr. Fraser was his usual thorough self. His current conclusion: I have a bacterial infection and a virus. I might also have a fungus too. Ew! How gross! Does this mean I have athlete's chest?

I have been on a very powerful oral antibiotic since Tuesday, so now we sit tight and watch to see how things change—what started out as a few red spots on my chest this past weekend is now thirty-plus-yucky-looking spots. He will see me again Tuesday of next week to reassess. He said if things are not much improved, then we call in another doctor. I seriously thought he meant an infectious-disease specialist and asked him as much. He did not even crack a smile, so I can only wonder what sorts of questions his patients ask. What he meant was he would get a pathologist to sample some cells just to rule out cancer.

So, we are much relieved and expecting that this is all because of a few cooties and not cancer. In the meantime, I seem to feel well and then not well for hours at a time. I think (as Joe pointed out) mixing a really strong antibiotic with chemo, while still being under the influence of some bugs, is not a recipe for feeling great. But I'm sure this 95-degree humid spell will perk me right up.

June 23, 2009

Hooray for me! The spots are just about gone. Dr. Fraser and Dr. White were both quite pleased this morning with the current state of things. I do still have some redness we are going to keep an eyeball on, but other than that, we are gratefully in good shape. And hooray for everyone else, I seem to be over most of my whiny spell! The whole ongoing (and I do realize how lucky I am that it is an ONGOING problem) cancer thing sometimes makes it tough to deal with all the other life stuff, like various parts of the house trying to break in major ways all at once.

July 8, 2009

Ahhh, can you hear that? No, me neither. It is the beautiful sound of silence (I suggested the boys and Joe go outside), and it is the reason I am finally able to sit at the computer and catch up on a few things. Last week was a bit of a tough one. The contractors, that long second week of summer vacation after school ends and before camp starts, another round of worry-fueled depression, and a bit of firework-related toddler terror has just about did me in.

But we started the week off right with a good visit to Dr. Fraser. He did not see any reason right now to do a biopsy on the aggravated areas of my chest near my "wounds." Once that was out of the way, my mind started clearing, and I'm in a good place once again. Now, I can ponder many important things like, is eye gouging an instinctual defense move? Rocco attempted this in response to very hard bite on the butt cheek by Luca. Also, just how far can the pinky toe get wrenched out towards the outside of the foot before breaking? Apparently, it's less than ninety degrees. Why have there been so many MJ memorials (sure, he was a ground breaker, but come on)? And will Lance be able to do it again? I want to LiveStrong just like him.

Better go, Joe looks a tad tired. Thank you for all your support!

July 13, 2009

Hi, everybody ("Hi, Dr. Nick!"), not sure why this little Simpson's gem popped up in what's left of my brain. We now seem to be over most of the craziness at our house, thank God. We saw what we hope is the last of the repair men and contractors this morning. Our basement is once again functional, my toe now stays in place without tape, and there are no new scary spots on my chest. Sweet!

I can finally now resume looking ahead, and I'm really excited about our first Go Jen Go event for 2009. On Sat, July 25th, we are having a kick-a** pool party to kick-off the 2009 Komen race season. Come get some sun, eat some bar-b-que, drink some beer, and do it all for a good cause: healthy, happy boobs!

Thanks a bunch for keeping Jen (me) going. I wanna be like Lance!

July 21, 2009

We've been busy Pagani's lately. Summer can be so very, very much fun (when the threat of death doesn't loom large), and we've been enjoying our time of late. We had a few ups and downs last week, but one of the week's highlights was a photo shoot at Panther Stadium (in the Top Cats locker room) with RB D'Angelo Williams, his mom, and our family. D's mom is a survivor (his three aunts are not, which was a bit sobering), and he is lending his celebrity to help Komen raise breast cancer awareness.

We had a good time on the shoot, even though Joe and I are rather camera shy. We were really excited for the boys. How cool is it to get a stadium tour and then a personal photo shoot with a star? D'Angelo was very nice, down to earth, built like a brick house, and not too hard on the eyes (not at all!). Joe and I seized on his looks and demeanor to have him deliver some parental propaganda about eating your fruits and veggies so you can be a football player when you grow up. D fed (get it?) the boys the approved lines and then asked Rocco what he wanted to be when he got big. Joe and I (and I am sure D, too) were all expecting a manly answer like football player (the obvious), superhero (the cool choice), or fireman (the old standby). Instead, Rocco replied that he was going to own six cats when he was big. What? Where did that come from? And what a proud moment for mommy and daddy! D musta been thinking, "Is that kid's name really Rocco?" We all had to stifle smiles (at least I think that was what Joe was doing). At least he didn't say he wants to own lots of fancy shoes or work for E! TV ....

JULY 26, 2009

Wow! Wow! Wow! What a great weekend (minus the over-tired toddler drama this evening)! The Go Jen Go party was totally amazing! I am still a bit beyond words. It was just phenomenal to see so many people out to support us and Komen! Quite frankly, I am still a bit blown away. The planning and giving (from the raffle donations to smoking the yummy bar-b-que) from so many of you touched my heart in the most tender of spots. THANK YOU!! And the support for us from so, so many of you was absolutely fantastic. I hope I was able to say hello and thank everyone in person.

Tommy and Judy's backyard proved to be the perfect backdrop for the band, food, beer, swimming, games, and activities. Rocco, Luca, and their cousins are still sporting lots of temporary party tattoos! I think fun and happy boobs were had by all! Thank you for such an amazing party, and let's keep this momentum going strong!

JULY 30, 2009

We've been in party mode since Saturday. Rocco turned four on Tuesday, and we celebrated all day with Gammy and Papa. He now has enough Bumble Bee gear to star in the next Transformers' movie. Yesterday, we pool partied (I stayed dry) again with a dear friend whose daughter turned three. Whew, the boys are starting to look like raisins.

Today, I did my usual Thursday CMC circuit. I had some good news and some bad news. The good: my PDT wounds are healing up nicely. The bad: my weight is at an all time high. It seems I missed the summer swimsuit shame season (try saying that three times fast, or maybe just once) and have now found myself in the middle of summer as fat and sassy as I have ever been. It seems like it's time to buckle down and get back to eating right and eating less. Maybe I should start by putting down the M&M's? I think I'll start Monday ... I might as well finish this bag first.

Time to go, can't type and eat. GJG

JULY 31, 2009

Tomorrow is the two-year anniversary of my diagnosis. It's weighing heavily on me. I can't quite put all my thoughts and feelings into words. I've been on a rollercoaster ride since 11:30 last night when I pulled out Luca's baby album. The pictures tell the story. It sucks that the story unfolds in the baby album. At first, there's a pregnant, happy mom, a dad, and a son waiting for the new arrival, and then baby Luca comes, and all is well. The smiling, tired, normal family adjusts to life with a new baby. Rocco turns two, and the baby three months ... and then the rug gets pulled out from under everyone. Life changes for us all, forever. The new life (at least there is one) is a string of treatments, side effects, doctor's appointments, fear and stress, wondering how much time I've got, whether or not this recurrence is the beginning of the end, etc. Staring my disease in the face everyday makes it so hard to ignore. It is not at all what I had imagined life would be like with our new addition; it's not what any of us imagined.

The last two years have been so hard, but what is to come? The statistics suck. Screw the stats, some of you say. I say that too, but sometimes it's so hard to look past them. Some things in particular about my journey haunt me, wake me up at night, and make me wipe away tears in hopes that my sons don't see. The post-mastectomy pathology report said I had eight out of fourteen positive nodes, even after six months of the initial chemo. That, combined with the fact that I've already had a recurrence indicate very low long-term survival rates .... These statistics screw with my head from time to time.

But (I did say this was a rollercoaster ride) for every negative thought, there is a positive one. I am still here. I have two years of precious moments with my incredible family. I have amazing friends, new and old. I have incredible doctors and nurses. I have so many people praying and supporting me. And I am finally able to get the ball rolling to give a little back.

My life has not turned out to be quite what I thought it would be, but it is mine, and I don't take any of it for granted.

Thank you.
-Jen, extant

August 5, 2009

I am over the anniversary hump and movin' on. Thank you, everyone, for your extra prayers and messages.

I also have some news to report. I had a chest scan Monday (it was supposed to be late last week, but it took the insurance company a while to get their act together) to assess breathing difficulties/chest pressure that began a week or two ago. My scans looked good: no metastases! The scans can't detect the presence of disease in the skin and some other tissues though, but we knew that, and that's why we watch it so closely. I still have the post-radiation and Tykerb swelling/scarring from before, but that hasn't changed either, which is also good news! Gary thinks that most likely the breathing problems are a combination of the old lung changes and the new (not improved) increase in humidity, with a few other factors. He decreased my Tykerb dose, so hopefully that will help.

Please start training/sign up for Komen if you haven't already. It is in two short months!

August 14, 2009

I was going to blog about it being "the most wonderful time of the year" (back-to-school time, for those of you without kids). We've managed to have lots of fun the past two weeks, but Mommy is pooped and ready to have some downtime when she is not napping (gosh, that sounds so spoiled). School starts Monday for the Paganis!

But while we've been blessed with normalcy (or what passes for it in our house), others have not been so lucky. My friend, survivor, and fellow mom of two boys (almost the same ages as our two), just found out her breast cancer has come back again (she had two previous brain surgeries for it). This time, it's in her chest in two spots. She and her husband have some difficult decisions to make this weekend and more challenges to face. Please pray for them. My heart aches for them, and I feel like they could use some extra support.

Also, I have heard of two other women, women I don't know but whose stories have been passed on, who were diagnosed recently with stage 4, with cancer in multiple organs. Please pray for them, too. Sign up for our Komen team, or someone's, please. So many women need help. This disease sucks and can be so devastating. We need to find a cure.

August 21, 2009

There just simply aren't enough hours in the day. Now that school is back in session, I thought I would be catching up on errands, the growing mountain of paper work, emails/phone-calls/letters, and maybe even get in a non-hurried workout or meditation, or (God forbid) just sit and relax. I had visions of myself as this super Martha Stewarty cancer-surviving, ass-kicking mom. I was gonna do it all. Ha! Reality check time. In actuality, I have a few hours Monday and Wednesday mornings to try to get it all done. As another mom at school said, when we were both lamenting the other day, "It looks good on paper." As I sit and write this, my "babysitter" (what we fondly call the TV in our house) is failing to keep Rocco entertained. Time to wrap it up.

But before I go and deal with a now obstinate boy, I had a pretty good appointment with Dr. Fraser yesterday. He cleared up some concerns I had and told me he was 75 percent sure the redness on my chest is in not malignant. I have some more specific items to address with Gary and Dr. White in the next two weeks, and then we can decide whether or not another biopsy is needed. This is really helpful, and I feel good about the appointment. I am not looking at my chest seven or eight times a day now and wondering if I am watching my death approach with my head in the sand, which doesn't help me in the getting-stuff-done department. But I have a plan and odds I can live with!

Thanks so much for everyone who is supporting Komen and Team Go Jen Go!

August 31, 2009

The weatherman said today was gloomy. I suppose most would agree with him. I don't. I love the rain and clouds. They seem like a time for quiet, reflection, and renewal. I savor change. I thrive in these conditions. My preference for cool and cloudy (or cold and snowy, as the season dictates) puts me in the small minority. I suppose it makes me unique, but often it makes me feel alone.

My disease is another matter though. It is also unique in its presentation, but with it I feel isolated, lonely. I have no peers. And of late, I have been keeping my feelings to myself. I've been locking things away in my heart-shaped box, but now my box is full. And as my husband and mother will tell you, I am not too good at suffering quietly. I have been largely silent on things of the heart. This is for a number of reasons: I couldn't manage two seconds of uninterrupted thought with the boys around; when I do have the time, I need to rest not reflect; I'm not sure if anyone has the time to listen of late; and whenever I voice my fears, frustrations, and concerns, it is difficult and perhaps tiresome for those that love me.

My therapist suggests that I keep a private journal, which, in theory, is a great idea. In practical terms, it's not happening. Two years ago, when I was first diagnosed, I made a decision to open my heart and my head on this site, but somewhere along the road I seem to have lost my way. So, I've decided to set out once again on my original path. The journey's far from over, and I wanna get back to writing "old school" style, authentic and real, not fluffy "tweet" stuff. We'll see what happens. Despite being a "glass half-empty" kind of gal, I think it will be good for me (and hopefully, for everyone else too).

I feel better already, and I will roar once again!

SEPTEMBER 9, 2009

Rocco and I had a visit to Total Drama Island yesterday, a.k.a. the doctor's office. He was due for his four-year checkup, and I conveniently scheduled it during lunch hours. That was my first mistake. He also refused the yummy snack-bar I brought to tide him over until the appointment ended (low blood sugar does make for happy Paganis). Not bringing an enticing backup choice was my second mistake, and unfortunately, not bringing toys for distraction during the wait was my third. Oh, and did I mention it was the first day in the practice's new office? I found the new décor bright, cheery, and delightful, but Rocco found it unsettling and suspiciously unfamiliar. So, by the time the doctor arrived, Rocco was not too charming and only moderately cooperative. After the doctor left, Rocco was practically beating down the door to get out. But somehow, I had missed the nurse's request to go over a four-page packet of developmental tasks with Rocco (to see if he was progressing in an age-appropriate manner). So, I had to make the best of the situation.

Our conversation:
Me: "Can you describe three things about the chair you are sitting in?"
Rocco: "NO."
Me: "Okay, how about the doctor's office?"
Rocco: "Yes, I hate it. I want to leave now, and I am never coming back!"
Me: "Hmmm, I guess that is three things."

I managed to do some improvising and extrapolating, but thirty or so hostile, semi-answers later, I think he is developmentally right on track.

After we finished the questionnaire, I practically had to restrain him to stay in the room a few more moments until the nurse returned. When she reappeared and whipped out the syringes, things definitely took a turn for the worse. I really did have to restrain him—good thing I have resumed lifting weights. He went berserk: screaming, shaking, and generally acting like he was having limbs pulled from his body. I, on the other hand, sat as calmly as I could with a thrashing boy on my lap. I've been poked more times than a pincushion, so I am not a mommy who gets hysterical. But the drama must have been pretty intense, because we got several questioning looks from the staff as we walked out of the office. Rocco was so shaken that I had to drag him into to Chik-fil-A for a milkshake and nuggets. His arm (the one that got the shots) was hurting too bad for him to walk (insert mommy eye-roll here).

All this was good though for me though. I love doing what every other mom gets to do. I love dealing with the ups and downs of being a mom and wife. It keeps my head on straight and thinking about the here and now. I don't wanna dwell on the question marks surrounding the skin on my chest and the possible progression of disease. I want to kiss away boo-boos, play with my kids and hubby, and yes, even get some things done around the house.

Please help other women to do the same. Please join or donate to the Go Jen Go team. We have a long way to go to meet our goals and just under a month to do so.

Thanks, Jen the Mom on the Go

September 12, 2009

The kid can really hold a grudge. "Moody" doesn't really do him justice. Rocco was still so pissed off and traumatized by Tuesday's doctor's appointment that I kept him home from school on Thursday, after he informed me that morning that the shots I made him get at the doctor's made him mean. It was a bit of a long morning for Mommy (and perhaps for Luca, who was also home), but I figured I'd take the hit for the team and spare his teachers some drama. Thank God we have one "sweet" one. Luca just has to throw a few toys, hit someone, or clear a table with an arm sweep, and then he is totally over his mood. Damn that Irish/Italian blood coursing through my children's veins!

But mommy woes and laughs aside, life has been blessedly normal. I've been feeling good and strong (as much as one can for the circumstances), and really getting a chance to experience my life in a different way. It has been wonderful! Some days I even forget about "things." But that's not as good as it sounds; it's both a blessing and a curse. When the gravity of my situation comes rushing back, I almost drop to my knees. The realization is brutal. My world tilts, my heart rate skyrockets, and anxiety and fear come rushing in. It feels like getting diagnosed all over again. Somehow though, I manage to regain control and refocus on the gifts of the here and now, but it does wear my soul a bit thin. I get rescanned on October sixth, three days after Komen, and I'm sure that is driving up my anxiety level a bit. But God willing, I will get good scans once again and be able to continue with the good quality of life we've been experiencing of late.

Thanks for listening and supporting us!

SEPTEMBER 23, 2009

I had a good reason for not writing last week: I can't type and hold my breath. We were due to leave on a much-needed vacation (last family trip was May of 2008), and I was so worried that my health might screw it up again that I dared not write for fear of jinxing myself or worrying my family over my stress. So I stayed somewhat quiet and opted for grumpy instead ... or was that just the normal pre-vacation stress/moodiness as a trip approaches?

Well, long story somewhat shorter, we made it! We have been at the beach since Saturday and are having a blast. Souls have been soothed, spirits lifted, family enjoyed, and nature appreciated. It's just what we needed. I've even managed to not think about "things" most of the time. It's glorious!

OCTOBER 2, 2009

Wahoo! Tomorrow is the big day! Thank you, everyone, for your incredible support—emotionally, spiritually, financially, and physically. Team Go Jen Go is going to kick some cancer booty tomorrow! THANK YOU ALL FOR HELPING US HELP OTHERS!

See you soon, Teammates!

OCTOBER 5, 2009

I keep waiting to bounce back after all the cancer ass-kicking and celebrating life this weekend, but so far it hasn't happened yet. I was so tired last night when I tried to blog, it took me about fifteen minutes to write what little I did manage. I couldn't even think of words let alone form sentences (and it didn't help that my computer was acting like it was on acid).

But today, I'm feeling a bit more rested, and this weather (cold and rainy, my favorite!) is definitely helping. I am still rather pooped and am suffering from scanxiety (I get scanned stem to stern tomorrow, and that never, ever helps me think straight), so I hope my ability to express my gratitude and appreciation for all the support doesn't fall too flat! You guys rock! Thanks for being part of finding a cure, supporting so many women (including myself) and their families and friends, and helping to kick some breast cancer ass!

I hope I managed to speak with each and every one of you over the course of the weekend, and I hate that my time with each of you was limited, because I am so thankful for your emotional, spiritual, physical, and financial participation and support. I am sure you all noticed I am rather poor at expressing these things in short conversation and just plain awkward in the quick conversation department.

I am starting to get a bit rambly, and before I get too nonsensical again: THANK YOU! Oh, and please pray my scans come out clean (results should be in by Thursday for my next appointment with Gary)!

I am nervous (like always), Jen

October 8, 2009

Rated M (for Mystical)

With the scans behind me, in the system, and awaiting analysis, my stress level hit about a nine out of ten yesterday morning. Once the kids were finally out the door and to school, I decided it was time to walk off some anxiety, regain some perspective, and let the wonders of nature soothe my soul. Of course, I was out looking for omens, too. I thought my friends and spiritual guides (the crows) might whisper to me again of my destiny.

I hit the bricks with my iPod blasting and found turbulent skies, an erratic wind, and warm, sticky weather (which, in my book, is never, ever a good sign, especially in the non-summer months). As my heart rate climbed, some of the fear, anxiety, and stress started to leach away. God, how I miss my old muscle-burning, lungs-panting, heart-pounding workouts! The music helped too. I was almost out of the neighborhood and onto Carmel, and not one bird (the other animals don't ever have anything to say to me—

nothing I can hear, anyway) had spoken. Then I looked up, startled, as a turkey vulture flew down to about twenty feet in front of me. He didn't say anything, but I knew what his presence meant: that some dead thing was nearby. I stopped to watch as the big bird settled in a tree and then took flight, circling on a thermal just above and around my head. It made me wonder if perhaps I was the dead thing the bird took notice of, but my heart knew this was only the fear I felt in my head, and so I continued my walk wondering which part of me was more perceptive: my soul or my mind?

A few blocks further, I turned back into my neighborhood when something caught my eye, a single crow alone on a branch. This turned my heart cold and my blood icy, despite the sweat on my brow, until I looked up in the tree and saw two more crows sitting side by side on a branch just a bit higher than the solitary crow I first spotted. I knew these three crows were there just for me—a triumvirate message from God of good news.

But despite the sign, my head and heart continued to do battle. Later, thanks be to God, what my heart heard and knew was right: MY SCANS ARE CLEAN! ALL OF THEM. Let us hope and pray that my skin (disease here does not show up on scans, as some of you have asked) is clear as well.

Thank you all, Jen

October 19, 2009

*A*s part of my seize the day, suck the marrow out of life, live in the now and celebrate the moment game-plan, I came home with a boxer puppy last Wednesday. This is one reason for my lack of posts lately. Now when I have a free second to write (i.e. Rocco and Luca are not around), it is spent either playing with, reprimanding, or pooper scooping for our newest family member. She seems to have three modes: sleep, play, poop. I know some of you must be quite surprised and wondering what the hell I'm thinking, and I must admit Joe was/is too, especially since I really only gave him about twenty-four hours notice before bringing her home. But to the nay-sayers, I say this: if the Paganis can survive cancer, we can surely survive one small, occasionally poop-covered puppy! Besides, boxers make my heart sing, and I feel like singing loud. So, say hello to Sophia Pagani (Sophie) next time you're in our neck of the woods!

-Jen, smiling wide because Sophie is happily trying to disembowel a stuffed squirrel.

October 22, 2009

*T*uesday morning, I marched in, friend by my side, to Dr. White's office for an official state-of-the-skin update. I was quite nervous. Life's been so good lately, normal even, and I just didn't want the bubble to burst. A new red area (at the edge of my treatment fields and below my PDT wounds) threatened to do just that: ruin this relative normalcy that I've been enjoying and desperately want to preserve.

Well, I was examined. And then after I patiently explained to him how to do his job correctly—"look at it from this angle," and "touch this spot very gently like you're reading Braille"—he examined me again. In conclusion, there will be no biopsy, and we are still on a wait-and-see plan. In four weeks, we'll revisit, reassess, and go from there.

This is both good news and bad. The good part is obvious, and the bad part is that this is not the definitive answer I was looking for (the area is still there afterall), and so began my mind games. By last night I was in stress overload mode, which is not pretty and called for some extra pharmaceuticals.

This morning, my stress level peaked at the DMV (surprise!). People who are busy fighting for their lives should get a pass on this visit. I sure as hell didn't want to squander some of my precious time waiting in DMV hell, so I smartly drove to Monroe (even tolerated that blight on the state of North Carolina known as Highway 74). I walked right in, and they were ready to take me, just as soon as I forked over my current license and my thirty-two dollar "cash or check." What!? Come again? I must have missed that important tidbit of info (and unfortunately, I am one of a small few who don't carry my checkbook or a debit card around with me).

So I marched right back out to the car seething. Unbelievably mad and frustrated—not with mad at the DMV folks (heck, there was no line), but with my freaking disease. I don't just happen to have moolah on me anymore. Since the diagnosis, all of my cash goes to sitters so I can nap, and my checks all go to CMC. I hate this damn disease!

Well, after a few phone calls, exceeding the speed limit multiple times, and one illegal U-turn at a red light (the boys were obviously not with me), I met Juju, who sweetly drove part way to the boonies to meet me with some cash. Day saved. I passed the test, and there was only a fifteen-minute wait. And for some reason, my fear of the unknown is now a bit more tolerated.

October 27, 2009

I am currently curled up on the sofa out on the porch, enjoying the cool weather, listening to the rain, and trying to type around Sophie, who is cuddled up with me and napping on my arm. The rain that started this afternoon seems to have soothed my soul a bit and eased down my (rather high) level of stress. It's a great way to spend my last night as a thirty-something.

So tonight, instead of mourning the passing of my lost "youth" (okay that was a stretch) and contemplating the inevitable forward march of time, I am thankful for my forty years (despite the sometimes overwhelming challenges of the last two years). I am trying to live in the moment as much as I can, and I'm praying like hell I live to see fifty. It's funny how cancer changes things.

Feel free to make all the over-the-hill jokes you want—I got a jump start on my downhill slide, so you won't hurt my feelings.

But please do be nice to my oldest son. He was the innocent victim of a Mommy's hair-clipping abilities, and he is now under the mistaken impression that his new hairdo looks "cool."

November 1, 2009

Chaos reigned supreme yesterday in the Pagani house. The boys were beside themselves in anticipation of trick-or-treating and just about drove Mommy and Daddy crazy with their enthusiasm. To liven things up a bit, we added an extra two-year-old, a baby, and some adult friends to the mix. By the time we finished dinner and waited out the rain (which conveniently started around five o'clock), we were all slightly nuts. I know the menfolk breathed a sigh of relief when we finally walked out the door.

Even though it was too hot for Mommy, the mist and fog totally added to the flavor of the season. The boys had a blast, and Rocco couldn't wait to get back and eat some of his loot. Of course, you have to let them indulge a bit, so we enjoyed some record-breaking energy levels until about ten. They were record breaking because not only were the kids all whacked out on sugar but football was blasting (damn that gorgeous, perfectly-mannered Tim Tebow) and the dogs needed to unleash some of their pent-up energy as well. Sweet little Sophie has finally and completely come out of her shell and now barks incessantly at Seether to try to get her to play (Seether, despite her advanced age, has finally given in).

This morning, we suffered through some serious post-sugar psychosis fall out, and thus, we had a few time-outs, some thrown away sweets, and lots of drama—all before nine. But all in all, we had a great weekend!

Please pray that we get some additional treats and no tricks tomorrow. I see Dr. White for some skin biopsies at 3:00 p.m..

November 5, 2009

Despite one long, fear-filled, shock-inducing afternoon yesterday, I was still able to go out to dinner with some friends for a belated fortieth birthday celebration last night. I had a really great time. I ate lots of delicious food, enjoyed laughing and talking with my friends, managed two cocktails, and of course, sampled three different desserts. It was quite frankly a perfect evening.

Somehow, I truly managed to enjoy myself despite finding out that my biopsy was positive just a few hours earlier that day. That means the tissue sample was positive for the presence of tumor cells. The area Dr. White chose to biopsy (out of the three choices I offered) was in the middle of the treatment fields for radiation and PDT, which is definitely not too good. His call confirmed my suspicions and what I knew in my heart to be true all along. But despite the relief from my imagination the results did provide, hearing my worst fears (at the moment) confirmed was not easy. I hit about a 9.5/10 on the stress, anxiety, and sadness scale. What was even more difficult was having to call Joe, my parents, and JuJu. Hurting people you love, even when you can't help it, totally and completely sucks.

We will see Gary today. We are not expecting to hear about any miracle options. Hopefully, we can come up with a good plan to continue to keep my scans clean. Please pray for our whole family today. I want to live to see my sons graduate from high school, and that is a long time from now.

November 6, 2009

I managed to keep my nerves at bay yesterday until we were on our way to see Gary. My dear friend Susan met us there and joined us for the appointment. Her presence soothed and comforted both Joe and me, and she lent her medical eyes and ears to the proceedings. She is awesome. I can't quite sum her up in one word, so I'll just borrow a favorite of Rocco's: I *love* her.

Anywho, Gary reassured us that we still do have a couple of options. The plan is to meet with Dr. Fraser on Monday. He will determine, in conjunction with ECU, whether or not PDT is an option again. If so, we will rescan, and if those are still clean, we will start PDT as soon as possible and tweak my current therapy a tad. If I'm no longer a PDT candidate and/or my scans show spread to my organs, then I will begin (most likely) four to six months of a new IV chemo drug. The drug being considered will come with all the typical chemo side effects. I can deal with the hair loss, but I don't care for the nausea, germ concerns ….

Please continue to pray for us. All your prayers and words of encouragement mean so much, especially during uncertain times. We will feel so blessed to have options and two potential plans.

November 10, 2009

As usual, it's been completely nuts since my last post. A Friday night out with the gals from my old neighborhood turned into a surprise party for my fortieth birthday. I fell for the cover-story hook, line and sinker. I was shocked and thrilled. It was a great night, one to be remembered (except by my husband and another male attendee who celebrated a bit too much)! I've got some pretty incredible friends.

So, after partying, a poor night's sleep, and one insanely stressful week, I decided to forge ahead and go to the corn maze, as I had planned, with my good friend and all four of our boys who, combined, have a total age of nine years. We managed a 10:30 a.m. departure and then spent the day playing, petting, munching, and of course, wandering through the corn. Another great time! I was totally on a roll … until I wasn't. It was Sunday when all the fatigue (think ridiculous exhaustion coupled with some major anxiety), stress, and emotion hit at once.

It wasn't pretty, it was contagious, and it was one of the worst days we've had in a long, long while. Monday morning wasn't much better. I quite frankly was not even functioning well, although, somehow, I managed to get the kids off to school. Joe and I were both stressed over my appointment with Dr. Fraser at noon, when (to finally make a long story somewhat shorter) we found out that PDT is an option, and even a good one. This is great because it is by far my best, safest choice for my current condition. So we left CMC more hopeful but still quite worried about logistics, timing of treatment (no time to wait), etc. And shortly after arriving home (to a kiddie-induced chaos), we received a call from the ECU RN. She told us they would take us this coming Monday. Wow! Talk about God at work!

So, we leave for ECU this Sunday. The hope and prayer is that the treatment kills the remaining disease this time, because the amount present is less than it was before. To say we hope it works is an understatement. Please pray it works. Pray for me and my family to find peace and comfort—Rocco is having a hard time with this news, even though we gave him the four-year-old version. And while you're bending the Big Man's (or Woman's?) ear, thank Him for providing us with this opportunity.

Looking for peace, joy and healing, Jen

November 17, 2009

From the American Cancer Society's Hope Lodge, Greenville, NC (home of the Pirates and Parker's BBQ):

Please forgive me, it has been six days since my last confession (not poking fun of Catholicism, but it just seems aprops). Last week, on the evening of my leak discovery, I had a bona fide mini breakdown. Joe pulled me back from the edge, and I have needed some time to restock my mental and emotional stores. I'll spare y'all the details (I whined enough in the last post), but I may have hit a new low. It's been a rough few days. Every little hiccup in my life is threatening to push me over to the point of no return, but I seem to be a bit more stable now, perhaps due to a day of sleep and no real responsibilities yesterday. All I had to do was show up at the cancer center, get injected, and come back to the Hope Lodge and crash. It wasn't even hard to stay out of the sun. All I did was sit, rest, and snooze.

Tomorrow morning is the laser treatment. We had a few questions about efficacy and duration this time, and Dr. Allison addressed our concerns. I was majorly fuzzy as to why the last treatment didn't do the job a 100 percent. We found out that for this treatment to work, the cancer cells need to have their own blood supply (I think they must be sufficiently clustered to do so, like in tumor). Apparently, the cancerous cells can also exist on their own (and aren't large enough to be detected) by obtaining nutrients through their own cell walls without a vascular connection. These cells don't croak when treated because they don't take up any of the treatment drug (and in this case, don't subsequently get fried by the laser). So, please pray that every single cancer cell gets zapped and killed. I am tired of fighting this.

Tomorrow should go fine, I start early and should be done by early afternoon. I get a morning cocktail of pain meds and an Ativan to help pass the time with three lasers, two physicists, one radiation oncologist, and one radiation nurse. Oh, and several ice packs and some really funky glasses that look like they're for a 3-D movie. I will spend my time trying very hard not to look at my chest while they slowly march three cones of laser light across it. All while trying to hold very still and make occasional conversation with folks whose combined IQs probably total 1,000. Please pray this goes well. Please pray for peace, strength, comfort, and healing for me and my family. And thank you very, very much for making this time easier on us all.

NOVEMBER 18, 2009

Hello All, Joe here. Jen has finished her procedure and is back at the Hope Lodge resting uncomfortably. Everything went well, and the doctors and physicists were all pleased. The treatment area was close to the same size as last time, although her disease was not as pronounced. Because of that, she should have less damage and smaller wounds this time. The initial few days, however, will be as painful as before because of the area of treatment. Jen is in good spirits, due in part to the inspiring and supportive messages you all are posting. Thank you for those notes; they help more than you can know. And thank you for the many, many prayers that are being lifted up on her behalf. More info to follow.

-Joe

November 20, 2009

We met for my follow-up appointment yesterday morning with Dr. Allison. It looks like several areas (ones which concerned me) responded favorably to the treatment, even though the total treatment effect takes months to mature. Hopefully, we zapped every last cancerous cell back to hell or wherever they came from. If not, the possibility exists for another go or two with this treatment. I don't want to say we've given up hope, because we haven't, but Joe and I kind of get it now. I will most likely always be battling this, trying to stay in front of distant metastasis and trying every new, reasonable treatment that comes along.

So, with that constant fight in mind, and with a tender, swollen body with just a bit of nausea, we packed up and headed back to Charlotte. We were very thankful to get the official okay to depart, but I was also rather reluctant to leave the peace and quiet. Ready or not, it was time to dive back into the chaos we call home. Well, after a long, uncomfy (but at least cloudy) drive, we walked into a tidy (thanks, Gammy and Howie) and quiet (thanks, JuJu) house, and we had some time to unpack, unwind, and watch a bit of adult TV. We both even slept in until nine! Aside from the cancer treatment stuff, it was really luxurious.

Then, karma decided to give us the finger once again this morning. Our dishwasher was full, so I ran it. It naturally leaked and started dripping through the drywall ceiling and into Joe's shop directly below. I'm not sure whether to laugh or cry. As I am writing this, the repair guys are ripping out drywall in the basement ceiling and are running super-drying fans in the kitchen. They have already pulled out our dishwasher. The last time this happened, it was much worse. A pipe broke in the same area and flooded the kitchen and down below. It required months to repair and happened when I was pregnant with Luca. It marked the beginning of our troubles.

I wonder what it portends this go-around? I can't help but wonder, just a little bit, if my fate and the state of our house are somehow one and the same. It reeks of something Poe might write. And I know it is irrational, not practical, and certainly not economical (especially since I am a one-woman health-care money pit), but I can't help but see the parallels. I am tired of treading water (this figure of speech seemed appropriate given the leak) with my health and with the state of the house, and never taking a step in the right direction.

Laughing, crying, trying not to lose it, Jen

November 23, 2009

Suburban bliss, or what passes for it in our house, has pretty much returned once again. In short, the industrial fans and dehumidifiers are gone from our kitchen and Joe's shop, the contractors will most likely not start until next week, and I should have some quality days this week to focus on my health.

I am currently tired and not thinking straight at all (thank you, pain pill), so I think I will write a bit more tomorrow. But despite inability to express myself right now, please know that I am sustained by your prayers, thoughts, vibes, and deeds. You all have made a very, very difficult couple of weeks doable, which is really saying a lot.

November 25, 2009

I've been too tired and fuzzy-headed to write. I am most definitely struggling to stay in the moment, but my mood is changing as frequently as the skin on my chest, which is about as constant as the sky at sunset (but not nearly as pretty). I find myself worrying about whether or not we bought more time rather than a cure, and that's a really crappy thing to ponder. There are certainly more pressing issues to concern myself with, like why the boys can only talk about "poop and wieners" at the dinner table and finding out what Sophie was up to when she disappeared earlier.

Better go, Rome is burning.

November 30, 2009

My entry will be short and sweet today. I've got "homework" to do with Rocco.

Despite getting off to a rocky start last week, we ended on a high note. The holiday weekend was just what I needed to get my mind off the disturbing "what ifs" and refocus on the present. We ate, laughed, decorated, and lounged in front of a real fire. It was wonderful and like pushing a reset button for my brain. It was just what the doctor ordered.

December 13, 2009

So much has happened in the past two weeks. There's too much to tell. After the great Thanksgiving holiday, my spirits dipped very, very low. I was struggling just to keep it together, and I knew I wasn't going to be able to hold on for much longer. But mountains were moved, and I was able to get away, once again, to the Well of Mercy. I cleansed my heart and soul in the waters there, and I have regained the strength, joy, and determination to move forward.

If you are looking for a worthy cause to support this holiday season, they provide peace, comfort, and healing for those who need it!

December 17, 2009

Jen and I are on our way to meet with Dr. Frenette for Jen's first post-PDT checkup. Please pray for a good meeting with Gary, and please pray that some spots that have Jen worried are not breast cancer. Thank you all for your prayers and meals and notes of love.

-Joe

December 17, 2009

I'm feeling a bit pukey and quite tie-yerd, but I'm very happy. We were a wee bit anxious earlier this afternoon but then we got a good report from Gary. He thought the spots that obviously had disease and got blasted are healing well, the existing spot that was treated but isn't going away is not disease, and that I don't need scanning until around March. Awesome! Then I came home to an incredible and generous surprise package from "Santa" filled with gift cards. Awesome again! And for the tri-fecta, Luca pooped on the potty three times at home totally by himself. What a fantastic day!

Thank you for your prayers and your generosity!

Merry, merry,
-Jen

December 23, 2009

Okay, so I celebrated Christmas with a bit too much enthusiasm on Friday. No, I was not hungover; I went to the boys' school lunch and the choral program at church. I ended up in bed all weekend feeling pukey, shaky, and exhausted. But thanks to the concerted efforts of both grandmas and a break from chemo, I seem to be feeling better each day. Hopefully, I'll be 100 percent by tomorrow evening. My ill feelings were a bit compounded by the fact that it has been an all-out battle to get my chemo sent—it comes from a specialty pharmacy in Raleigh and is not available elsewhere. I spent many, many hours on the phone with many people, and finally it is due to arrive today, one day late. How ironic that Zappos, with about one minute of effort, ships shoes (for free) to your door within twenty-four hours of your order, but something that is literally life or death (now, I know some women will argue that new shoes fit this bill too) has taken about five hours of phone calls and two weeks of stressful effort and anticipation.

Better go, Rocco is literally climbing on me.

Have a beautiful, joyous Christmas!

December 30, 2009

We had "the best Christmas evah" according to Luca. And he knows, after all. This is his third go-around. It was a holiday to remember. It was everything I hoped it would be, and we are so thankful for that.

I will have to wait to share the cute stories later.

Two boys beckon.

P.S. I had to reschedule a checkup with Dr. Fraser yesterday due to a sinus infection, so please pray we get a good report. The ever-shifting landscape of my chest looks a bit different than it did when Gary saw it last week. Thanks!

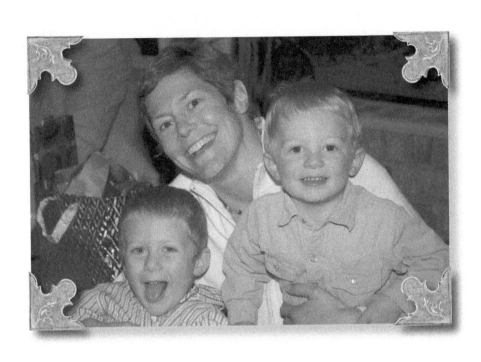

2010

January 5, 2010

PG-13: Language

Yesterday evening, my cell phone finally met an untimely end. The little piece of shit deserved it. It had been functioning at 100 percent only ten percent of the time (weak *Anchorman* reference) for a couple of weeks. So after a most stressful day, I decided to send it on its way to cell-phone heaven (or maybe, I think, hell). It turns out, flip-phones aren't that hard to rip in two, after all. I was that mad, but not that strong. The funny thing is, after I rendered it into pieces and had strewn it about my dash, it actually rang (one last "screw you" from the little beast). I was stunned and even more pissed for a second, then I picked up the largest bit, mashed the receive button, and laughingly explained my situation to whomever might be on the other end. I didn't think it was possible that they could hear me, because it didn't work properly before, but it turned out Joe was there and was not too amused with my story.

No, I didn't finally succumb to two weeks of no school and cooped-up boys, although that is quite possibly enough to push any sane person over the edge. I had a very rude awakening from the dream I was having over the holidays that included pretending I didn't have this monster living on my chest. The ugly bastard reared his head again right after Christmas, and yesterday was the day to get it officially checked out. After a look-see by Dr. Fraser, I was hoping to get the "let's wait and see" line again. Instead, he made several phone calls and sent me directly to Dr. White's office for a biopsy. Read between the lines here: PDT was not 100 percent effective, and Tykerb is not working. Joe and I marched (it felt a bit like I was going to the gallows) over, waited possibly forever in the waiting room because they had to work us in, and then we definitely waited forever in the exam room. That must be what hell is like. There, my very important doctor friend, Dr. Susan Bliss (yes, that is her real name, try not to be jealous) joined us. It turned out that even Gary was around (I have never seen him for an appointment at this location) and so was Dr. White's very capable PA. So, I had the pleasure of sitting on the exam table with a room full of white coats (very compassionate, dedicated ones) and one very stressed-out looking husband while I recounted how the events unfolded: when I noticed the new areas, other changes, blah, blah, blah. I explained it while they all peered at me, examined my wrecked chest, and pondered the implications of the news. It was a Munchausen sufferer's wet dream and practically my worst nightmare; it was definitely not the kind of attention I wanted.

The ironic thing about the "cure" for me, Tykerb, is that it causes lots of skin side effects, many of which can mimic (or mask) the exact presentation of my particular brand of disease, which is insidious and nebulous, to say the least. So, during the great meeting of the minds (and perhaps the meeting of the great minds), it was jointly decided to stop my Tykerb for about two weeks to see if any of the suspicious spots change. If they get worse, I'll get a biopsy next week, I'll stop this chemo, and then we'll move on to the next one. That would be like our forty-seventh choice of treatment, which doesn't exactly make me feel too good for the long-term picture. If they get better and actually go away, we'll thank God for the miracle.

Please pray, and ask everyone you know to pray, for that miracle. My sons need it, my husband needs it, and I need it. And if we don't get one, please pray that my new chemo is liveable and goes "cellular" on my cancer's ass. Thanks.

P.S. Don't bother with trying to ring me on my celly until after January 17, when our contract is up. Then I will have a new, non-rippable, fully functioning model. Oh, and if you call my home phone, give me some time to call you back. I have three more appointments today to look forward to: big fun!

JANUARY 8, 2010

Yesterday's Herceptin treatment was uneventful, thank God. I was most definitely due. On Monday, though, I have a biopsy scheduled for three in the afternoon, and we are expecting to see disease (I don't need a freakin' microscope to visualize something I can see, very easily, in the mirror from across the room). Scans and restaging will follow. We should know the exact nature of this beast next week. Please pray we can douse the wildfire on my chest and that it is not burning anywhere else; that would change things dramatically, and most likely not for the better.

Stuck in the twilight, trying hard to focus between the "spots,"
-Jen

P.S. "Spots" are a bland euphemism for a varying array of visual disease, not at all representing what the word really hints at (something colored and maybe cute like on Sophie). These are more like spots from hell.

JANUARY 11, 2010

I'm pooped, it's late, and I've just come from having a tequila or two. I went directly from my biopsies to meet a friend at Cantina. It was just what the doctor ordered.

Tomorrow I get scanned and then restaged. Let's hope the spread is limited to my chest. Then on Thursday, we will meet with Gary to get results. Should be a fun week.

Off to bed and hopefully some sweet dreams.

JANUARY 14, 2010

Well, we're back from Gary's and a week's worth of extraordinary, unparalleled anticipation is finally, thankfully over. The results are in: both biopsies positive for disease, but ALL scans NEGATIVE! This is quite fantastic news in light of everything. We were totally expecting cancer to be present in the skin (I can literally see it all over the place), and I was sweating the scans like never, ever before. I've been to hell and back about forty times this week, and this is a truly a gift from God.

The suspicion, once again, is that my disease is biologically different (I'm going to make for a great case study and presentation some day) and is most likely responding to the chemo because it has not spread systemically (i.e., to my organs) but is limited to my skin. Gary is postulating that for a variety of reasons. The skin on my chest is not well vacscularized (doesn't have good blood flow), and therefore, the previous therapies (which require blood for transportation into the cells) have not worked on it. So, we will continue with some chemo (a new one, more about that later). Pray that maybe something will work locally and focus on our systemic success. The fact that it is not spreading beyond my skin is awesome.

I will begin a Gemzar (see ya later, Tykerb) IV regimen weekly, three weeks out of every month, on the 28th. It is well tolerated, and I won't lose my hair, which I think is most important for the boys, especially Rocco right now. So, in addition to the awesome scan news, I have two more bonus weeks of NO chemo. Sweet! Look out, tequila, here I come!

Thank you all for all your earnest prayers, meals, cards, calls, playdates and distractions over the past week or so. I am still here because of all of you, and we can't possibly thank you enough. Oh, and please say thank you to the Big Guy next time you talk to Him.

January 17, 2010

*T*omorrow, Joe and I head to Jackson Hole for a much, much needed getaway. I can't wait. It is the place that makes my spirit soar, a source of inspiration, and where I feel and see God's presence everywhere I look. It's just what the doctor ordered.

Laus Deo, Jen

January 26, 2010

*A*fter a ridiculously long travel day, thanks to the stormy weather in and around Hotlanta, we made it back from Jackson around two o'clock in the morning Monday morning, which is apparently four or five hours past my physical limits. I actually had a difficult time putting one foot in front of the other to walk from our plane to baggage claim. But at least we made it in one piece.

I am still swooning from the trip. Jackson Hole, to me, is like going home. The drive north of town toward Yellowstone, in particular when you arrive in Grand Teton National Park and see the park sign, is like going home. I have an intense connection to this place that resonates in my very bones, the very essence of my being—this place where the vast sagebrush-covered grass plain meets the Aspen tree-lined Snake River at the foot of the majestic Tetons on one side, and rises to meet the elevated plateau leading to the Gros Ventre (pronounced "grow vant") Range on the other. It is, to me, the most mystical, magical, and wondrous place. It is THE place where my soul feels connected and at home, the place I truly believe where my soul was born.

This is more than just a thought or a conclusion I have reached, it is something that resonates in every cell of my being. It is a truth my soul whispers to my mind each time I visit. After all, what do we really know of where our souls reside before the moment of conception? Where do they reside after? I know that this place is a part of me, and after my soul is free from my body once again, I will return here, for it is heaven on earth.

In addition to the existential moments of our trip, we also managed to have some serious fun. We snowmobiled for two days, and it was incredible. It was a physical treat combined with unbelievable, only accessible by snowmobile or snowcat, vistas. It was exhilarating, completely engrossing, and a fabulous physical release. In short, it made me feel ALIVE (versus just surviving). It was a true gift. And when we weren't doing all that, we managed to see bison, elk, bighorn sheep, pronghorn antelope, coyotes, bald eagles, an osprey, a golden eagle, moose, and lots and lots of crows. Well naturally, I've plenty more to share, but the wildlife inside is starting to stir and call out.

Time to go, Jen

JANUARY 27, 2010

I'm a bit tired and quite a bit anxious about tomorrow. It's the day my chemo vacation ends and the day I start my new weekly IV regimen of Gemzar. I have a wee bit of concern for the side effects. They are supposed to be "well tolerated," but that's a relative statement. The main reason for my anxiety, though, is that once we start this drug, we'll actually see if and how well it works. And it better work well. You see, while I was enjoying my chemo vacation, it turns out the cancer was enjoying it too. My spots look much more prevalent, more nodular, and they have shown up in lots of new places. That is not too good. I tried to ignore it as best as I could in Jackson (I needed to LIVE a little) because I knew we would be getting back to business when we got back to town. Well, tomorrow it's time to clock back in, and I am dreading it and needing it at the same time.

Say a prayer that the Gemzar kicks some major cancer ass. We got to get this skin thing under control soon.

JANUARY 30, 2010

Ugh! This new chemo, Gemzar, has totally kicked my hiney. Even though I was tired and not feeling a 100 percent going into treatment Thursday afternoon, I really didn't think it was going to be so tough. They give it weekly, after all, three weeks out of every month, so I figured it couldn't be too bad. Wrong! After some intermittent nausea, false post-chemo pep, and shakes from the IV steroids, I figured I was over the worst of it. And I may have been, but Luca started with a rather realistic *Excorcist* impersonation last evening, approximately twenty minutes after getting home from Juju's. Poor little guy. It's a good thing Mommy had taken a no throw-up pill about an hour before the spewing started, because that smell is hard enough to take when you're healthy. So after lots of outfit changes and loads of laundry,

Daddy and I were spent. Daddy had to pull throw-up duty last night, but I still woke up exhausted. Luca (who hasn't thrown up for twelve or so hours!) and I spent almost all day in bed. Neither of us has even ventured outside to just see the snow. Rocco, on the other hand, has had the "best day of his life" (how quickly they forget about Christmas) playing in the white stuff.

Hopefully, Luca and I will feel like getting out tomorrow and, more importantly, that I will not feel this bad several days of every week for the next six months.

February 1, 2010

Joe here. Luca's viral battle looked like it had passed, but at two thirty a.m. Sunday morning, Jen was violently ill. By five o'clock, she knew she needed to go to the hospital. I rushed across the frozen street to the neighbors' house to rouse our friend out of his warm bed so he could come and wait for my boys to wake up while Jen and I rushed to the ER. A frantic pounding at your door at five o'clock in the morning is not a wonderful way to start the day, but he sprang into action without a moment's hesitation, which is a quality that we have counted on from every member of that household for the past three years.

I got Jen out of bed and into the car, and tried to balance the speed of a frantic husband taking his wife to the hospital and the prudent speed when driving at night on completely ice- and snow-covered roads. When we arrived, her blood pressure was dangerously low, and she was minimally responsive. Excruciatingly long hours went by as they tried to pump her full of fluids and get that BP back up.

Since this is Jen's journal, I will let her go into the details. She is doing okay right now. They think she will be in the hospital until Tuesday, if all goes well. She is very worried about the chemo schedule, but Dr. Frenette hasn't made a call on that yet.

Meanwhile, Rocco was the next recipient of the virus. He spent yesterday with JuJu and got sick in the evening. He seems to be recovering this morning. I guess I am in line for that bug next. Yippee.

Life does throw us all some curve balls from time to time, doesn't it?

-Joe

February 4, 2010

(PG-13) Gross, frank content—after two kids and the past two-and-a-half years of being a medical oddity, I have little to no modesty left.

(OMGIL) Oh My God It's Long

I'm home; I got here Tuesday night but just have not felt up to logging on until now. Here's what happened:

Not that I ever suspected otherwise, but chemo and the stomach flu just don't mix. I felt about two or three pukes short of shuffling off this mortal coil on Sunday morning. I did not evah, evah think we were going to get to the hospital. It was literally the first time in my life I was unhappy to see snow and ice on the roads. But make it we did, and after four or five liters of IV fluids, lots of IV nausea meds, a whole lot of TLC, and only enough pee to fill a sample cup, I finally (ten hours after check in) had blood pressure high enough to be transferred to a room. It was a very long day for everyone.

After finally getting the puking, passing out, and pressure problems under control, I had high hopes of getting some rest in my room that first night, but naturally, explosive diarrhea decided to kick in from the witching hours of two to five in the morning. More fun to be had! It was a damn good thing I was strong enough at this point to get up and go to the bathroom on my own (although definitely on wobbly legs). What followed was a day of very thorough care, a day I spent listlessly in a dark and fairly quiet room just waiting for time to pass and to feel better. I also stressed a fair amount of time over my next round of chemo, which was supposed to be today.

For some reason (I guess I thought I was due), the optimist in me still prevailed, and I was really looking forward to a good night's sleep (or what passes for it in the hospital) by Monday evening. The virus, however, had other plans. It struck again in the early hours of the morning. Gary rounded at five o'clock. I looked stunned—because who the hell rounds at five o'clock? Oncologists, I don't care what they make, don't make enough— and (of course) stunning. He said some stuff, some of which I retained, but basically, I got the gist that I would be most likely get to go home that day (Tuesday) and chemo was out of the question for Thursday (now today).

Blah, blah, blah, one more full day in the hospital, and I am finally home. I'm tired, I'm still fighting some nausea/GI after-effects, and I'm weaker but rather slim (which of course, almost makes all this worth it). So, to cut a very long story a bit shorter, I am working on getting ready for Monday morning's chemo (damn, now I'll only be able to drink a six pack during the game), Joe did not get it but Gammy did, and we are all very, very grateful for the prayers and help.

-Slim Jen

FEBRUARY 8, 2010

We skipped the Super Bowl ta-dos and spent a night home with the boys. Mass and dinner the night before just about did me in, so we thought it best. It was a good choice. I got a good night's sleep, at least until about six o'clock when I woke up with a case of nerves. I definitely was feeling gun shy about Gemzar today. Is a repeat puke fest in the cards? I hope not.

We saw Gary, and he thought I looked much, much better than I did a few days ago (I've showered!). He gave his final go ahead and said he didn't think we could've gone any earlier than today (we concurred). He said getting treatment today was the aggressive choice, but I told him surviving cancer is not for sissies. Let's get back to kicking some cancer ass. So, despite the chemo hangover, nausea, head pounding, and weakness, I feel pretty good and probably a lot better than some Super Bowl watchers I know.

Thanks for helping us survive this, Jen

FEBRUARY 14, 2010

Why I'm Not up For Mom of the Year

Luca has completely flipped his lid. He woke up on the wrong side of the crib Saturday, despite the snow, and hasn't looked back. Yesterday morning, when Mommy walked out of the den for about two seconds to go make beds, Daddy announced it was time to go outside. And within two minutes, he and Rocco were out the door and playing. I, on the other hand, was left with a very contentious Luca, who was not at all pleased by this sudden announcement. So, after several trips to the big-boy potty, several of what I am now calling "costume negotiations," one sullen, partially-dressed boy clad in *Super Hero Squad* jammies and I went downstairs to find my snow clothes so I could play too. Well, after rooting around in the basement closet and carefully selecting an outfit that would keep me warm and looking good for the video and pictures I knew were to follow our morning in the snow, I headed back upstairs to see what the very quiet Mr. Luca had been up to. I had the momentary, false, and high hopes of any mother of a "terrible two" that maybe, just maybe, he saw the wisdom of my argument for warmer clothes and had gotten himself dressed. What I stumbled on, however, was something all-together different.

He was indeed in the process of dressing, but instead of adding some clothes, he had stripped off his big-boy underwear and pants, and colored his penis and the palm of his hand (I wondered why he decided on that combo) with a bright orange marker. He was in the process of doing some other decorating in the boy-parts area when I interrupted him. I wasn't mad, I was, though, most definitely surprised. I figured no glue was involved, so it wasn't really too bad. They were washable markers; thankfully, I had the foresight to buy these particular kind in case the kids drew, I was thinking worse case scenario here, on the walls. Quite frankly, I had to give him an A for creativity and coloring in the lines, but he got a C for color choice.

Meanwhile, forty-five minutes have passed, and Joe and Rocco are blissfully unaware of the events that have unfolded in the house. They've had a grand time and are just about done with the snowman by the time we finally get out door. We get outside, snap a few pictures (and despite my outfit, I am in none of them), and then Luca announces to me that his feet are too cold and demands to go in. Well, Mommy is way, way pooped by this point, but determined to enjoy the snow, damnit, because she missed the entire last snowfall thanks to the flu she got from none other than Luca! So I immediately caved (that's some quality parenting) when he wanted to watch *Super Hero Squad*. This is a show the boys and I watched for the first time the day before, and I had told Joe that under no circumstances should we ever, ever let them watch it again because it is utterly inane, teaches absolutely nothing of value, and is even more annoying than *Bakugan* or *Pokémon*. Well, I planted him in front of the TV and popped in *Super Heros*. Then, without a backward glance (the markers were at this point out of reach), I went back out the door to play for a bit.

At this point, I was too pooped to play, so I managed about fifteen minutes in the great outdoors before joining Luca on the couch. The morning's events pretty much set the tone for Luca's weekend behavior. And by nine o'clock this morning (Happy Valentine's Day, Mom), he had peed all over the bathroom floor, pooped in the big-boy potty twice ("I need some privacy!"), gone through three pairs of different *Super Hero* underpants, and went through five costume changes. Looks like it's gonna be another busy day at our house. But honestly, I don't expect any different. His father is a pistol, so naturally he's a son of a gun. Better go do some laundry.

SuperMom, Jen

FEBRUARY 17, 2010

I'm not a doctor, but I play one online (and occasionally at CMC).

Pretty much every mom I know with multiple little ones is tired, so I figured my recent dragging around was partly due to being the mom of a "terrible two" and an intense and challenging four-and-a-half-year-old, mixed with some residual after-effects from the flu/chemo combo. However, at treatment on Monday, I found out otherwise. The first question posed to me by my favorite infusion room RN after my labs were back was, "Have you ever gotten a transfusion before?" This was immediately followed by "Have you discussed getting a shot for your white counts with Gary?" Hmmm, not really off to a great start. Apparently, my counts are at an across the board all-time low. Red blood cells are for energy, white blood cells are to fight infection, and platelets are for blood clotting. My numbers sucked, to put it bluntly and brashly. Discussions were had, calls to Gary were made, and then we decided to go ahead with treatment. I've never, ever even been questionable for treatment before, aside from the recent flu thing, but we just rescheduled for that.

So this explains why Mommy is getting pooped during costume negotiations and potty time (for Luca, not me). I basically feel like I've been out in space and come back to the hard, exhausting reality of gravity. I'm light headed, have a numb feeling, and get winded walking up the stairs. I am, however, very, very, very sick of sitting on my ass all the time. Since I seem to be on an accelerated aging program, I don't want to waste my time on the couch. I crave the outdoors. I need it to see and feel God, to reconnect with some of the old me, and to get my mind and spirit pointed true north again. So yesterday, in between the sofa and lying in bed, I managed a walk with Sophie. It was fabulash. The temperature was just right, the sky brilliant blue, the sunlight warm and generous. It was a bit of a physical challenge though. I did at times feel like I was trying to summit Everest and had to focus on just putting one foot in front on another, but it was so, so good (and absolutely necessary) for my well being. It made me feel a bit like I did a few times during the peak of Ironman training, which of course made me smile and feel like I was indeed still the same Jen of days past.

Basically, my counts will continue to drop this week as Monday's treatment continues to take its toll. If I can tolerate the symptoms and don't feel too much worse, I don't have to go to get labs until this coming Monday. So, let's pray I can continue to function this week and that they can straighten my counts out by whatever means necessary so I can continue on.

February 23, 2010

Well, I fell on a few dark days last week. The extra gravity that seemed to have settled on my body finally dragged my mind and spirit down along with it; it was a week of a pitiful existence. I was barely participating in my life, let alone that of my family's. It sucked (sorry, that word keeps popping up), but I'm over it. I've been feeling better and better since yesterday morning, so I don't want to waste any time looking in the rearview, especially when the view's not that good.

Despite my being a sorry, little shell of myself, we did get some really good news last Friday. At an appointment to discuss starting some local therapy (which ironically, would need to be done in Durham) in conjunction with the chemo, Dr. Fraser was very pleased with how hard the disease on my chest is getting hit. It seems the Gemzar is kicking the cancer's ass right along with mine, which is a pretty good consolation prize for feeling so crappy). The thought is to zap the skin with a special type of radiation therapy done at only Duke while the disease load is small, so it won't (hopefully) be able to grow back/spread. Basically we'll kick it while it's down. Sounds good to me! Let's stomp that shit back to hell where it belongs!

Later, Jen

March 3, 2010

I feel a bit uninspired in writing this, a bit flat. I think it's because I am in the one-day post-chemo fog ....

Last week passed, and I was able to progress from the bed/sofa shuffle to going out with Joe and some of our friends over the weekend. We had a great time, and God knows, it was great to get out and have some fun. Gammy and Papa had the boys, and though I missed them terribly, it gave me some time to feel pretty good and relax like an adult (and not have to wipe any hineys but my own).

We saw Gary yesterday before chemo. We discussed the fact that the Gemzar was really, really beating me up. We went through the long list of my side effects (including my lovely lab values, which are in the crapper), and I told Gary this was about the longest I have felt this bad in two-and-a-half years of chemo, which is really saying something. After some consideration, Gary decided to reduce my dosage by twenty percent. He said that it sounds like I have Grade Three toxicity (I'm guessing Grade Four is six feet under). Apparently, I am most likely deficient in an enzyme needed to metabolize the drug, so I don't require as much to do the same job someone else would. I think this means I will get all the benefits and hopefully a lot less of the side effects (i.e., I will be able to function; that would be nice). He also gave the go ahead to meet with the Duke folks about discussing the possibility of the hyperthermic treatment.

And today, after a brief chat with Dr. Fraser and asking if he would request an appointment from Duke on my behalf, I have an appointment in Durham this coming Monday. All I have to do is call there tomorrow and find out what time. Sweet.

Better go. I am running out of steam.

March 10, 2010

Apparently, I have a lot to say ....

Life just doesn't slow down long enough for me to type about it. Let me catch you up to date a bit on the recent medical stuff, and then hopefully I will get to share another excerpt from my upcoming book, *How to Ineffectively Parent in 90 Days or Less*.

The Duke trip had me really, really stressed out. The thought of potentially starting another treatment for an extended stay away from home, and with potentially devastating skin side effects, was a bit too much for me emotionally. Durham is rather depressing, and our previous trips to the Duke clinic have been far from uplifting. But with all that being said, we got off to a good start, the radiation waiting area was pleasant with a nice view, and we were the first patients of the day, which meant no six-hour wait in the world's most depressing waiting room this time! The doctor was very, very thorough and explained that he thought I was responding excellently to the chemo, my skin looked far better (remember, this is relative) than he expected, and that we have this hyperthermic radiation treatment as a backup option if and when we need it in the future. There is no need to stop the Gemzar and start his therapy now. In fact, the risks (the worst being total devastation of the skin in the areas treated) far outweigh the benefits of doing his therapy now, and he also said (which we suspected, but I always hate to hear) that the hyperthermic treatment is palliative rather than curative. But it is an option we weren't sure we had, we don't have to make any tough decisions about what the right course of treatment is, AND I don't have to miss Luca's birthday (last year I was in Greenville getting PDT). I'll get to spend spring outside with the boys. AWESOME!

That brings us up to yesterday. I went to get Gemzar, and for the first time evah, in two and a half years, my counts were too low to get chemo. I have really, really been dragging, struggling with very dark thoughts, and in general not feeling like myself at all. I figured it had to do a lot with my red counts, but I was really shocked to hear my bone marrow is taking a beating. My white counts, which are low and have been steadily dropping over the past month, are a quarter of what they were a week ago and by far the lowest they have ever, ever been. Blah, blah, blah. I got an injection to boost my bone marrow and will be getting two units of blood on Friday. Hopefully, I will get my Gemzar as planned next Tuesday.

Well, this little hiccup was a surprise, and I couldn't help but wonder if my life was unfolding like the pages of some great novel and that I was the tragic figure in it. Was my body finally starting to crumble under the weight of these past years of treatment like my mind and will seem to be of late? But so as not to star in a tragedy of my own making, I questioned several of the nurses, and they put my fears of foreshadowing largely to bed. Apparently, Gemzar frequently wreaks this kind of havoc, and besides, one of the RNs I really like said I look "too damn healthy" to be heading in the wrong direction. After twenty-two years of oncology nursing, she said that "definitely counts for something."

I am thrilled to be getting some blood Friday. I am overdue. I've been dreaming, strangely realistic, about blood off and on for two weeks. So, my thirst will be quenched in two days' time, and hopefully by Saturday morning, I will feel like a new woman.

MARCH 15, 2010

*A*fter weeks of dragging around and dreaming about blood, I finally received the two units of packed red cells on Friday. It was a bit disorienting, going to the infusion room at Dr. White's office. Despite my numerous visits to that office, I had never set foot in the infusion room or even seen any of the staff there. I have been a bit of a nervous wreck there of late, so the excitement I felt was a bit unsettling to say the least. It was also a bit of a surprise not to feel like crap after leaving (I guess I am so used to chemo). In fact, I didn't leave there feeling like Superwoman, but I felt noticeably more peppy by Friday evening.

By Saturday morning, I felt like a new woman. And (total bonus) I was no longer on germ-alert code red because of the Neulasta shot I got earlier in the week, so I was able to go AND participate for an event I have literally been waiting for since I was pregnant with Rocco: our very first soccer team practice. It was awesome! We signed up for Park Sharon, and the participation of one parent is required. I was lucky enough to be that parent and hope and pray I will get to do a lot more participating over the next eight weeks. The rest of the weekend was active and normal, which given the way this year has been going, is really saying a lot.

Today I even braved the germs (took some serious precautions) and went for a swim at the YMCA. I haven't been there since diagnosis (this is only my second lap swim in a year), and it was rather bittersweet. I'm happy to say that after all this physical abuse of the last couple of years, I am still not the slowest person in the pool.

Tomorrow (assuming my counts did rise, and if not, it is panic time), it's back to the weekly grind. And even though the Gemzar is working (though unfortunately, I can tell the cancer enjoyed the break), I really just don't want to go.

Trying to get my head back in the game,
-Jen

MARCH 22, 2010

We had another normal (translation: GREAT) weekend. Soccer, birthday parties, etc ... it was heaven! And the boys were surprisingly well behaved, considering the vast quantities of sugar and corn syrup they consumed. Although, I did suffer a bit of a blow to my ego when Rocco informed me that I don't really look very much like a girl—that's just what a tomboyish chick with one boob wants to hear to make hear to make her feel good! But after a few investigatory questions, I realized he said this because of my short hair. Whew! I thought for a second I was going to have to step up my around the house wardrobe and my a.d. (after diagnosis) lifestyle is more slouchy rather than stylish.

I am trying to make the most of my week off of treatment. Today I went back to the YMCA (no teary eyes this time) for another swim. It is definitely good for what ails me. I was more mentally prepared to talk to the many peeps I hadn't seen in ages. Sometimes catching up is a bit tough ....

And because good news comes in threes, I don't have chemo tomorrow (no post-treatment poisonous thoughts to deal with), the Burnette's (my brother and his wife) are expecting their first baby, and I was recently the humble recipient of the Brown Cup by the City Track and Tri club!

APRIL 1, 2010

In recent months, my muse seems to have been largely absent. My mind longs to hear her sweet murmurings, but it finds the dull void of silence instead. I spent these past few days at the Well of Mercy. I was able to revel in the quiet, reconnect to my soul in the midst of God's great playground (the South in the spring time), and at long last heard the ...

I didn't get to finish. I ran out of time, and now I am post chemo and sitting on the couch with Luca trying to mash computer keys while I type. I have decided to use one of my parenting "cheat" cards and turned on *Bakugan* to buy some time.

Chemo went well on Tuesday, thanks to my third dosage reduction. I can still feel the physical effects, but my brain and soul seem to have fared quite a bit better this go around. Thank God, because I can't even tell you how much I was dreading the blackness again.

We have a busy few days ahead. I have an ultrasound today to rule out a blood clot—we're ninty percent sure the symptoms are left over from the clot from a year ago and have just re-surfaced as they can do. Then we have an opthamology check up for Rocco's scratched cornea tomorrow in Belmont (could they make it less convenient?), a choral thing at St. Gabe's tomorrow night, Easter egg hunting first thing Saturday, and a party immediately following that. Then of course, Easter Sunday, the day of rebirth, joy, and hopefully rest.

April 9, 2010

*L*ately, I keep falling so far behind in blogging that I find myself with too much to say, and thus have to gloss over everything to keep from having to write a novella, and I don't have the opportunity be my usual witty self. Hah! Part of this absence is due to the fact that Rocco missed the two weeks of school prior to spring break, and Luca missed one week (great timing on their parts), partly due to the fact that I have really been struggling with depression of late, which is, hopefully, in large part due to the effects of Gemzar, and partly due to how hard it is to manage life with a chemo regimen spaced like it is. I only have a day or so of feeling decent, and that day spent quite depressed and dreading chemo like nevah, evah before. Then I get hit with the crap all over again. If I were an artist, I would most definitely be in a black period, or at least very dark blue.

It has been an odd time. I don't look too sick (what, with hair, eyebrows, eyelashes, and decent skin color), apparently, I have a good appetite (as was noted by an astonished, fellow guest at the Well who was shocked at how much I could put away while on chemo), and I am still managing to function somewhat decently in my various roles of mother, wife, and daughter. But despite my best efforts, there are cracks in my façade that are threatening to bring the whole thing down. I have not ever felt quite like this before, or for such a long time. I pondered yesterday, while at counseling—why am I like this now, after fighting so long? Has some fundamental part of me changed? Is the Gemzar causing most of this? Or am I finally succumbing to almost three years of unbelievable, unremitting stress? Will I have the will to continue treatment when the next recurrence hits? And very much on my mind is this one: how long of a break will I have after Gemzar ends before we scramble to find something else that doesn't kill me but keeps the cancer at bay for a bit longer? I am consumed with these questions. What I want is to be consumed with being a mother and wife and well, the old me, the one that existed somewhere a long time ago.

Perhaps I won't find the answers to these questions. Life is full of great, unanswered mysteries. Maybe what I should focus on is regaining an acceptance of my situation. I'm not sure how to go about this. I told my counselor that she should have the answer to this dilemma (that's why she gets paid the big bucks), but she, of course, said I had to figure it out for myself. So, if the boys actually go to school next week, that is exactly what I am going to do with my "me time."

Going out to talk to some crows,
-Jen

April 17, 2010

A week in the life...

Sometime early last week, the boys finished all their pink eye drops, and by the time Friday arrived, everyone was still healthy! Uh-mazing! I had one of those joyous, "It's the most wonderful time of the year," moments, because all we had to do was make it through the weekend (seemed easy enough at the time), and then everyone would be back to school come Monday morning.

Friday and Saturday were uneventful until, while at a party for Juju's birthday, Joe and I noticed that neither Rocco nor Luca finished all their cake and ice cream, a Pagani family first. Initially, we were highly suspicious but soon forgot all about it. Then, Rocco took an unexpected nap in the middle of everything, and we became a bit uneasy. About an hour later, it looked, according to my sister-in-law, a bit like New Year's Eve. At least he managed to do most of his puking in the bathroom. Luca, thank God, did not get the throw-ups but suffered some lower GI problems.

Surprisingly, we made it through the night without any more sickness (Joe and I both went to bed wary, and praying I didn't succumb to the bug, but both boys were fine by Sunday evening. I even took them to see *How to Train Your Dragon* in 3D. I had promised to take them during spring break and was determined to follow through. Despite the fear of stomach problems, being out-manned, and just plain running out of steam, it turned out to be a great night.

When Rocco woke up Monday morning with more pink eye, school was obviously out of the question and I suffered a mini breakdown (which might come as a surprise to some of you; I have either been up or down, light or dark, depending on which me you encounter). The thought of dealing with the needs of sick, sequestered kids while on my third in a row and worst week of chemo was just too much. I had been burning the candle at both ends for a while and was absolutely counting on recharging my battery while the boys were at school.

On Tuesday, both of Rocco's eyes were icky, but the Rx drops seemed to be working. The boys spent the day at Juju's, thank God, because I was approaching crisis mode, while Joe, Susan, and I jumped through lots of hoops to get an appointment to get my head straight. I talked to Gary that afternoon before chemo about our options, and we decided to go up on the dose of my antidepressant. What I needed was a timely appointment with a psychiatrist (preferably on my health care plan) to manage my antidepressant meds. What we found instead is a gaping hole in the mental health care of cancer patients in our community. There exists no in-hospital network that specializes in helping people cope with a cancer diagnosis. I just assumed, when and if I was in need of someone to help manage this, I would be able to pick up the phone and get them. And get them without a five-week wait or without the combined efforts of my husband and two friends that just happen to be doctors. Let me also add that Charlotte is not without resources: CMC has one MSW for its entire cancer center; and Presbyterian has the amazing Buddy Kemp Caring House, a fabulous resource open to everyone in the cancer community, no matter where you are getting treated. Buddy Kemp has several counselors, all of which I believe are MSWs, so they can't perscribe meds either. Buddy Kemp is an incredible place and offers so, so many valuable and needed things. My counselor there is literally a life saver, so please don't think I am saying otherwise.

Wednesday, the day after chemo, was not bad. By Thursday night I had a fever, so we called the twenty-four-hour oncology number, and Joe had to make a late night run to the drug store. On Friday morning, I still had a low temp but was feeling better. So while the boys were at school, Gammy drove me to Gary's office. What we found was a bit surprising. My white counts were fine, good actually, but my hemoglobin (necessary for oxygen delivery by the red blood cells) was at an all-time low. I of course, knew it was low, and I thought that I needed blood prior to the labs. But I guess I lack a little thing called a medical degree. Naturally, the only immediate option to get blood was to do a twenty-three-hour admit to the hospital, which I flat out declined. So now I am in physical limbo: I feel like crap and am wasting time on the couch because I am not able to do more until tomorrow morning when I go in for two more units (and sacrifice five or six more hours of my week).

I am currently trying to play with the boys and referee from the sofa until my transfusion tomorrow, and I can't help but ponder the state of things. Why doesn't CMC have a group of psychiatrists (to manage meds) and clinical psychologists and more MSWs dedicated to the needs of its cancer patients? Doesn't anyone see the need to give a referral to an easily accessible, mental-health worker to everyone newly diagnosed with cancer? Why can't you leave that initial, life changing appointment and head directly to another floor to see a professional to help you cope? What happens to the thousands of newly-diagnosed people in Charlotte that don't have the support and resources I do? And if money is the answer, is there a way we can start to fix this problem?

April 19, 2010

*T*hank you so much for all of you who continue to support us in so many ways. Reading my blog (I am sure is no easy task of late), writing in, praying, fixing meals, helping with the boys .... The strength I gather from all of your efforts on my behalf has been a literal life saver. For lack of the appropriately articulated verbiage, a simple THANK YOU will have to do.

I received my two units of packed red cells yesterday. After a brief, tense ten minutes of not being able to get in the building, and wondering if I really got the day right and whether they really work on Sunday at Blumenthal, God intervened and Susan just happened to be post-rounds over at the hospital and just happened to call me while we were out front of MMP, continually trying the after hours call box and not getting a response. She came over and let us in with her ID badge and saved the day.

So I am already feeling much better, still nowhere near 100 percent, but nowhere near zero percent, either. I can already feel the darkness in my head starting to brighten. I am looking forward to a week of being more of the mother, wife, and woman I know I really am.

-Jen, extant

P.S. Donate blood if you can; the infusion room had lots of other cancer patients who were getting it too.

MAY 6, 2010

$\mathcal{S}$ aturday, the much-anticipated day of Luca's birthday party, finally arrived. He had been asking about his special *Ben 10* party multiple times daily for two weeks. When he woke up and realized we weren't immediately leaving for Mickey D's, I noticed a sour look on his face. So I cheered him up with some waffles and bacon and suggested we go on an "outdoor adventure," which is Pagani-talk for poking at bugs with sticks, hitting things with said sticks, and jumping off our retaining walls. I even pulled out a new (Target dollar bin) butterfly net and showed him how to use it. Ahhhh, crisis of impatience averted ... or so I thought. The second we were out the door, I heard him mumble something about his net. It caught me a bit off guard, and for some reason, I repeated back to him what I thought he said. "Did you say something is wrong with my net, damnit?" With a big, big scowl, he said, "Uh, yes, I did." Hmmm, I wonder where he got that little gem? Mommy? Or Daddy? Or perhaps both. I wonder if we'll get a note home from school ....

Well, what ensued was a very, very difficult lesson about the progression of time. I'd forgotten how hard of a concept this is at age three. And of course, I had originally wanted to have the party at 11:00 a.m., but was informed by McDonald's that this was the start of their busiest time of day, which didn't seem to bode well, so instead we opted for 5:00 p.m.. Well, this was an eternity to Luca, and he expressed his displeasure with a very foul mood, constant scowl, and a full-on meltdown late in the afternoon (followed, thankfully, by a nap; all that disappointment is so exhausting). Perfect. Happy Birthday, Son!

I was a bit scared to wake him up, and rightfully so, but I don't think it too polite to be late to a party you are hosting (call me old fashioned that way). He woke up seething, feisty, and refusing to go. Eventually, I managed to soothe him (the promise of presents helped), and off we went. He had a great time but was holding a bit of a grudge. He played nicely with all his friends, loved his cake and food, but scowled and looked away for all the pictures. I find this amusing and think it makes for great stories when looking at the photo albums. He would not talk to a single adult. Oh well. Naturally, I was wondering if I let him down in some way, but as luck would have it, the minute we were back in the car and driving him home, he gushed the whole time about what a great party he had. Whew, chalk that up as a parenting success (we were due).

May 11, 2010

"Balls or Testicles?" An excerpt from *How to Ineffectively Parent in Ten Days or Less*
PG -13, Frank Content (or at least not totally watered down)
Read this at your own peril, especially if you don't have young kids

We've reached that odd, precarious time in Rocco's development where he still needs help washing, wiping, and the like, but he also needs to be doing this more and more on his own (after all, he is "four and three-quarters," just ask him). The problem is how to go about this transition so that all the icky stuff is actually, successfully removed and not left to "fester" or worry Mommy constantly about potential suspicious hygiene. I think you get my drift.

A couple of months ago, when I was struggling with how to take a bit of the battle out of bath time, I decided to make washing their "boy parts" (this did not really elicit any cooperation, let alone enthusiasm) sound a bit a bit more intriguing. After several weeks of rather unsuccessful attempts (including detailed explanations of what all was down there, because Rocco is big on science), clever (or so I thought) euphemisms for what those areas are called (whilst trying to avoid the standard slang), and multiple reasons why it needed to be thoroughly cleaned, I got really desperate and told them, God help me, about their "t'aints."

Now, please realize that I, myself, had never, ever even heard this term until about ten years ago. And at the ripe old age of thirty, I was so bewildered by the reference I had to ask for an explanation. So, I was promptly told, and for those of you who haven't had the (mis?)fortune of hearing this Southern gem, "It's that spot that t'aint your balls and t'aint your ass," Well, desperation sometimes forgoes reason (my mantra). And besides, what the heck else do you call it?

For whatever reason, that term was not memorable to them. Time marched on, and I finally settled on "wiener wash." They had been zealously using the "w" word at that point for a bit, and so it just popped right out of my mouth. It of course, was a hit. And even though we (okay, me) were scrubbing down more than just "wieners," it worked.

Since then, I have been instructing Rocco on how to do his own, "wiener wash," but we've yet to achieve the necessary level of success. But as I mentioned before, transition time is upon us. So, we are still, despite a lack of cooperative participation, working on it.

Well, the thing I didn't really consider was the post-bath towel off. I know how quickly you get cold after getting out of a warm water, so I accommodate by pulling them out of the tub and wrapping them in their hooded character-towels and then again with a regular bath towel. I usually proceed to rapidly rub their bodies and extremities in that up and down manner you do for someone quite chilled. It is an assembly-line job: face Mommy, Mommy rubs sides, turn, Mommy rubs front and back, then on to the next boy.

Then, about a week ago, when I was drying Rocco's sides off and was about to request the turn, he looked me in the eyes (so I knew this was bound to be an important statement) and told me solemnly that he would dry his own balls. Unfortunately, I had the wisdom, or what passed for it at the time, a few weeks prior to address all the remaining slang that I know he had been privy to at school and playdates. I figured it would be like sex ed: address it in the home to avoid some of the questions, mystery, or subsequent naughtiness. It seems that I was not being appropriately delicate (I did mention this was an assembly-line operation) and was no longer "allowed" to do that.

For a brief moment, before I really even acknowledged that perhaps, despite being wrapped in two towels, I should be a little more cautious in certain areas, I had a raging internal debate over whether to correct him on his choice of the word "balls" and instead instruct him to use the word "testicles." And despite running through some rather unsavory scenarios, uttering this loudly at Mass, for example, I went with "balls." So, "balls" it is.

Being the loving, tender mommy that I am, I told him I was sorry and that he was a big boy, was getting more grown up every day, and that he needed to dry off his own "balls" (and his ass and t'aint, for that matter. Okay, I didn't say that last part, but God, was I thinking it). He then dried off said "balls," gave me a little crooked smile, and left the bathroom so I could deal with his brother (who had unfortunately heard this entire exchange).

So that's my story ... per my usual M.O., I am obviously not up for Mommy of the year, but I feel much better for getting that off my chest. Wish me luck, I still have one more to break in (and now probably some agitated grandparents to deal with).

May 14, 2010

It is Friday eve at six o'clock, and I'm sitting at home by myself convalescing from my third chemo in three weeks. I go from feeling fine (in the quiet and dark) to feeling rather icky. And I am a bit sad. Joe is at the school carnival with the boys, and I wish I was with them. I hate missing so much, so often.

But good times are, hopefully, only a few days away. We are going to take our very first family-of-four trip ever! We are beach bound thanks to some very generous friends who have offered their home! And thanks to the universe, which has allowed us to go. My counts are bizarrely up (this is not normal for this time in my treatment), we are all relatively healthy, we have a sitter arranged to help out a bit, and Luca is out of his crib and diapers. We might just hit the road without as much as a glance in the rearview.

Let's hope our luck holds and we have a great, normal family vacation.

May 25, 2010

The beach was ab-fab! It was just what the doctor ordered, pardon the pun. We went stressed and somewhat broken (me, anyway), and we've returned renewed in mind, body, and spirit. The house was perfect, the beach beautiful, and the water a healing, vibrant mix of clear green and blue. We played, contemplated, relaxed, and enjoyed. Life was good and seems a bit sweeter still.

June 2, 2010

Okay, so early last week, I was trying to recover from our fab beach vacation (it seems you always need a vacation after your vacation), and I was actually driving to chemo, feeling like it would be a good place to catch up on some rest (obviously, I was pretty pooped). I had a meeting with Gary beforehand and figured I'd get through that, and then it would be lights out while the drugs dripped in. Well, I didn't get my nap. Gary decided to surprise us with some terrific news: it's time for a chemo break!

Joe and I were a bit stunned to say the least. We started the Gemzar with the intention of most likely doing four to six months of treatment. But when we broached the subject at the previous meeting with Gary (the one right before we left for the beach), he shut down the conversation, which put a wee bit of a damper on the start of my trip. So, we asked all the right questions and even decided to wait on scans (!). All I had to get was my Herceptin, which I will still have every three weeks.

Instead of a long, holiday weekend feeling like crap, I was a normal mommy (okay, not quite, but close), and we were a normal family doing things. It was and is heaven! I am still quite pooped, my red blood counts are still low. Obviously, one does not go from three years of treatment to 100 percent quickly, so I still need my afternoon comatose naps, but I am one happy momma!

We do not know how long the break will last. We are keeping a close eye on things. But in the meantime, it is time to seize the day, suck the marrow out of life, and I hope soon have some margaritas!

Thank you for your support and prayers! They work. Please pray our break lasts a long, long time.

June 14, 2010

*A*side for the need for my daily nap, I've hardly given cancer much of a thought this past week, and it's been mahvelous. We've already been to the pool more in the past two weeks than all of last summer, and the boys have only been out of school for two full days. Now that I am feeling the best I've felt in a long time, I plan to pack a lot of fun in. The kids are actually pooped at bed time, which is yet another chemo break bonus. And Luca said just this morning that the "summah vacation" is awesome. I agree, but it's the break from treatment that makes it incredible.

Oh, and please pray for us tomorrow. We see Gary for a checkup, and I want my summer of fun to continue.

July 6, 2010

*W*ow! Chemo-free time flies by. I'm full of life, roaring forward, full steam ahead. What a change of pace from that oozey, Dali-esque treatment time that has occupied so much of my last three years. Has it really been almost a month since my last blog? We've played at the pool and at home, been to birthday parties and two lakes, did Taekwondo, went grocery shopping, did laundry ... and every last thing has been wonderful to do, experience, and enjoy as a "healthy" person.

I don't want this domestic bliss to end. But we see Gary this Thursday, and I think the time for scans and restarting treatment is probably upon us. The spots on my chest have enjoyed the break too. Keep us in your prayers, if you will, for a favorable report from Gary and good, clean scans. Next week will most likely be stressful as we go through all that again. We've got to keep this stuff confined to my skin if I'm to be in it for the long haul.

Lots of stuff to cram in ....

July 9, 2010

By the time yesterday afternoon rolled around, I was totally dready (I just made that one up: a combo of dread and ready, in case that wasn't obvious) to go see Gary. Naturally, I was running late, stress has a funny way of making me procrastinate. After frantically taking a shower, I took a few deep breaths and tried to calm myself as I dressed. But instead of quiet, an internal melodrama followed (queue the dramatic music). I imagined myself a soldier donning my uniform (in this case, a scoop-neck T-shirt (for port access), fashionably scruffy white shorts, and flip-flops) to once again march into battle, not knowing the strength of the enemy, only that it was out there, waiting for me.

I still feel a bit like that today. You see, we've been following the progress of these new spots on my chest for a few weeks now, and yesterday Gary took one look, a few measurements and photos, and announced that it is time for chemo once again. And since there is no better time that the present, we started yesterday. I'm on Navelbine. I was on that one before, paired with another drug, but it didn't get a fair shake because the other drug caused some lung edema, so we stopped both. It is weekly for three weeks out of the month, but it should be way easier on me than the Gemzar, thank God—Gemzar proved to be one mean bastard. The plan is to do scans in one month. (Gary felt confident the scans would be clean and that the breast cancer is still confined just to my skin.) We'll also check to see how the Navelbine is working, and if it is not doing the trick, then I'll switch back to the Gemzar.

Let's keep our fingers crossed this works, that I feel decent on this treatment, and that something really good is coming our way.

July 23, 2010

*A*fter reviewing photos at Gary's yesterday, we decided the Navelbine is not quite doing the trick and has allowed a slight spread. So, I will be starting up the Gemzar again in two weeks (next week is my week off). I'm trying to get my head around that while I'm cooped up, post-chemo, in this horrific heat. It's proving to be a bit of a challenge.

I want to thank everyone, including Anita's Prayer Warriors, for all the prayers and good vibes! Please keep 'em coming.

July 28, 2010

*T*oday, we had a great day. Rocco announced last night that he was going to run the show. It was his fifth birthday, and he was the man with the plan. We started off with pancakes topped with chocolate sauce and whipped cream, and we ended the day with a Silly String fight. It was perfect, and I am so incredibly thankful I was a part of it. I get a bit emotional around his birthday because it was on his second birthday when I decided to go to the doctor again—despite all assurances to the contrary, I felt like something was very wrong with my breast. August first is my three-year anniversary. Unfortunately, it has not been three years without recurrence but rather three years of a constant fighting. But I am still here, still fighting, and I am very, very grateful for that.

Tomorrow we leave for our second family-of-four vacay. We are off to see friends in Maine, where it should be a thousand or so degrees cooler than it has been here. It'll like stepping into an L.L. Bean catalog: gorgeous, cool and, lobstah everywhere. It should be heavenly.

We return next Tuesday night, and then I have to wake up from my beautiful vacation dream and head to scans first thing Wednesday morning, which will be followed by chemo (the old icky one: Gemzar) on Thursday. Yuck. Please pray my scans look good and that the Gemzar will work on this stuff on my chest.

August 5, 2010

R-Language, good news, but a bit edgy with the adjectives

KA-LEEN SCANS!!! Per Gary, they are perfect (remember, the mets on the skin don't show up). I have lovely bones, and all that! Whew, I was really sweating them because I have a swollen node in my left armpit that was worrying me. My anniversary date definitely compounded my stress.

I was SO not relishing the start of Gemzar again and, huge bonus, I don't have to. I started a new chemo combo today that Gary thinks will be more effective and much better tolerated. I will not suffer from the weekly mind-fuck (sorry, I can't think of a better way to describe it) that I felt within hours of getting the Gemzar infusions. AND I only get it every three weeks. Sweet! The big, obvious drawback (to other people, not me—I don't mind it much) is that I will lose my hair. But as long as Rocco and Luca aren't too bothered by it, I am all good. Bald is beautiful, and of course, I have "a lovely shaped head."

More on our visit with old friends and lobstahs tomorrow. I am already looking at the computer screen sideways due to all the drugs.

Thank you for your earnest prayers and encouragement!

August 9, 2010

I am in the mood to wax poetic, but my brain can't quite seem to flow. It is almost exactly twenty-four hours since I first sat down to start this entry. The chemo and multiple doses of steroids (I need the steroids to keep my body from over-reacting to this new chemo cocktail) all seem to be stifling my ability to relate, which leaves me edgy, tired and, unable to follow a thought to its conclusion. So, readers beware! There is no R-rated language though!

Our trip to Maine was spectacular. It is such a rare, sweet gift to have friendship that neither time nor distance can diminish. It had been three years since we had last seen our friends. Their daughters, whom I somewhat expected in that absentee way not to have grown since our last visit, have made that transition from beautiful girls to lovely young women. But as astonished as I was upon seeing how much they had grown on the outside, it was just as reassuring to see their good, loving natures hadn't changed on the inside.

It was like we didn't skip a beat. What a joy! I have honestly never met another group like them; they are so cohesive, engaging, joyful, loving, and genuine. It's very good stuff, and I am honored that they just welcome us right back into the fold whenever we manage to make the trip. And the joy of coastal Maine in the summer is not to be underestimated. The windows stayed open, fires were had indoors (no, I am not making that up), fleeces and blankets were worn while boating, very thick wetsuits were needed to swim. Brilliant blue skies with wispy clouds topped vibrant conifers that sat atop sun bleached rock that seemed to float just above its darker, water-soaked base. Lobstahs were plucked from the water, lots and lots were eaten—okay, Luca spit his out, but Rocco managed to swallow his. Crabs and urchins were picked from amongst the kelp and held up for kids to see. It is most definitely a slice of heaven on earth. It is a rare combination of natural beauty, quaint architecture (there is no fast-food or even a Starbucks for miles and miles and miles), incredible weather, and a rare gathering of people. Ahh, Maine ... I miss you dearly already.

That's not to say we were totally at ease during our travels. Hitting my third diagnosis anniversary was harder emotionally on me than I thought it would be, and coming home to the immediate stress of scans and the chemo was certainly no picnic either.

We did manage to weather the travel storms well—it was Luca's first airplane trip, after all—and we flew into Boston, which meant a three-hour drive each way. It as a bit of a headache, but it turned out to be a bit tougher on the flight home. We just took advantage of boarding the plane first, and Luca, who had literally just been taken to the bathroom moments before, announced he needed to go again as soon as were seated. So, I popped up and accompanied him to the tiny little lav on the plane, where he had the pleasure of being the first on this leg of the flight to pee everywhere but the toilet. Lovely. Needless to say, I risked dehydration, and we stayed in our seats the rest of the way home.

Okay, Rocco is now up and on my lap, explaining in detail his plans to have a "sailing, pirate boat with 10,000 motors" on it. Better go.

August 12, 2010

I finally came back to life yesterday afternoon. Think of a '50s horror film with Rocco, Luca, and Joe screaming, "It's alive!" and running away from a lurching, crazy eyed, splotchy-skinned zombie momma. Ok, maybe it wasn't quite that bad, but it did pack one hell of a wallop. The chemo kicked my ass, but *major bonus*: it is kicking some cancer ass too. I can actually see the nastiness getting smaller in spots, and I most definitely felt the cell death. Yeah, that's right—cancer cell death. It is the good kind of hurtin'.

After judiciously managing my germ exposure, we went in today for labs and for what was gonna be one of the several-thousand-dollar white-cell boosting shots (Neulasta), but I didn't need it yet! Sweet. I will go in seven days to get rechecked, so I will need to watch out for cooties next week.

August 30, 2010

The Go Jen Go pool party was a blast! It was sweet to be out and partying so soon after chemo. Okay, maybe it was more like me mingling from the horizontal comfort of a pool chaise lounge. I was truly honored and humbled by the day. We had a great turnout, broke in our friend's lovely, newly-renovated pool with style, and raised money for a good cause. Many, many thanks to our co-captains, our party hosts, our coordinator, Chris Pagani, the many businesses who donated so generously, and to all of you who came to support us and participate in the raffle. We also had a number of folks sign up for Komen. Yeah! Together we can make a difference in the lives of many women and cure this disease!

All that excitement did put a little shuffle in my step yesterday though. I pretty much moved from the bed to the sofa and back. But today is better, and I am in the process of perking back up and getting past the icks. I hope to be back to sassy in a few days.

Thank you for helping us beat this,
-Jen

September 3, 2010

I woke up this morning thinking about these words: perspicacity, loquacious, and insouciant. I figured it was definitely time to blog. Waking up with words on my mind is a big improvement over recent mornings. I have been opening my eyes with a start after an all-night-long freak-show dreams that are as intense, densely populated, vibrantly colored, and bizarrely themed as a hallucination. They have been so real and vivid, it would take all morning to shake off their effects. My perspective gets slightly askew, like I'm drunk on their magic in a not all that unpleasant sort of way—with the exception of one night, that is, when I was under the spell of black magic, and was almost afraid to get out of bed to see what I would find, wondering if perhaps my dreams were in fact truth. Because after all, what is reality? Don't worry, I haven't gone around the bend, these "sleeping hallucinations" are clearly a result of the myriad of stuff that drips into my veins for five or six hours every third Thursday.

So, I've officially been "outted" as a person on chemo. My hair, which I shaved rather short about two weeks ago, had, up until a few days ago, still given the impression of a choice of style. I pictured someone thinking, "Hmm, her hair's rather short, but she looks too healthy to be sick, so it's probably just an edgy, pixie cut. I like it; she has a lovely shaped head." Well, it started falling out, and I pictured each individual strand jumping off a sinking ship and someone, somewhere in the background, saying, "Women and children first!" I got tired of it and shaved it with a number-two cut in the front yard yesterday (yes, I am that classy). It looks like I have mange, which, at first, I thought was because of a bad shave job, but then I realized lots and lots of hair is gone. I've taken to wearing a scarf or hat since then.

Yesterday, when I picked up the boys at school, one little charmer asked why I had that "thing on my head" (pink scarf). I told him I was a part-time pirate, and then he asked, "Why are you wearing that?" Well, thank God I had on a cute tie-dyed, ruffled pink skirt and a peasant blouse (you have to make more of an effort when you have no hair) instead of my usual big T-shirt and gym shorts, because I realized right away that it was the kid who had the problem, not me, so I told him they were my pirate clothes. I told him I was a part-time pirate and a full-time mom to Rocco and Luca. Rocco overheard this exchange and seemed pleased with my answers. But this morning, I decided I really didn't feel like wearing a hat at seven o'clock, and he told me I was "more bald" and then stuck his head in the couch and said, "Not again" when I explained it was all going to fall out. So much for the chemo pep talk a couple of weeks ago. I freakin' hate how cancer stresses my boys!

So, I wore my scarf for the first time ever to Harris YMCA this morning. I most definitely felt outted. I got the whole range of looks (empathy, sympathy, dim wittedness). It would make a fascinating sociology or maybe psychology paper to follow around a woman with no hair. But anyway, I popped on my iPod to avoid some inevitable conversation (it worked!), went to the locker room, put on my bikini, and made everyone in the pool feel really bad that the chick with cancer kept passing them. And just because God wanted me to feel a bit better, the pool was packed with triathletes (men and women) and lap swimmers alike. Hah!

In the midst of all this craziness, I would like to welcome Parker Brown Burnette into this world. He is already five weeks old, and he is a perfect expression of life and love. I can't wait to see him again soon.

SEPTEMBER 10, 2010

I started this entry yesterday, before my computer (which is apparently in self-destruct mode) started acting hinky, the internet went out for no apparent reason, the oven decided to not work for the first time ever, and the downstairs TV refused to even power up. What the ... ? If I was a bit less confident, I would think it's somehow all my fault. The boys then had a rough time going to bed. Luca kept creeping out and lurking in the hall everytime I put him down, but he finally fall asleep at 10:30 p.m. (I'm sure he'll be in a lovely mood this evening). Rocco had a night terror at 10:15 p.m., but at least Luca was up watching *Johnny Test*, so he didn't get caught up in that very scary drama. I may have forgotten to mention that Joe is OOT, so he wasn't there to fix all our bad household karma.

But despite the usual challenges, we've been up to our usual tricks here at the Pagani house. Typical boy stuff: Legos, *Johnny Test*, "ripping the cheese" (what Rocco very fondly calls passing gas), *Superhero* puzzles, that kinda thing. And true to their love of icky, gross things, we have already decorated for Halloween. We have skulls, skeletons, giant spiders, bones, and ghosts everywhere. It's awesome, and a very special thing that the boys look forward to doing with Mommy every year. Rocco can remember us doing it for like three years in a row; they must be some of his earliest memories. It is really cool.

Before I prattle on too much, I do have a few humble requests: Please pray my current chemo regimen is working, I'm not sure it is, but we will find out soon. And please sign up for our Go Jen Go team for the Komen Walk/Run on Saturday, October 2. We need your help beating the shit out of breast cancer.

Thanks for all your love and support,
-Jen

P.S. My laptop prevented me from posting this twice when I finally finished. So now, I have a philiosphical question for you all to ponder. If I toss my laptop out of my third-story window onto brick pavers, does it really smash into a million pieces if I don't watch it hit? It might be time to raid the coin jar for an MacBook so I don't resort to violence.

SEPTEMBER 13, 2010

What is hope anyway? A thing with feathers, a tune without words, this ethereal thing that supposedly springs eternal, something that floats? Or is it just a series of wishes, a thousand lies, a multitude of rationalizations that we tell ourselves to make the unknown a little easier to swallow, especially when we are choking down a jagged little pill?

For me, it changes moment by moment, like clouds shifting shapes in the sky. We'll see what tomorrow's visit with Gary brings. I will get biopsy results I don't want, and there are a new host of side effects to figure out and deal with. It's time for Gary to pull another rabbit out of his hat and for me to see if the scales tip toward resignation or summoning hope for a future with my boys and Joe.

SEPTEMBER 14, 2010 3:43 P.M.

Just now home from a full day at the hospital. It was almost an eight-hour affair, so I'm spent. The biopsy, as expected, showed the disease has spread to my back. So, Gary's new rabbit is a chemo cocktail of Carboplatinin and VP-16, which I started today. I'll get it three days in a row every three weeks (and I was bitching to myself yesterday about all the time I already spend at doctor's offices, hah!). We'll pray it works and that I won't feel too bad or have too many icky/serious side effects. We'll see.

I'm not really thrilled about having to go back the next two days, but on the plus side, neither boy has pink eye. They were both checked out by their pediatrician while I was getting infused.

Please pray this stuff works and that my quality of life (and thus my family's) is good to boot. Also, please add my psycho home appliances/TVs to your list, if that is not too petty. It stinks to be home from chemo but not distracted by a bit of quiet TV. I'm not always up to reading.

SEPTEMBER 19, 2010

Where was I? Last week passed in an IV drip, drip, drip blur of chemo pulsing through my veins. Time oozed, and I was in a hazy fog of side effects, both physical and mental. I battled the demons of fear, dread, uncertainty, and indifference every day. I was grumpy, bitchy, incomplete, a stranger in my own skin. Friday finally came, and I was able to begin the process of healing and recovery, both physically and emotionally. I made some serious headway but am most definitely still a work in progress to say the least.

And in the midst of my physical and emotional assault, it seemed the universe (or at least what passes for it from my perch in the den) was conspiring against me as well. Appliances were breaking left and right; the whole house seemed under a black cloud to match my mood. But times they are a changin'. Joe got the den TV working again, a friend came over to see about the one in the basement, and so many of you generously offered your help. Thank you. It always helps to know and feel the love of others when things look kind of bleak. It leaves me in awe and with a smile on my face, and it helps me reconnect with the good, sweet part of life that I sometimes overlook when I'm overwhelmed.

Thank you for sharing our journey, our battle. Please pray this treatment does the job and that in the upcoming week none of the delayed nausea that can happen on Carboplatinum hits. I just want to get back to being me. Thank you, Jen

September 24, 2010 8:18 p.m.

Wow, what a week! I escaped the potential delayed nausea (whew, was holding my breath about that!), the storm striking all our household appliances has passed, and we had a surprise visit last night at dinner time. I opened the door to a crowd of smiling faces singing a cheer song written just for me, complete with pom-poms and Go Jen Go signs. I was totally shocked and a wee bit embarrassed (thank God I got a shower; that's not always a given). It seems Newk's Eatery has teamed up with Komen to honor survivors, and I was this month's lucky gal. Apparently, a few peeps nominated me: thank you, whoever you are! The food was awesome. It seems they were in cahoots with Joe on this, and they brought some super yummy stuff! The grilled portabello sandwich and the four-cheese pizza are not to be missed! And the group of supporters was fantastic!

Among the enthusiastic crowd was my old bud DeAngelo Williams, his wonderful girlfriend, and their beautiful, new baby girl. Sweet! They are super nice, and it was really cool that they hung out for like an hour. He is very obliging with my pic requests too; I had to get a few snaps of us on my couch.

So, things look much better than they did last week. And to top it all off, the temperature is going to drop out of the nineties on Sunday!

Many, many thanks to everyone who has signed up and donated! I can't believe the race is next Saturday.

September 29, 2010

The past few days have been crazy and fun! I just now watched the Go Jen Go interview (we forgot to tape it, and I was on the go yesterday with doctor appointments and boy stuff). It was good. Ann was great, all my boys looked too cute, and I didn't look too bad, (although, I have the most terrible, nasal whine). All in all, it was a pretty neat experience despite my being much more comfortable in front of a keyboard than a camera. And hopefully it encourages more folks to support Komen. It also shed some light on the Go Jen Go Foundation and how we are trying to provide financial assistance and support to local women going through treatment. This is our way of paying back all the incredible support we've gotten and get from all of you.

I saw Gary yesterday, and he thought it looked like the disease hasn't progressed and my skin even looked better in some areas! Whew, thank God. Some days going in for a checkup is like walking the green mile, never knowing until the last second if the governor will call in a pardon or it is off to the gallows. Thankfully, I got my call! I also got a shot for my white counts, which are low (what a perfect time to be susceptible to germs: right before I join a crowd of 15,000). My red counts are just a smidgen too high to get a transfusion. I am dragging, to say the least. Really, I feel like I've been hit by a truck, wiped out. My energy level should rebound a bit before Saturday though. Maybe Luca can hold me while he walks this year, instead of the other way around.

Thank you so, so much for all the incredible, generous support!!! Our Komen team is as strong as ever. I look forward to seeing everyone for the T-shirt Pick-Up Friday evening and then for the race on Sunday. We have a tent in the team village, so look on the website for that spot (unfortunately, it is in the far corner). And hopefully tonight, we will hammer out some of the other details. Thus far, we've been way too tired, by the time we get the boys down at nine o'clock p.m., to even think.

I hope you could follow all of this. Muddled thinking is a side effect of low hemoglobin. I still can't wait for the big day!

October 3, 2010

Wow, what a fabulous race weekend! It was simply incredible, but I'm going to have to wait to tell y'all about. I'm so tired that I can't see straight. Have a great night, and I'll talk to you soon.

Happy and tired,
-Jen

October 4, 2010

I've been crazy tired (as you may have noticed from my entry last night). The weekend was just fabulous. Channel 36 even did a surprise visit and covered a bit of the T-shirt Pick-Up celebration on the evening news.

Britt, you were a very good sport to do the interview; it's too bad you didn't make the cut.

We had a bit of a harried departure from our house Saturday morning (did I mention there was a keg of OMB at the Friday evening bash?), but that was really the only hiccup all weekend. The race and the weather were both picture perfect. It was so fantastic to see and visit with everyone, and I must say, we looked fetching (been on a British author jag of late) in our retro pink and green GJG tees.

I was totally swept up in the pink tide; I was awash with love, support, and power, buoyed by hope and inspired by all those around me. What an extraordinary day!

And to top it all off, Joe and I were both honored at the balloon-release survivor ceremony. We were surprised (especially when the crowd broke out into a spontaneous Go Jen Go chant!) and deeply, deeply touched to receive the first annual Lynn Kennelley IMPACT Award for our "passionate and strong-willed drive to make an IMPACT by supporting and empowering those around us." Lynn was a member of the great team Circle Up, and she lost her fight before last year's race; what a tremendous way to honor her. Wow! I was speechless (not to mention way too shy to speak, although in hindsight, I wish I could have pulled it together), but Joe managed to say a few eloquent words. I am so extraordinarily proud of him, because without Joe, there would be no blog, no team, no T-shirts, no tailgate, no Go Jen Go Foundation (not to mention no Rocco and no Luca!). Thank you, husband. I love you.

And thanks to all of you for supporting Komen and the Go Jen Go Foundation, because without you there, would be no impact.

Better go—Scooby Doo has lost his charm

OCTOBER 18, 2010

*L*abs on Thursday at Gary's confirmed what I already suspected: my lowest hemoglobin evah. I got two units at CMC Main the next morning. I came home to find that our almost fourteen-year-old dog, Seether, was not doing well at all. She'd been on a downhill slide for a while and decision time had arrived. She went to puppy heaven later that evening. It was a difficult thing, but it was best for her and us. I hope she's having fun up there.

Needless to say, I wasn't in the best of moods Friday morning, but I arrived at 9:30 a.m. in the main lobby ready to get my room, to catch up on emails and phone calls, and to nap while getting blood. I spent three-and-a-half hours sitting alone in the main lobby waiting room (this was my fault—I had offers of company, but I thought this would be more of a "spa" day. My pampering standards have clearly fallen since getting diagnosed). I was expectantly waiting to get called, so I was afraid to go to the bathroom, get food, or wander out of eyesight to use my cell phone. My phone was getting a whopping one to two bars of intermittent coverage by the loud fountain. I was unable to send emails because of the hospital's internet. I ended up killing time reliving (not on purpose, of course) the experience at the vet's the night before. Also, watching this wretched state that passes for the human condition filter in and out of the hospital took its toll, too. On a different day (on most days, I would like to think), I might have been more grateful for all my blessings, especially after witnessing all the people who really, truly need help, love, and care. But on Friday, it didn't go that direction.

I won't call it despair, because I have experienced that more than once in its most pure, devastating form. It was more like frustration and futility. Why do so many of my days have to pass like this? Hours and hours of my time are spent waiting to receive or getting treatment that doesn't cure me, that knocks me down day after day, that requires a constant fight and positive attitude. Treatment that so far hasn't cured me, most likely won't ever. Treatment that is buying me time, but how much? Treatment that still allows this freaking monster to march across my chest, back, and into my soul.

It obviously wasn't a good night, and unfortunately, I unleashed (shared might be a better word) my demons on my husband. It is always hard on the other when one of us cracks (or should I say when I crack; he usually holds me up). I hate the toll cancer takes on my family.

I am still not quite right in the head yet. I am still battle-worn and weary, but I am still here, and for that, despite everything, I am very thankful. And the blood did boost my energy to a more acceptable level. I was able to spend the weekend with Joe and the boys doing some normal, fun stuff, the kind of stuff I want to get back to sharing (the boys are both a riot) and hope to soon.

Sorry for being such a drag,
-Jen

October 25, 2010

*M*y babysitter is only available a few more minutes before I must turn this off, so I'll have to make it quick. My whiny, foul mood has finally gone away, and it was the Go Jen Go Foundation that did it. Last week, we received an incredibly uplifting and touching email from one of the women we support about how the donations she recently received from GJG are making a wonderful, positive impact in the lives of her and her daughter. I can't wait to share some of her email (I have her enthusiastic permission) when I have a bit more time. Hopefully, I'll be able to do it from the infusion room this week. And GJG has begun assistance to a family of four in our area. They are post-foreclosure, without insurance, and also battling breast cancer. They are extremely thankful, and so am I! Together we are making a difference, and damn it feels good!

We ended up having a great weekend. It was picture perfect, and I can't wait for more! Please say a prayer or two for a good appointment with Gary tomorrow.

October 29, 2010

I've got a wee bit of a hangover today, just not the kind you should have after your birthday. But chemo is ovah, and now I can focus on Halloween weekend with my vampire and my Frankenstein/Spiderman/JetRay. Luca, true to form, is currently in costume-change mode, and I expect he will continue to be up until we walk out the door to trick-or-treat. He does, after all, change clothes multiple times on any given day. I'm hoping and planning on feeling good enough to enjoy the festivities and the weather, which is finally going to be seasonally appropriate.

It will be a great weekend, full of life and fun, to keep my focus off of Monday morning, which is when I get rescanned. Gary and I both suspect the disease is currently spreading a bit, and he wants to make sure it is still confined to the skin. The visible diseased area is now roughly the size of one-and-a-half car license plates, which is distressingly big to me. So, I'll report to Mercy bright and early Monday morning, kill a few fun hours in the waiting room, and then try to keep my head on straight until we see Gary for scan results and another look to determine if this week's treatment had any visible effect on the skin. My guess is that we will be switching treatment yet again. I'm trying not to go down the path of "what ifs," but occasionally I lapse and find myself treading down that rocky lane.

I'd Better go, my post-chemo brain is at it's limit. Please say some prayers for clean scans, an effective, livable treatment (that is available to me NOW) and for others fighting too. Oh, and if it is not too much to ask, that UGA beats the Gators this weekend (now that Tebow is gone).

Thanks,
-Jen

November 2, 2010

We spent the weekend running from one activity to the next. Rocco received his yellow belt Saturday morning, and then we went to Trunk or Treat at Taekwondo later that night. It was a huge push for me that soon after chemo (I can officially say I am in a dark mood the Thursday, Friday, and Saturday of treatment week), both Joe and I were stressed, and the kids were seriously pushing our buttons. Luca, my very fussy dresser, adamantly refused at the eleventh hour to dress in the Frankenstein costume he had been talking about for the past six weeks, and we forgot to bring Rocco's fangs and black lipstick for his vampire costume.

It was not the Hollywood version of the Halloween I was determined to have, but the kids got lots of candy, and I got to go in a haunted house—I love being scared, but I'm not sure how my unsteady ticker was going to take a jolt that soon after treatment. We waited in line for the haunted house (we had secured a place in front, and there were several hundred people behind us) just long enough for both boys to chicken out, but I knew Rocco would regret not going in, so I convinced him to join me. My line of reasoning was that it was going to be "kid scary," not "adult scary," because it was, after all, hosted by a dojo that taught mainly small kids, and the families in front of us had gone in with some toddlers (who are most likely in for a lifetime of therapy). Well, it was totally "adult scary," *Texas Chainsaw Massacre* type stuff. There's nothing like a madman chasing you down with a power tool to make you forget about the possibility of dying from cancer sometime in the future. It boosted my mood, though I was a bit worried about PTSD when neither boy said one word the entire ride home.

Halloween night was much more fun. We went to a friend's house for the festivities, and it was great. Luca went as Spiderman—he actually refused to put any costume on at our house, but I packed several, assuming he would change his mind when we saw the other kids. He did. And this time, we remembered all of Rocco's vampire accouterments. Rocco was quite keen on applying his own black lipstick, which turned out to be great because we could see him clearly, even in the twilight, from about 100 yards away, as he applied it rather liberally. It was a late night followed by an early morning, but it was all worth it.

CLEAN SCANS! Wahoo! Gary's got it down to a science; he blurts it out without preamble the second he walks in. It is perfect. That way I don't have to read into the hello and small talk, teetering on the edge of the abyss, as I wait for the verdict. He also thought my skin showed some improvement, which I swear I did not notice until last night, so we are staying the course with this chemo. Sweet! I am ecstatic but wiped out. I've got a week of chemo, a really busy weekend (even for fully functioning mommies), and what seemed like an eternity of waiting for scans and today's results to recover from. Whew! Thanks to the Big Man and to everyone else who is rooting so hard for us.

November 11, 2010

It has been life, full steam ahead, ever since we got the scan results. We've been busy doing fun boy stuff (poking things with sticks, riding scooters, playing "follow the leader," and terrorizing the dog). Just plain, old fashioned-type fun. It has been a true gift from God, and I am thankful for every second of it!

In the midst of enjoying and savoring my life, I've had the privilege to devote some more time to The Go Jen Go Foundation. We are currently providing monthly assistance to two families who, in addition to dealing with numerous financial and personal challenges, are bravely battling breast cancer. And, we've also been able to provide one-time financial help to a few other breast cancer warriors in need.

To be able to do this is such an incredible, extraordinary feeling! It makes my heart smile and my soul dance. It is life the way God intended: reaching out to your fellow man with compassion and love.

November 17, 2010

I woke up, after a night of very fitful sleep, reeling like a drunk and kind of staggering around the house. I haven't improved much since then. I tried to turn on the TV with my phone and had to check the microwave to see if I accidentally nuked my iPad. Thank God I did not. I'm currently writing by looking at the screen sideways and taking frequent breaks. I had the second lowest hemoglobin ever in my years of treatment, and by far the lowest ever on a treatment day. So, I will go directly from chemo tomorrow to get a couple of units of blood. Let's pray my body can take the two treatments before then.

Enough about me. A big thank you, THANK YOU to all of you who so generously donated to Go Jen Go last week!!

November 19, 2010

I'm a couple of eggs short of a dozen right now. I got chemo Tuesday with my lowest hemoglobin evah. I was glad they did not withhold treatment. My counts continued to drop Wednesday, followed by a long, ill feeling, horrible dream-infested night of tossing and turning. Oh, and plenty of nausea, a pounding headache, and some major muscle weakness. We left at 7:30 a.m. Thursday for a chemo I was wondering if I was strong enough to take. But my counts were even lower, and the infusion RNs commented on how bad I looked. I was picked up by Gammy and hustled over to Blumenthal Cancer center, where I considered asking for a wheelchair ride up to the office.

Hours passed as I slept and blankly stared …. Then the blood started, and a friend brought me lunch. The food and blood started to work. Another friend stopped by too. It was nice, so distracting and uplifting, even though I am far from good or coherent company. I was home by 6:30 p.m. I'm better today; I showered and then walked a bit in the front yard, but now I'm pooped and spent again. I'm shakey, stupid, zoning in and out. I'm hoping to get it together so the boys won't notice too much.

Hoping I feel stronger as each day passes,
-Jen

November 27, 2010

Well, a week and a coupla units of blood make a heck of a difference. We've had a great holiday, got to love the low-key time with the fam. We decided to fly by the seats of our pants, something the four of us rarely get to do, and it's been wundaful! We've had no particular plan, and its turned out to be perfect. We had some major good times running around on the tree lot, playing "git chu," and picked out the perfect tree and even got it decorated. The boys and their mama LOVE to decorate together for the holidays, and this year they both totally get it and are really into it. "Not the mama" (Joe) has been crazy busy working on a total reno of the boys' bathroom. Why, you ask? Because we are apparently used to chaos, because, yes, he is that capable (nuthin, better than a man who can bring home the bacon AND knows his way around a tool box), and cuz there really is no better time than the present. The boys and NTM (Joe, in case you're drinkin' and couldn't figure that out on your own) will do the outside lights sometime soon.

We also managed our first fire of the season, complete with show (Pagani production) and refreshments (burned but tasty) marshmallows. And Luca and I went even went shopping on Black Friday. Kudos to the ad folks at Macy's and Kohl's who manged to brainwash me—in the midst of a chemo regimen that is kicking my ass and in the recent mindset of doing less buying and more giving for the holidays—into dragging along a three-year-old to the point where nothing was going to stand in the way of me and the Early Bird Specials. We saved some big bucks ('course, you gotta spend 'em to save 'em) I reveled in the crazy consumerism happily for a little bit, and Luca got treated (bribed) to lots of sweets. He was perfect, much better than Joe woulda been had he come along, and I loved the time with just the two of us. The only hiccup in my plan was not knowing where to hide Joe's gift when I got home. Where to put it so that he wouldn't stumble upon it, especially since he seems to be in every nook and cranny in the house now that he is playing contractor? A-ha! Got to put it inside the dishwasher (too big) or in the laundry room. Got it stashed. And if the past fifteen years are any indication, there's not a snowball's chance in hell he'll see it before Christmas.

While we've had a mah-velous few days, there are still plenty who need your prayers. Please pray for the family of K. Higgs, who was killed in a car accident this past week, and the family of our friend Omondi, whose brother died suddenly. Also, please pray my brain scan Monday goes without hitch and that my skin check up with Gary goes well on Tuesday, 'cause I am concerned my skin looks worse. Thanks! Jen

November 30, 2010 12:03 p.m.

Brain scan is clean! Echo good. Overall, a positive vibe from the appointment! My skin seems a bit more nodular to Gary too, so we are going to recheck it next in a week ('cause it changes in color and texture as often as the clouds shift in the sky). If it seems the same, we are going to most likely change up my chemo regimen. And most likely I will get a break from treatment next week 'cuz my bone marrow has had it with these drugs. I feel good about this news, that he is in agreement with me about the changes (reassuring to know I am not imagining it) and that he considers a slow spread unacceptable (i.e., we can still fight it). Nice to know. He also wants to see if Dr. Fraser thinks maybe radiation is an option again to kick the stuff in the skin, since that seems to be where the cancer is staying (thank God!). Thanks for your prayers! Off to nap; the stress and the holiday fun have wiped me out.

-J

December 4, 2010 5:39 p.m.

It's only the first week of December and we've already had a Christmas miracle! Last night while figuring out what to wear for the Mountain Khakis Holiday party, I managed to squeeze into a size 6 pants. Obviously, all my years of triathlon and strength training gave me the courage and mental toughness to stay the course and get 'em all the way zipped, no easy feat for my 161.4 lbs. (sometimes the weigh-in at Gary's is worse than the chemo). In the end, though, I went with another pair of pants so I could sit in the car on the ride over and actually breathe at the party. I even had fun, despite being tired and my normal reluctancy to ever leave my house after dinner (even, or maybe especially, for social occasions). And they had cupcakes!

Thank you for your support, prayers, and for making The Go Jen Go Foundation a reality. GJG just purchased requested items to help make a woman undergoing treatment, and her family, have a more joyous Christmas.

-Jen

DECEMBER 8, 2010 10:37 A.M.

*T*hank you for all the thoughts and prayers, and so sorry I haven't responded till now. Monday was extraordinarily tough. We met with Bob and confirmed what I expected: radiation not really an option. Basically, there's no way to stop the spread of the breast cancer in my skin by treating it locally with radiation as opposed to systemically with chemo. Didn't really want to hear I'll be on chemo the rest of my days. It sucks, to put it mildly. But Bob did mention the possibility of trying the hyperthermic radiation combo that's only available at Duke. I had completely forgotten we checked into this before (if I recall, I was not a good candidate then because the risks out-weighed the progression last time), and I think it might be an option now, only because the heat allows for the delivery of less radiation and the disease in the skin has grown so much since we were there last. Apparently, the big risks are permanent, non-healing skin ulcers and rib fractures. Super. The implications (no more swimming, no more wrestling with the boys, no Taekwondo, no snowmobiling ... the list seemed endless— just more stuff to add to what breast cancer has already taken away) of dealing with these two game-changing side effects, combined with more chemo, pushed me over the edge. I broke down a few times. Then I settled on numb. The only really good take-aways from the appointment were:

1. The disease is defying all odds and continuing to stay out of my vital organs,
2. I seem to tolerate treatments better than most and,
3. I don't have to rush off to Duke right now to start (assuming they think I am even a candidate, so I won't miss Christmas, which was gonna be a deal breaker for me—got to draw the line somewhere).

Tuesday we saw Gary. He'd been briefed by Bob and was totally on board with starting a new chemo regimen now. The new drugs he's chosen are taken orally, which is nice. The downsides are diarrhea (sorry for the TMI), the usual fatigue, zits, and other stuff. The upsides are no hair loss and that it's much better on my bone marrow. Somehow, as a visit with Gary often goes, we left there ready to start the new drugs, ready to see Duke in January, and with hope in our hearts that this treatment combo might actually kill it all. He doesn't fill you with false hope, just the facts and a never ending sense of optimism, and a great, goofy sense of humor. Maybe he is angel and not just a man. Whatever he is I am so thankful he is in my life.

-Jen

December 14, 2010 4:58 p.m.

I've only got a few minutes, so I'll make this quickish. Physically, it was great to get a few days off of treatment last week. Mentally, it was a bit tough because I can see the spread. But we had a big weekend—Mommy and Daddy got to go out Friday night with some friends (even managed a few margaritas!), I had lots of fun play with the boys during the day Saturday while Joe worked on the bathroom, and there was a visit with the neighborhood Santa and then Juju's party.

On Sunday, the boys and I "made" (from a kit I foolishly bought at Michaels—which did actually require some frosting assembly and delayed the actual decorating for hours while the sugary stuff dried and the boys waited impatiently) our annual gingerbread house. I let them eat lots of the decorations, and we also whipped out some of our own. When we couldn't cram one more carb on that thing, I deemed we were done. Naturally, it was the "best house evah"! Due to the construction delays (the kit, not Joe—he is right on schedule for a spring-ish completion), the boys ate tons of sugar right before dinner-time, then refused to eat a proper meal (no big surprise) and ran around like crazed maniacs, followed by some abundant, rather poor behavior despite multiple threats of bad reports to Santa. I was totally pooped. It was a great family weekend.

It is such a treat this year to see how excited the boys are about all things Christmas, Rocco especially. He's fascinated with our Elf on the Shelf (appropriately named Watcher). Every morning, he runs out of bed and looks to see where he landed after flying back from his nightly trip to give Santa the lowdown. He even tells him about the good things he's done and occasionally reports Luca's transgressions to him too. Luca loves looking for him too in the mornings, but other than that is not too impressed.

After days of impatiently waiting, two mornings of phone calls and a trip to a specialty pharmacy, I finally have my new chemo drugs. I started last night, and so far the side effects are tolerable (not much chemo in the system yet) and will hopefully stay this way. I must admit, after such worry about not being treated, I had a few teary moments last night before starting back. Sometimes it is hard to swallow (pardon the pun) that my life is a constant battle and most likely will be till the end of days (the end of my days, that is).

I am off to the Well of Mercy to get my mind and spirit cleansed and to gear up for whatever comes up next.

Thank you to everyone who continues to support us through prayer, meals, playmates .... And also a big thanks to all of you who have donated to The Go Jen Go Foundation.

Thanks,
-Jen

December 27, 2010 3:09 p.m.

It has been so long since my last blog, I am goin' to work my way from the present back in time. Christmas was fabulous! The boys were thrilled and overwhelmed. Santa did not disappoint, Mommy and Daddy are very pleased and happy. I absolutely can't believe it snowed and stuck— what an incredible treat! We've had gobs of great family time, we were able to celebrate with all the grandparents, aunts and uncles, and cousins in town. The day before Christmas Eve, I saw Gary and was Thrilled with a good report. We both agree the disease in my skin looks less vigorous with just one week of the double doses weeks behind me! Thank you, God! The boys and I were even able to squeeze in a few pre-Christmas few days with Gammy and Papa at their house and up in Blowing Rock. We hit the trifecta there—sledding, snowball fighting, and snowman making. It was blissful, a very special time, and the icing on the cake was I did quite well even though it was my heavy chemo week (take oral Tykerb every day, then seven days off / seven days on of Xeloda).

Sweet! Prior to our mountain trip, the boys had their annual Christmas Program at Christ Lutheran. It was precious, and true to their promises, both boys actually sang this year (last year they both had the deer-in-the-headlight thing going on). Luca was in full Santa gear, including beard, and Rocco was a very enthusiastic "golden ring." I drove straight from the Well of Mercy, where I had spent two days trying to get my head around more chemo, the upcoming trip to Duke (this Monday the 3rd), and it's potential impact on my life. I went there with a heart full of fear, grief, and resignation. I returned with a heart open to possibility, full of joy, light, and hope. I can't find the words to express my love for the people there and the for place itself. Amazing ... a gift from God.

That's the past two weeks in my life, from despair to joy and celebration, from resignation to new healing and hope. Thanks to all of you who continue to support us in so many ways, who support Go Jen Go, and also the Well of Mercy, you make my life better.

-Jen

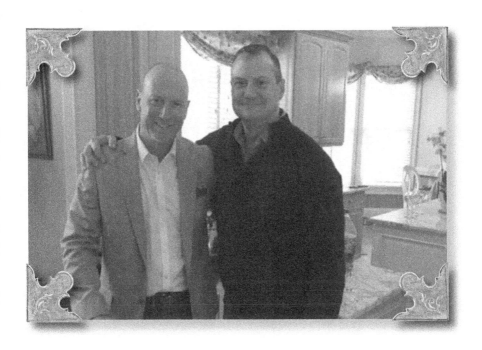

2 0 1 1

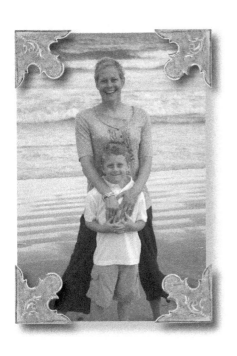
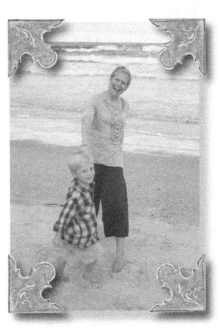

January 4, 2011 9:50 a.m.

Happy New Year! We hit the ground running as usual here at our house. Joe was sick for about a week and was on the mend (thank God, he is a rather unpleasant sick person, unlike me, I am always a joy to be around) enough for our trip to Duke yesterday. It turned out to be a marathon day, which we did not really expect. The short version: we will start the hyperthermia/radiation/Xeloda therapy THIS Thursday. I will get treated every weekday, in Durham for a total of three weeks. I will come home on the weekends.

They are estimating with this trimodality therapy that I have a fifty-fifty shot at a "durable cure," one which can last years. Dr. V (full name way too complicated for English speakers) was a bit apologetic for these odds when he watching my reaction. But I am quite excited at this news! We have a fair shot at kicking some cancer ass for the long haul. Wonderful! He also estimates the odds at having non-healing skin problems at 10 to 15 percent, normally it is around 1 to 2 percent, but my post PDT skin is a bit more delicate.

So, I am scrambling to find lodging, confirm pre-authorization by my insurance, organize childcare/playmates, find someone to basically adopt Sophie for the next few weeks (weekdays only), coordinate rides to and from Durham at the beginning at end of each week (most likely won't be able to do that on my own-but still need a car while up there), and a whole host of other stuff. Fun.

Please say some major prayers that this KILLS the cancer for the long haul, that my skin stays intact so I can still swim, for me and for the boys, and that it all goes exceedingly well! Thanks! Got to run (not literally—I am covered in stickers and marker that the docs use to outline radiation treatment fields, and sweating is a no-no 'till after Thursday).

-J

JANUARY 8, 2011 11:59 A.M.

Whew, a bit more craziness than usual. Just back from Durham late yesterday (thank you, Neel), and heading back tomorrow after nap. I managed to get a room at the Caring House there, which is basically ideal—all cancer peeps, quiet, no check in/out, shuttle, right off campus ... but big thanks to so many of you who offered accommodations!

Going from explanation (on Monday) to application (Thursday and Friday) was intense.

JANUARY 10, 2011 5:35 P.M.

Fried, frazzled, seriously fatigued, discombobulated; that about sums up my past couple of days. I think the past three and a half years is seriously trying to catch up. I drove up here in somewhat of a haze, went up 77 'till exit 25, realized my mistake and then had to make my way over to 85. The rest of the trip went without incident. I got checked in, unloaded, food labeled and put away, but couldn't quite settle down. A long restless night followed. I couldn't get outta bed, rushed to my appointments in a haze. I did manage to prepare for hyperthermia, though; I wore shorts and flip-flops. Dr. V (manages hyperthermia) popped in, gave me a look-see, and seemed pleased. I hustled on to radiation and was told that Dr. Blietzblau (manges my radiation, specializes in breasts) would see me today.

At this point, I am in a complete fog, nearly weepy, exhausted, hungry and desperately in need of caffeine and some water. I met Dr. B's RN (can't quite think of her name at the moment). She is wonderful, caring, intelligent, and compassionate. She also has a lovely Irish accent. She and Dr. B spent lots of time with me—answering my questions, addressing my fears/concerns and worries over my current anxious/uber fatigued state (basically, it is not just me, this is what happens when you get chemo, radiation and heat all at the same time—it is aggressive, but they wouldn't do it if there wasn't a decent chance of success). I felt validated and just better when I left. I then stumbled back to Caring House, ate a quick bowl of soup, and fell into bed.

Woke up at 4 a.m. (obviously, I set the alarm), went out to get supplies (apparently, I cannot navigate worth a damn in my current state), took an accidental tour of this side of Durham. But the Big Man was looking out for me; there is a Super Target with a Starbucks about a mile (turns out) from where I am staying. Sweet.

So, a bit of caffeine and some food later, and I am feeling better (a bit more like me), like I CAN DO THIS. Like I can still mentally, physically, and emotionally take this triple beating, despite the beating I've already taken.

All the while, I've been OOT; my email and celly aren't working too well (I will hopefully address that, with help, tomorrow).

Please also say some extra prayers for me. This is tough. I need to get rested while I'm here, despite the treatment effects. I need to be back in that place where I think, "They (the cancer cells) Can't Stop Me."

Thanks,
-Jen

PS. Just now starting to snow here!

JANUARY 18, 2011 7:32 P.M.

Of late, I have so much to say, so many stories to tell (like the most recent exploits of my two monkeys, what it's like to get microwaved, and a bit about some of the characters here at the Caring House); and I find myself so far behind when I actually do feel like blogging, that I feel like my entries are a bit lacking in charm and are reading more; like a rather dry narrative. Sorry 'bout that ….

The weekend flew. Fantastic seeing my three boys! I alternated between fun Mommy (trying to cram a lot in and on the verge of exhaustion) and very cranky cancer patient (poor husband, he got to see Jenny Rotten). This weekend, Gammy and Papa are bringing the boys here to see me, less travel should help keep the exhaustion factor to a minimum.

Treatment continues … I continue to slog forward. Had a good checkup with Dr. B today following my therapies. She is pleased with the skin reaction so far, which is tremendous news. Still way to early to know how things will turn out, it's a kinda wait and see how things develop over time type deal, but it's looking good at this point in the game. And she gave a huge thumbs up on my continuing to work out, saying absolutely to stay the course. One more doc to add to the pile of MDs of who determine my continued ability to run, walk, bike, lift and/or swim (I am praying these will be an option again sometime in the future). Despite all the treatments, my athleticism is a big reason why I am still here.

Sometimes though, like this afternoon, when I am so tired and just feel like sitting on my hiney, it is unbelievably tough to get up and move. But I did, I do, and I will. I figure when I am moving the cancer can't catch me. I get up for my husband, my kids, and myself. I get up because it clears my mind (although briefly), brightens my soul (it is when I am closest to God), and strengthens my body. When it's hard to lift my legs; when my lungs burn because of damage they suffered (and continue to suffer during radiation); when my skin is so irritated and sore I just want to rip my shirt off; when my skin breaks open and bleeds in the weirdest spots from all the chemo; when my pec keeps cramping because of the scar tissue; when I know I am gonna want another nap even though I just got up from one—I still keep going, with a knowing little smile on my face, because in these moments, I am truly alive and truly free.

Thanks for all you do for me. Without your hope and prayers I would not be able to do any of this.

-Jen

JANUARY 25, 2011 8:52 P.M.

Whew, still recovering from all the weekend fun. I miss the boys so much it hurts. I spoiled them rotten with all kinds of sugary food, "Duke Devils" (what Luca calls 'em) gear, and a toy or two. We spent lots of time just hanging out, playing "hot and cold," running around a bit (after making sure we weren't bothering any of the weekend guests), and snuggling here in the great room of the Caring House. It was bliss. It was so damn hard to watch them go ... Sunday night was tough. I was sad, tired, and worried about my upcoming eval with Docs B and Z. I could not get outta bed (unfortunately becoming a real problem of late) yesterday, so naturally, I was running late, but the checkup turned out great. Both docs were surprised and very pleased with how my skin is handling the radiation, AND it looks like it is making quite a dent in the disease. Sweet! So the decision was made to continue on, give me the full dose of radiation (shoot for 40 gray (Gy) instead of stopping at 26, for those of you that speak medical physics), despite the fact that the extent of my radiation reaction is still unknown (there is a lag time of three or four weeks from the start of treatment and skin effects). But I am so excited to be able to press on. It means they still see the potential for a "durable effect." It means we still have reason for hope! Thank God!!

JANUARY 26, 2011 7:10 P.M.

Thanks for the outpouring of love, prayer, and concern. Every bit of it helped and continues to do so. This evening I am in a much better place. And tomorrow I get to see Husband! It has been eleven days since I saw him last, the longest we've been apart during fifteen years of marriage.

God bless,
-Jen

JANUARY 31, 2011 8:22 P.M.

Jubilant! Joyful! Just down-right happy! It was amazing to see and be with Joe, here, after such a long absence. His tender embrace made me feel whole again and rekindled the light I was losing sight of. And it was so good to have him accompany me to treatment and my appointment. It eased my burden in a way I didn't quite know I needed.

The weekend at home was perfection. I was pampered and quite spoiled. I obviously deserve it (made myself chuckle with that one). It was restful (the effects of this treatment are getting more and more noticeable—I practically need a spatula to pry my ass off the recliner in my room at Caring House these days), fun, and just really what I needed. Laughing with the boys, holding hands with my husband and getting some sweet kisses from Sophie made my spirit soar! My dear friend Britt drove me back yesterday. We had a grand time catching up and even went out for a great meal at a Turkish restaurant (awesome food and oodles of cool atmosphere) in Chapel Hill. We really needed the quality girl-time. It felt right; it felt "normal."

We did have a bit of an issue to contend with when we arrived back at the CH, my SUV was the victim of a smash and grab, as was another car in the lot (and according to the police, lots of others cars around Durham this past Friday and Saturday), over the weekend. You following all this? Cuz I am painfully aware that the combination of my crazy train of thought (stream of consciousness, if I wanted to sound smaht) and poor grammar is hard for even me to follow (I fancy myself a bush league Philip Roth). Initially, I was a bit ticked (I mean, who steals from cancer patients?) and quite worried it would be a massive headache to get replaced and yet another thing to add to our rather long list of "Things That Need Taking Care Of." But the new window was replaced this afternoon, it works, and it was a "Stuff" problem, not a "Health" one, so water under the bridge. The bandits did, however, make off with my canvas Duke Radiation Oncology tote bag (a patient perk) and a treasured, vintage (glamming it up a bit—but they were twenty years old!) pair of gym shorts (wore them to hyperthermia every day because it is a seventy-minute sweat-fest). So I figure the perps are pissed with their booty (instant karma), that I am extremely lucky nothing of value was in the bag (except sentimental value, that is), and that the cops in Durham must have promptly issued a BOLO (Be On the Lookout, for those of you who haven't watched fifteen seasons of *Law and Order*) for suspicious characters of obvious poor moral character, clothed in hospital gowns, and wearing mesh Vanderbilt gym shorts.

Have good night,
-Jen

P.S. The docs still very pleased with my skin, AND I get to go home Thursday!!!

February 2, 2011 8:28 p.m.

Today was graduation day! Wahoo! Mixed feelings a bit. Can't wait to be home, but at the same time, this treatment option is ticked off the list. Hopin' and praying the docs remain pleased for a long, long time. On my way home tomorrow!

-J

February 8, 2011 7:11 p.m.

Soooo good to finally be home! Ahhh, my little slice of heaven. Snuggling, cuddling and loving on, and playing with my three Pagani boys is what makes my heart sing. But I did hit the ground running (though my body is starting to scream for some serious lie around and rest/recuperate time, the cumulative treatment effects are really kicking my hiney at the moment). Luca has been on and off with a fever since last Wednesday (though he is now finally well and acting happy and silly) and home from school since then (which has been both wonderful and exhausting). I kept Rocco home Friday too—not because he was sick—but because his tears that morning really pulled at my heart strings (got to spoil 'em some, especially in our situation).

I've had an on-and-off fever, aches (all over—joints/ muscles ... but I think it is a combo of the cooties and the major strain of three types of concurrent cancer treatment), and a horrific amount of green goo in my sinuses (finally started an antibiotic yesterday). I need some cheese with my whine. Gammy has confirmed flu and pneumonia. Juju has been suffering from sinus stuff, too. Thus far, Joe (I think he paid his dues last month) and Rocco remain well. Fingers crossed, God willing, no surprises—tomorrow I'll drop 'em both off at school and peel outta the parking lot. :)

-Jen

February 13, 2011 7:10 p.m.

My mood is all over the place today. Not looking forward to a return trip to Duke for a follow-up appointment tomorrow, as it seems too soon to know much of anything. I suspect for the most part, I'm good, but a few spots are concerning, and unfortunately, I always seem to know .... Right now, it's a mind game every time I look in the mirror, because the treatment side effects are basically the same as disease progression symptoms. Super. And I am crazy, bone-tired but I don't look it, which almost makes it worse. There are plenty of positives in my life to focus on, but sometimes it's just tough to do.

-J

February 15, 2011

Well, yesterday at Duke went better than I had expected! I was beaucoup stressed about some areas on the upper part of my chest and under my collarbone, and I was increasingly preoccupied with the whole, "Is it the disease or the treatment?" question. After a very nice reunion with some of my Duke peeps, I went through my list of concerns/questions with my nurse and doctors and a sat through a very thorough examination. The verdict is in. Duke feels that my chest looks great! All things considered (after all, they basically burned the crap out of me), I'm most likely just experiencing some major treatment effects which, due to a variety of reasons, are peaking now and will stay like this for a bit. I should still expect more blistering, oozing, and itching, but the fatigue should now be at its highest level—thank God, because I am like an 8.5/10 on that scale. Of course, the whole "worried about life and death" thing is rather stressful, but my current level of tiredness is not really acceptable as a mom. I still wasn't quite getting why I am as wiped out as I am and was very worried my body just wasn't recovering anymore. One of the doctors got it and managed to dumb things down a bit for me (I'm not the sharpest knife in the drawer when highly stressed and missing my nap). She told me to remember that this trimodal approach works synergistically, and the (bad) side effects are synergistic too (why this never occurred to me, I honestly don't know). She said, "Rest, rest, rest, eat well, and get your hind quarters back on the couch." She told me not to spend my energy on anything other than healing or playing with the kids and to, "concentrate on the doing with, rather the doing for." Sage advice. So basically, I am under doctor's orders not to do any housework of any kind! I knew there had to be an upside to this whole cancer deal. It's almost worth it ....

As far as my skin goes, they think it'll probably heal (yes!), that it will most likely take months of waiting and watching to know the extent of the healing, and even longer to know whether or not the treatment had the durable effect we are shooting for. To "wait and see" is a tough game for me to play, but I'm working on it. I also found out that if these areas are actually disease progression rather than treatment side effects, "it would be very bad," especially given that I have just finished this most aggressive therapy. I will continue to storm the heavens on this one.

All in all, it was a very good report and a great day with my dad, despite the destination. I'm still not out of the woods yet, but I think I'm sitting in a very pretty spot. Thank you for all your prayers, love, and help.

February 23, 2011

PG: some gross burn details

*A*hhh, this was a weekend made in heaven. We had perfect weather, and I had plenty of help at home, which meant lots of good rest and thus, good, energetic time spent with my boys and Joe. We romped, swung, scooted, tickled, and laughed. We even made it to Mass, dinner, and then out for yogurt. It was domestic bliss! It was what I dream of nightly, what we lack frequently, and what I pray for all the time. God willing, we will be blessed with many, many more such weekends. We managed all this despite the fact that I am still on my pre-treatment chemo regimen and my skin is looking and feeling noticeably worse daily. The treatment effects (and hopefully not the cancer—still in "wait and see" mode on that) continue to increase. Almost the entire treatment area is an angry red or a burned, crispy brown in some spots, and it has gotten tons more sensitive. I apply Aquaphor three times daily—it rubs off pieces of skin and then leaves my shirt sticking to my chest, which is rather icky, but I have found the alternative intolerable. This process leaves me frequently shaky and nauseated afterward because of the pain. I was prepared for these side effects and have over the years found I have a high tolerance for physical discomfort, but it is cramping my style (literally).

My wardrobe is limited to oversized T-shirts, which have greasy stains all over them and bits of skin stuck to the inside of them (gross), but I cover them up with a long-sleeved shirt. My bra with my chicken cutlet (i.e., fake boob) is out of the question, and quite frankly, I wouldn't be surprised if that is a permanent deal given the fragility and sensitivity of my skin. This bit is frustrating and caused me some stress about going to Mass, since I don't currently go anywhere else that I need to look nice for. And I do long for the days when I wore tight, frequently scanty tops that showed off my upper body. I thought maybe I could hide my situation in one of those fitted, women's oxfords with front pockets that are so popular right now, but after trying on a few, I realized I couldn't have looked more like a lesbian if I tried; it's not that there is anything wrong with that, but it's definitely not the look I'm going for. So for now, I'll just have to make-do with looking like one of those disheveled, train-wreck looking people on *What Not to Wear.*

Oh well, you can't have your cake and eat it too. I can deal with some wardrobe disappointments as long as I get many, many years to get over it.

February 27, 2011

It's been a great week. We've played and romped. I've seen a few friends, and I managed a little shopping and a trip to the farmers market. Ahh, it is so good to be out amongst the living. I've decided, no matter how this whole cancer deal pans out, I'm going to try to seize the day whenever I can. It's not as easy as it sounds (to live the life you've imagined) when one must constantly battle fatigue and is not feeling well daily. But it can be done, even for just bits at a time, and that is my current focus (along with the healing, of course). It has taken me a few weeks to arrive here mentally and emotionally, but here I am, and there is no better time than the present. My mission, and I have already chosen to accept it, is to find some JOY, have some FUN, and do it NOW!

All that being said, a battle is still being waged on my chest. My skin has gone from bad to worse, but it seems to be treatment related, which means that the cancer is dying, and judging by the size and amount of destruction, there was A LOT of cancer—like whole big areas of my chest, underarm, and flank. We seem to be past most of the oozing, and now it is mainly very angry red, purple, and brown, blistered, sloughing off in spots, open in others, and sensitive enough to make me nauseated and very shaky for hours (after coating it in lotion) or from just general moving around throughout the day. I told Joe last night that I now know I am truly one tough cookie— this shit ain't for the faint of heart—and that most people would never have any idea of what is going on with me, even at my worst.

I must admit it has taken me a few days this week to put it together that the nausea, shakiness, and at times extreme fatigue, are burn related and not related to my current chemo. Duke confirmed this by calling me Thursday afternoon. It was unexpected, so it concerned me a bit at first, but they told me that they reviewed the pictures we sent (Joe sends weekly photos of the treatment area). The doctors review them together in HD and from multiple angles. Well, I got a little lecture about not calling them and had to answer a lot of questions about the pain and the treated area. I told her this is pretty much what I expected to happen after they gave me radiation, microwaves, heat, and chemo to an already heavily pre-treated area. I've been playing "suck it up, buttercup" and eating Advil by the handful, and I figured if I was making cancer treatment history, it wouldn't be a walk in the park. Well, after some more lecturing, she said I had to get my butt up there, now. Naturally, I said no to Friday because it was already Thursday night when she called, so Papa and I head up there again tomorrow. I love Durham, but come on, let me stay away awhile.

So off we go for another long day trip. I am really looking forward to seeing the doctors again, as well as a whole host of other peeps, and to getting some special pain reliever patches for my burns. I didn't know they had those! I'm hoping and praying they like what they see and that all this destruction is cancer dying and not the reemergence of the disease from hell.

MARCH 1, 2011

*T*he news was good in Durham. My chest has experienced phenomenal changes since last week, and the mess of my chest is thought to be ALL treatment related at this time! Fantastic news, really; there was nothing they would even consider for a biopsy. The doctors were all big smiles and said they would say some prayers for it to stay this way. The largest areas have peaked in effect, thank God. Other areas, including my armpit and all the skin between my upper arm and side, are now just past peak-blistering. They are cracking open and are raw—bits of skin fall off and cling to my shirts. But I'm not weeping. I'm seemingly on the mend but very, very sensitive. My new pain meds take the edge off, but they disrupt my sleep and make my mood edgy in the evenings.

Slowly letting the good news sink in,
-Jen

MARCH 10, 2011

*L*ast week was rough and long. I was beside myself from discomfort every afternoon and evening, shaky and nauseated from the pain, and horribly uncomfortable in my own skin. BUT we still managed to pass some major Pagani milestones, and milestones for me are unbelievably precious—I just don't know how many I'll get to see.

Rocco spent the night over at a friend's house for the first time ever. I cried. Luca graduated to a big-boy booster seat (goodbye forever, five-point harness). I smiled, laughed, and maybe shed a tear or two. Rocco started practice on his first real soccer team. I beamed. It was ecstasy, a dream realized. We (Daddy) removed the bars blocking access from the backyard fort out to the monkey bars. I was nervous and proud. Luca took his first ever swim lesson. I smiled, beamed, and worried a bit. He cried for twenty-seven of the thirty minutes.

Health obstacles still abound. Other areas of my chest blister, seep, scab, and get rubbed raw. My skin is contracting as it heals, causing me to have to rip open wounds when I attempt to stretch. I moan when I finally relent in the wee hours of the night and roll onto my treated side, desperate to find a comfortable position, and the blisters pop and ooze and more skin rubs raw and sticks my shirt to chest. I know all that is going to happen, but I do it anyway. Showers continue to nauseate me. Tykerb disrupts my sleep further. The chemo side effects were getting the better of my body and my healing, so I took a two-week break, but I'm back on my seven-days-on/seven-days-off chemo routine. Tykerb and Xeloda continue to wreak havoc on my all of my skin in a multitude of ways. It's an endless cycle, sometimes one of misery. It's the cycle I tolerate and, on really bad days, dream of stopping.

BUT Rocco's first soccer game is this Saturday. I've got swim lessons, soccer practices, morning and evening snuggles, bedtime routines, smiles, and laughter to look forward to. It is the cycle I live for. I can't wait.

-Jen

MARCH 16, 2011

I've been having a hard time trying to blog the last few days. I'm either interrupted by the boys or just the fifth day in a row chemo. I go from not bad to feeling terrible in less than a second. I'll see Gary bright and early in the morning. He'll be thrilled—I have a laundry list of side effects to complain about. It's the usual stuff, but the acne-like rash that is threatening to cover my whole body (and leaving scars) and the inside of the nose sores are pushing me over the edge.

But my weekend was bliss. Rocco's game was perfection! 'Twas a gorgeous Carolina spring morning full of anticipation and excitement: the smell of wet grass, the air full of energy, enthusiasm and pollen, parents and grandparents cheering on the sidelines. It was suburban parenthood at its finest. I loved every second of it, and judging by his grin whenever he ran with the ball, so did Rocco. The only thing missing was Joe, who was out of town on business.

The rest of the weekend (and leading right up to the start of the "icks") was great. The boys had a little "lakation" at Gammy and Papas house, and I had some time to rest, play with friends, and then rest some more. Gammy and I had a fun morning together, and Luca's swim lesson even went, well, swimmingly. He cried the whole ride to the pool and for the first minute or two, but then he pulled it together and even enjoyed himself. That's my boy!

Better get to bed,
-Jen

March 24, 2011

Lesson of the Day: DON'T Mess With Rocco's Brother

*L*ast Saturday at the soccer game, Luca and I were sitting on the sidelines, soaking up the fresh morning dew and watching Rocco. Luca looked a bit bothered, and when I asked him what was wrong, he pointed across the field to a group of boys at an adjacent game and said they had called him a "baby" during some pre-game playtime. Well, judging by his distressed look, at age almost-four this must be about the worst thing you could say to the poor kid (aside, of course, from saying, "It's time to turn the TV off now and go to bed"). Little did I know, Rocco, who was currently on the sideline rotation (they rotate in at five-minute intervals; it's like micro soccer) overheard the entire conversation. He was called back onto the field moments after the "baby" conversation took place.

My oldest, well, he's got quite a good memory. He's feisty, temperamental, dramatic, and is a world-class grudge holder. I was not concerned with these things while I was chatting happily on the sidelines as his group finished their five minutes and rotated back off the field. Apparently, the whole time he was running (sometimes toward the ball now!) around the field with a huge grin on his face, because his brain was formulating a plan for revenge. He was in evil mastermind mode, and from outward appearances, you couldn't tell a thing. He's prone to drama, but I can generally tell when he is trying to be sly.

The second he was off the field, he marched around behind the goal and over to a group of three boys who were eight-years-old and under. Due to the distance, it was impossible to hear what was being said, but you could tell he was giving them a piece of his mind. His face was red, serious, his finger pointing right in the face of the accused ringleader. He was six to eight inches shorter than the lot of them, so he had to stand on his tippy toes while reading them the riot act (the biggest probably had twenty-five to thirty pounds on him, too). Then, as we watched on slack-jawed, he proceeded to draw back his right leg and kick, as hard as he could, one of the boys right in the shin. At that point, I hurried over there, a mixture of pride, dread, and astonishment brewing. I found the kicked boy to be a bit quivery lipped but all right, and I made some quick apologies. When we got Rocco back on the sidelines, we asked him what in the world made him do such a thing. He calmly replied that those boys were being mean to his brother, and Daddy always said to look out for Luca.

With my serious Mommy face on (and while Joe was proudly texting some friends about what just transpired), I then gave a talk about how that was not quite what we meant. I told him to rely on words or notify an adult instead of using his fists (or feet). On the inside, I was secretly beaming but simultaneously a bit worried about the force to be reckoned with that is my first born. At the next break, we were chatting with some neighbors when I happened to notice that Rocco had tracked down another, even larger boy, and let him have it, too, but this time without the kick (obviously, I have fantastic parenting skills). I just kind of shrugged, smiled, and thought: *That's my boy.*

To make a long blog a little longer, my appointment with Gary went quite well last week. I got more of the "watch and wait" lecture, but he thinks things are looking good. And after this week, I'll be off Xeloda. Also, my skin has done some extraordinary (like a normal person) healing, and I am feeling much, much better. Yea!

Better go or I'm going to get carpel tunnel.

March 31, 2011

This week, I managed to get to swim and soccer practice, visit Gammy in the hospital (she just got a new hip and looks and is doing great!), buy some necessities, and rescue (hopefully) one baby squirrel. It was a helluva lot for a chemo week, but I wanted to do all of it, and I did, but now I am worn thin and way off. I need time for quiet, stillness, and rest so I can recover and stop the shakiness that undermines my sense of well-being. Instead, I had a terrible night's sleep, because the Xeloda causes sleep disturbances. I tossed and turned while I was pursued by an unseen, malevolent force in the darkness. I can never manage to get a light on in my dreams.

I finally got up around 5:30 a.m. and am not functioning too well. I'm fuzzy-headed from the exhaustion and the multiple pharmaceuticals I took at bedtime to ensure this very thing would not happen. My first impulse was to go to Target and buy some lamps, and I wondered briefly if I could get there and back before the boys woke up. Obviously, I am not on top of my game. I shook off a bit of the mental fog, peered out the window to see red skies through the darkness, and wondered if I am somehow in tune with whatever nature has in store for us today.

Before cancer, I found comfort in waking up from my nightmares, but for the past three-and-a-half years, I frequently don't. The monster that threatens me is real. It has shape and form and sometimes an insatiable appetite. It eats people alive, usually from the inside out, but in my case, the outside in. Sometimes it just scares the shit of me, and my subconscious turns over phrases like "increases length of progression-free survival time." It doesn't discriminate, and it doesn't care whether you are a precious child, a parent, a spouse, or a friend.

I better stop now. Dawn is breaking, and the red skies have cleared. The dogwoods just feet from my perch are in bloom, and tender, vibrant leaves are beginning to shimmer in the gloaming. I have a squirrel to check on, boys to feed, dress, and get to school, Gary to see, and life to live.

Please take a moment today to say a prayer for all those fighting cancer, their families, and those whose battles were lost.

Thanks,
-Jen

APRIL 4, 2011

Gary was positively giddy with the healing that has taken place on my chest and back. He giggled, made some comments in his goofy Kermit the Frog voice, and just beamed. As for the cancer, we are still in "wait and see" mode, and we will continue my current chemo regimen of seven days on/seven days off. As long as it's working, and I feel this good (I really only have five rough days every two weeks, which is not too bad), I am good with this plan.

On Saturday, we had soccer, flag football, two birthday parties, and I did my friend Paula's 5K, the Sarcoma Stomp. It was fabulous! On Sunday, we did yard work, played and ate outside, and even managed some quality time with Vito (aka Bolt, Squirrleykins, Chewy). We all went to bed pooped. Vito just walked down our driveway and into our lives last weekend. The boys started petting him before I had time to scream, "NO!" in full blown mommy-panic voice. My head was calculating horrible kiddy/wild animal scenarios at the rate of ten scenarios per second for the first few minutes after s/he showed up. The boys were desperate to keep the animal, but I was very wary. Of course, after I got up close and saw that it was so darn cute, that it obviously had gotten away from it's nest prematurely, and that it would most likely be on its way soon enough, I decided to cave in. The boys and I built an outside "nest" from a shipping box and some shop towels. We left out some food, and I figured it would be gone come morning. No such luck. Morning came, and it was still there. The food had been partially eaten, but who knows by what? Well, a few days come and go, and s/he is still there. But now the temperature has dropped by quite a lot, and it is rainy. I felt like crap myself, but I just had to know if the darn thing was still out there in its box. Did I need to dispose of its little body. Did I need to make up a good story for the boys concerning it's whereabouts? So, I went out in the rain and sat about ten feet from its nest to look and watch for signs of life. No way was I sticking my hand in there, even with a glove on. Well damn, if the little critter didn't come out and hop over to me. It crawled up my leg and onto my shoulder before snuggling in between my chest and my arm. He was shivering and obviously desperate for warmth and comfort. I was stunned, shocked, and a little scared. It was surreal. But I thought, how often does the universe conspire to put a baby squirrel on my shoulder? Ignore the mind; listen to the spirit and the wind. Right then and there, my heart melted, my fear went away, and I decided to make what was most likely this baby's last few days on earth comfortable at the very least; a cause for which I feel great sympathy.

Well, more time has passed, and I find myself tending to Vito's apartment (a doggy carrier; he's moving on up), washing his linens (he prefers old fleeces), and washing anything I've had on when I handle him (because I need some bizarre squirrel-born illness like I need cancer). He loves to be held, comes to me when he hears my voice, and follows me around the yard. I slice and dice fruits and veggies and nuts, I warm up his hot water bottle twice daily, and I move his carrier inside at night and outside during the day. Did I mention I have gone around the bend? I have yet to enroll Rocco in school for the fall, book Luca's birthday party, call my insurance company back, work on my foundation, work my way through the ginormous pile of "stuff that must be tended to now," and buy dog food ... but I am working on Vito's squirrel skills. I try to stick to normal squirrel hours. I am trying out a more advanced diet of nuts that are harder to crack (he is nuts about avocado, though; pun intended). I am encouraging tree climbing and foraging, holding food on his own, and other basic squirrel survival skills. We are not keeping him long term. He is going to the Nature Museum. I worry about his vitamin and electrolyte levels, and whether or not he'll be accepted by the other squirrels .... I have lost it. I opened my heart up to a new experience and most definitely got one. I have to go. A friend brought dinner tonight, and we laughed at the irony as I sat and fed Vito while she fed my family—she's obviously a good friend!). I really am a few eggs short of a dozen.

If you want to meet him (he is precious and kind of amazing), come by soonish.

APRIL 14, 2011

Today was, well, shitty. We started with a high stress, low cooperation morning trying to get the boys groomed for school pictures. It was a bit tough for the first morning after a treatment week. Flash forward to Sophie puking up, at my feet, a huge pile of animal poop that she had been eating in the yard all morning long in an effort to erase any signs of any competing animals (i.e., Squirrelykins). Flash forward again to a building internal stress level regarding a mass I just noticed, just beyond the treatment area, on my back. Joe and my dear friend Britt convinced me to call Gary to see if I could get in.

Got in I did, right away. Britt dropped everything and drove me, because I didn't trust my driving skills at the moment. This was a good move because when I got home, I found I had left the back door and the screen door both wide open. Gary immediately confirmed that the area on my back is disease.

Now the shitty whirlwind winds up again. I'll get scans tomorrow. I'll go back to Duke Monday to see both the radiation/hyperthermia people and the medical oncology folks to see if there are any trials available.

April 15, 2011

Not one of my better days. At my unscheduled visit with Gary, he took one look at the mass on my back before saying it was disease. I also have some other areas adjacent to treatment margins that are questionable. Scans are tomorrow. I'll be back to Duke Monday to meet the doctors about possibly treating there again. I'm also seeing a medical oncologist while we are there to see if there are any trials.

Please pray my scans show it has not spread distally (i.e., to my organs) and that we have viable, effective treatment options that will beat the disease and give me a continued good quality of life.

And please, if you are moved to do so, continue to support Go Jen Go. We have made one-time donations to women in treatment and in need, and we've been providing monthly financial assistance to three families. We need additional funding to continue to help. As hard as it is for us, the battles the women we assist are even more difficult. Please pray for us all.

Thank you,
-Jen

April 18, 2011

I'm back from Duke and just got the kids to bed. I am crazy, crazy tired. 'Twas a good visit; I got clean scans (neck, chest, thorax), and treatment options still available. We go back on Easter Monday for some biopsies and to start the chemo trial application process. Thanks for the prayers, and thank God! Still more hurdles to jump, but we are still in the race!

April 26, 2011

It took me almost the entire Lenten season to realize what I had given up. My original sacrifice was that of "whites" (the overly processed sugar and flour, not the people) but that lasted all of four hours, until I succumbed to a slice of chocolate cake with extra frosting. Oh well. So all during the time leading up to Easter, I was soul searching and trying to figure out what on earth I could intentionally give up, or maybe if by chance, there was something I gave up quite by accident. Well, give up something I did! I gave up NOT cussing for Lent. And I did it with style, flair, and enthusiasm. When I suspected, and then Gary confirmed, that my cancer had returned two weeks ago, I went ahead and devoured several cupcakes, brownies, one chocolate, velvet brownie shake, and two jars of Nutella ... because I gave up "giving up 'whites'" (not the people) and had realized my sacrifice was all about giving up NOT cussing. So, to fulfill my promise, I dropped f-bombs everywhere: alone, to friends, to Gary, to my mother (gasp!), to Sophie, to Vito, and especially to my yard (whilst de-stressing with some very vigorous mulch hauling and rock moving). It was my most successful Lenten season ever!

And perhaps, or maybe in spite of, my enthusiasm for my Lenten "sacrifice," I was blessed with a great Easter with the boys, my parents, my brother, his wife, my incredibly perfect nephew, and my friend. Joe was the only piece missing in the equation. The fun ended a bit prematurely as Joe and I stressed and worried about the Duke trip. It didn't turn out too bad yesterday, though. I met with Dr. Markham (Duke's chief breast-oncologist) and another doctor. The consensus is that a trial drug called TDM-1 is my best option. It is not available at Duke, and they are checking to see if it is in Charlotte, but is most likely available in Charleston, SC. A biopsy (only one; I was expecting up to five because you can see disease in five separate areas) was taken to retest the genetic markers of my disease to see if they've changed. They can morph over time, and it would probably be good if they did, because that would mean more drugs would be available for treatment. It will take a week to a week and a half to see if I "get in." Fun! I love to wait and am a very patient person!

If I don't, then we use hyperthermia again as our backup plan. After that, there is not really a good choice available in a reasonable time frame, although another trial drug is in the works for the future.

Of course, we had lots of questions, especially since we've never been through the trial drug process before (never before had I been eligible). We asked about the side effects, dose schedule, treatment location, quality of life, and how effective the drug had been on other women in similar situations. Apparently, they don't know of anyone who has failed so many previous treatments and is still around—lovely. I'm trailblazing time and again. And as for the million-dollar question, "Are we talking about the possibility of a cure?" Well, Dr. Marcum gave me a funny, knowing, sideways smile, put his hand on my arm, and said "You know the drill by now; we'll try this until the next best thing comes along, but we can't rule out the possibility of a cure."

So, we left Duke tired, a bit soothed, and a bit anxious about the waiting and all the ifs. I was secure in the fact that my new Lenten habit of not not cussing would serve me well.

MAY 4, 2011

I am majorly under the gun. I'm in a big hurry to get the boys off to school in a few minutes but wanted to quickly blog. We've had another extraordinarily stressful roller coaster of a week. Rocco's school orientation (extremely emotional for me given the circumstances) on Thursday was followed by a very fun and long overdue trip to Hilton Head Island to see Big Daddy and Lillie. It took me the first two days to rid my brain of cancer fear and what-ifs (like the major, current one: what if I don't get into the trial in Charleston, which is our only good, new option for the time being?!), and then I finally unwound a bit and enjoyed myself.

The stress returned the moment we got back to town Sunday night. All the unresolved issues were not fun, given the most likely outcome for new treatment. On Monday, my stress was unbearable, and I almost completely cracked. You wouldn't believe how tough it is trying to get three separate medical institutions to coordinate information, tests needed, etc ... and that's even when they are trying to work together! But yesterday, following time on the phone with Charleston and a visit with Gary that included some reassurances, my mood shifted to be much, much better. Thank God! It looks more likely now that, following a few more scans and tests this week,

I will most likely get to start in Charleston next Thursday or Friday! Please pray this is the case, that the treatment works, and that it is covered by insurance—I will most likely be getting this treatment every three weeks until the next new drug comes out in a few years!!!

I'm still stressed, waiting to hear the final, "YES, you are in" and to get an appointment, but I'm feeling optimistic and ready for Luca's birthday. He turned four this morning!

MAY 5, 2011

*A*fter several days of lunging for the phone every time it rang, we heard late yesterday afternoon that, barring any unforeseen complications from my echocardiogram and CT scans tomorrow morning, I am accepted into the trial!! Thank you, God, and thank you all for your prayers!

This week nearly did me in. But the good news came right before we had Luca's birthday dinner, and the night couldn't have been sweeter, more fun, or more celebratory. I felt as if a giant, almost unbearable weight had been lifted. Now I'm worn thin but elated. I'm still a bit overwhelmed by all the logistics that need to be hammered out though.

Assuming all goes according to plan, I will be seen by my new doctor in Charleston next Wednesday and will get the infusion that day or the next. Then it will be back and forth every three weeks in perpetuity or until the next trial drug (nothing on the horizon for another couple of years) comes out. The drug is supposedly "well tolerated," but I've come to realize that when an oncologist utters those words, it's all relative (i.e., the cure the won't kill you, at least not right away). So, it's a bit of a mystery as to how it'll make me feel, but I am hopeful that my quality of LIFE will be good.

Better go, I've got to squeeze in some nap time before I pick my monkeys up.

-Jen

MAY 22, 2011

To borrow a phrase from a fellow survivor friend of mine, I'm "back from the dead." Two weeks ago, my disease was running rampant, visibly and palpably changing daily. 'Twas very, scary stressful times, and they just about did me in. All my hope hinged on the TDM-1 trial. And thank God it went off relatively smoothly.

Gammy and I had some good quality time together and even a bit of fun enjoying Charleston before my treatment. We had such an enjoyable meal and fun time shopping in the market, the seemingly ever-present specter of death disappeared completely for a while. It seems that we lost him amongst of the other shoppers (there were lots of elderly folks, maybe he got side-tracked). The Hampton Inn is surprisingly quite charming—which is very important to my outlook, given how much time I will be spending there in the upcoming months and hopefully years—and it is very close to where I get treatment.

I was full of trepidation at the thought of a new chemo doctor and nurse at this point, especially given my close relationship with Gary, but the new doctor, Dr. Keogh, is personable, caring, and lovely. I am only the fourth or fifth person they've had to start this regimen, with the longest being on it already for eleven months, so it is a lot of wait and see. Dr. K said his hope is that it would "work, and that I would be on it for a very long time." His concern over the disease's rapid spread during the trial which enforced a two-week period of no treatment was very evident, but he was hopeful.

I didn't feel too bad immediately following treatment either. But about thirty-six hours or so after, it began. It started with a bad headache and was followed by the "weepies" (lots of fun for Joe), and then there were several days of intense flu-like symptoms, but no nausea, and only one full day in bed this go around.

In the midst of a few hours of feeling decent Sunday morning, we up and went to the beach. Convalescing there was not too bad for me, and fun for everyone else. The first few days, though, were a constant, agonizing mental battle as I watched the drama—swelling, redness, shooting pains—that unfolded on my chest and back, and I wondered whether it was death marching, unchecked, full speed ahead, or whether it was inflammation caused by the drug. Is it the "cure" or the disease? What a freaking heck of a conundrum.

But the sun, the sand, the timeless nature of the surf and the sky, and the infectious laughter and enthusiasm of my husband and kids, helped me focus on the present. And the present was good, despite everything. We had a great time. The boys had gobs of fun crabbing, running and playing in the surf, swimming in the pool. We all had quality time to relax, de-stress, heal, and find peace and joy. It was perfection and an amazing gift. And my chest seems to have settled down noticeably, which means, most likely, I had a good reaction (i.e., cancer-cell death) to the chemo. Whew. And then, to top it all off, we came home to a surprise stocked pantry and fridge. Wow!

Thank you all!

June 2, 2011

We made it back from treatment last night, and my brain is still on the fried side. It was a bit like a mini-vacation, aside from the chemo bit. I think I've fallen for Charleston, Mt. Pleasant, and Sullivan's Island, even despite the heat (at least they have an ocean breeze). Since then, I've been stuck in limbo, purgatory, twilight, the gloaming, whatever-the-hell you want to call it, doing the bed to sofa shuffle all day now. I feel odd, off, shifted, weird eyed. There is no non-chemo experience to which I can compare it to. Does this makes sense?

What I do know, though, is that I got the drug. Dr. Keogh is as perplexed with the visible changes from this treatment as I am. My left breast could now be the poster child for Inflammatory Breast Cancer. purple-red beast, but it helps me fill out a top (okay, half a top) like I haven't done since I was breast feeding. The rest of my chest and back are a tough call. The plan is to continue on, at least for the time being. Dr. Keogh said if he had his druthers, he'd hang another agent with the TDM-1. This is not an option, since this is a trail, but I did pick his brain on which drugs he might consider. We mentioned some oldies and two new ones that they don't usually give to women with my kind of breast cancer. But he said my cancer is not behaving the way the pathology says it should, so we might try a different approach. I've heard this before, so it sounds like a potential, viable option.

But in the meantime, please pray the TDM-1 prevents the disease from spreading to my vital organs, doesn't cause any really life-altering side effects, and that if a better option is out there, we find it in a timely fashion.

Thanks.
Still hard to kill, Jen

June 10, 2011

*T*his past week or so has been nuts, starting the day after we arrived home from chemo. We had relatives visiting, birthday parties, high-school graduation parties, the mad scramble to buy gifts and write thank yous, an oncology appointment/labs, an emotionally draining yet good meeting with Rocco's new principal and school counselor, Luca's end-of-the-year party, an ice-cream social, and finally, Rocco's TK (transitional kindergarten) graduation and reception last night. I handled all of this while trying to physically recover from treatment, while dealing emotionally with the fact that it appears this chemo trial is most likely not doing the trick, and while watching what might be the only graduation of my sons' that I get to see. It has been a week full of extraordinary emotions, and my soul is worn completely thin.

I've got more on my plate than I can currently handle. I am going to be making some changes, putting things off or on hold, and stopping some things entirely. And it is going to have to start today. I am wrecked, spent. I ache like I have the flu. I've got muscle cramps, muscle tension, an eye that won't stop twitching, and a bitching headache in the works. I am shaky and just plain pooped. Everything is taking effort. I feel like running away and staring quietly at a vista, but it seems like too much trouble, so an afternoon in bed will have to do (the boys are at back-to-back parties today). God knows, I frequently find myself just suffering through things that should be enjoyable, because I just don't feel up to it, which is a source of frustration and guilt for me. Living life and my full-time cancer schedule don't seem to be jiving of late. Hopefully, a balance can be struck soon-ish, not just for me, but for the boys and Joe too. We've all been burning the candle at both ends, and now the boys need time to be at home so the four of us can spend time together. It will be interesting to see how it all pans out.

June 14, 2011

*N*ot the best mood, not the best language ....

I am very emotional, grumpy, and feel like shutting down, so I am surprised to find myself blogging. I live life around chemo side effects, so I tend to count on my "good weeks." Well, this week is my "good week," and it sucks. Gary confirmed this morning that the TDM-1 is not working. Tomorrow I go see Dr. Fraser, my radiation oncologist, to see if there is any possibility of radiating my previously untreated and newly diseased (since getting back from Duke) areas. On Thursday, I get re-scanned. On Friday, I suppose, some official decisions will be made as to what the best new plan is. I currently have appointments for chemo in Charleston and in Charlotte for next Tuesday, so something's got to give.

What a fun, low-stress week and a lovely way to start summer vacation. Trying to walk the tightrope between anger and sadness is leaving me flat and short tempered. I don't have patience for much of anything, including my family, which is ironic because they are the only reason I soldier on. I am really tired of this shit.

June 17, 2011

Hair today, gone tomorrow. Scans are clear of distant organ involvement, thank God, or whomever. The tumor in my left breast has stayed relatively consistent from my scan last month, holding steady at a size larger than a golf ball. The option of a mastectomy has been thoroughly discussed this week and decided against, because the skin is too widely infiltrated with disease to do any real good or allow healing. Radiation is an option at some point to give me relief from the pain and discomfort in that breast. It is palliative, as there are too many areas to radiate, and we can't re-radiate the recurrent areas that were previously treated anyway.

On Tuesday, I will start a drug called Halaven, which was released in November of last year and preciously given to women in stage 4. In these women, it increased progression-free survival time just shy of four months. Since I have a raging case of local/regional disease (stage 3c), rather than the metastasis to my distant organs (which is stage 4 and will happen eventually), Dr. Frennette and Dr. Fraser are hopeful that it will work, and work for a lot longer for me, since the disease is contained in just my breast and skin. This is our last option, and if it fails, we will revisit whether or not to retry a previously used chemo.

I am thankful my scans are clean, but I'm still in need of time to work through this all. I am in desperate need of solitude to sort this all out and become okay with everything. I need a physical release to free my mind, body, and spirit. I want to reconnect with the idea that I need to live whatever life I have left to its fullest. I am not returning emails, calls, opening mail … I am finding it tough to be around or talk to people anywhere. This includes my family and friends, who seem saddened and stressed, and are having difficulty dealing with this progression as much as I am. I am up and present for the boys as much as possible right now, but I can't deal with any bad behavior; the slightest problem threatens to send me over the edge, so I'm not at my parenting best right now. I am not mentally, emotionally, or spiritually in the right place for casual conversation, to answer when folks ask how I am doing, or to discuss much of anything. I feel like every time I talk about this shitty disease, it takes something out of me, and I have only so much left. I feel like that guy in Greek mythology who had to keep pushing the boulder up the hill, only to have it roll all the way down again every time he reached the top. There is nowhere to go to find the kind of aloneness I seek, nor the time required in which to find it. I hope I can find what I need anyway.

Thanks for your prayers,
-J

June 21, 2011

My mind and soul are in shut-down mode. I need every resource focused inward. I have not returned calls, emails, or written thank yous. I am not doing what I need to at home, and I don't care. I spent six hours in bed yesterday because I had sitters, and it was the only safe haven I could find. I am ducking out of public places where I might have to speak to anyone. I thought about writing something to that effect (or perhaps worded with a bit of an edge) on a T-shirt, but I decided it would most likely have the opposite effect or get the kids kicked out of Vacation Bible School, and the boys are busy getting their God on this month. I desperately need days or a week of time alone that is quiet, meditative, and restful. I need hikes in scenic, inspiring places or swims in cool, cleansing water to purge my physical being and reset my mind. In short, I need to go where the soul meets body. There are specific places this happens for me; unfortunately, two of them are not even in this time zone. And anywhere I might escape to in the South is going to be too hot or crowded or both. Summer time is a bitch for a cancer-caused existential crisis.

I will see Gary today at eleven o'clock and then get the first dose of Halaven after that. I don't want to go into the infusion room because of all the catching up to do there with nurses, staff, and patients I haven't seen all year. I am having a hard time with the unknowns of this treatment. Gary has no one else on it, so I don't know how my days will play out. It would be nice to have a little heads up, to know if my life will be tolerable or suck (or some combo of both) two weeks out of three, until we go off this drug. Currently, it is the very last rabbit in the hat, so maybe it will be some good magic.

I am rather reluctant to go, but my destiny awaits ....

June 22, 2011

First dose of Halaven is done. Not too bad so far. I called Well of Mercy, and I'm going as soon as I am packed. I'll be taking the vow of silence they offer, so I won't be communicating until I am back.

June 28, 2011

I have returned from the Well. It was a deeply meaningful visit. The silence and seclusion provided me the backdrop I needed to find what was missing, what had gone wrong. Amongst the beautiful hills and amid some extraordinary people, I looked within and found, once again, what I need. Somehow, I always find what I need there, and my cup runneth over.

Thank you for continuing to support us in deed and prayer, and also for honoring my communication blackout. I am back amongst the speaking and focusing on the present.

Yours humbly,
-Jen

July 7, 2011

The strength and peace I found at the Well did not last too long. When I went in for chemo last week, I found that my counts, in particular my hemoglobin (which is necessary to deliver oxygen to your tissues), had taken a huge hit. This was totally unexpected, and with it, my optimism for a good quality of my remaining life faded. I mean, what is the point of sticking around, feeling miserable, exhausted, and spending massive amounts of time in bed? I was in a total funk again, dragging everyone around down with me ....

But on Friday night, we managed to go out for an enjoyable family dinner and frozen yogurt, and my spirits lifted. On Saturday, Sunday, and Monday we went to the pool a couple of times, spent time with some friends (which we do way too little of as a family), went to a couple of cookouts, and saw two different firework shows. Luca, now four, is all of a sudden a big boy and loved the loudest fireworks that go "boom, boom, boom," just like his mama. Despite the fatigue—my fatigue is the deep-in-your-core kind, and the husband's is the, "I have been co-battling this disease and raising two young sons, supporting us all, and not getting any time for myself" kind (he never, ever complains though; I am not sure what is wrong with him. I complain all the time)—it was, at times, seemingly normal, suburban bliss. I savored it. I crave it. We desperately need it .... It was good.

On Tuesday morning, I was very tired from all the frolicking, and so were the boys, who were semi-whacked out on multiple days of non-stop playing, too little sleep, and too many holiday treats. So, I packed up the car, threw the boys and dog in, and headed off to get labs before heading up to see Gammy and Papa for a "lakation."

I was fully expecting, despite noticing a difference in mood in energy level, to get an appointment for a transfusion. Instead, we got a 911 call. But not for me! As soon as we checked in, I let the boys get a hard candy out of the jar in the waiting room. The three of us were sitting there quietly (how, you ask? Mommy had distributed her iPad and iPhone: priceless!) and alone in the waiting room, when Luca lunged at me, making these horrible straining sounds, clawing at his neck, with his face all purple and his eyes bulging. It was our first full-on choking situation evah. The front desk was blocked from view, and there was no time to get help, so I flipped him over and basically started pounding the hell out of him with the heel of my hand. Rocco, meanwhile, continued to play some golf game, completely unaware of the life-and-death drama unfolding an arms-length away. At first, it didn't work, and I had fleeting thoughts of starting the Heimlich, but I assessed him. His airway was still blocked, so I pounded some more. That did the trick, at least partially. He was gurgling, so some air was getting through. I ran to the front desk and told them what was going on, and they sent us immediately to the back. I yelled, in a voice choked with fear, adrenaline, and emotion, for Rocco to come on, and hearing the stress in my voice, he looked up startled and came running with us, iPad in tow.

A doctor, not one I know, looked and listened to Luca, who was by this time gurgling less and talking a bit, and said, "Call 911." Oh boy, I have never, ever needed to do that. I was picturing a full-on battalion with firetrucks, police, and an ambulance. I have seen this before at Gary's for chemo gone wrong, and it is beau coup stressful for everyone there.

We waited (the office manager took Rocco out for some snacks) in an exam room with two nurses until the medics came. If you want them to come immediately, tell them the airway is still blocked, because if you say "partial obstruction," which could change if the offending object is still in the throat, as was Luca's, you get pushed down the queue. Luca, pitiful and draped across my chest, was able to talk a bit and was gurgling less, but he was unable to move his neck due to pain from the still-lodged Jolly Rancher. The medics came, listened to his airflow, examined all sorts of stuff and, in the middle of the exam, got covered (as did Luca and I) by a huge amount of greenish throw-up. That did the trick. The Jolly Rancher was gone. They pronounced him to have a clear airway and told him not to eat anymore hard-candy and to eat only soft foods the rest of the day (he thought all the yogurt and ice cream was great). I was armed with a list of things to watch out for, and then he promptly fell asleep on my chest.

I had Terri do my port blood-draw and then give me a Neupogen shot. My hemoglobin had somehow gone up a half point despite the additional dose of chemo, but my bone marrow, which is necessary for fighting off infections, had really dropped. That produces a general yucky feeling and fatigue as well. By the time we got to the lake, Luca was totally back to normal, Rocco looked slightly traumatized, and I was pooped. But we've had a good visit. The boys are having a great time playing with and getting spoiled by Gammy and Papa, and I have gotten some much needed extra rest.

Whew, tired from all this typing.

Thanks for hanging in there with us,
-Jen

July 20, 2011

Caution-WUI (Written Under the Influence—not of anything good though) Time is such an elastic entity in my world, dictated in no small part by disease and treatment. Riding bikes with the boys, playing in the pool, romping, and laughing—these precious moments seem so fleeting. Days like today, when I'm reeling and flattened from chemo, just ooze and drip by. I am but a bit of flotsam tossed about in the tide. I am thankful, at least, that I am still floating. After the passage of these years, I should be used to this by now, but it still makes me lament. It's so odd to live in spurts, to have everything on hold while I recover from treatment, followed by a frenetic, sometimes frantic, cramming in of activities and to-dos before the tide knocks my feet back out from under me.

But the universe has conspired to give us a great, unexpected gift. Stars aligned, a butterfly flapped its wings, and we are going to Tuscany! It is still a bit unbelievable. I asked Gary to make it happen, because this is an extraordinary offer and opportunity, and he is totally on-board and taking measures to make sure it does. We are rather giddy and are focused on the bright, exciting idea of adventure and beauty. It is a precious, precious thing, to have something to look forward to, and we are truly savoring it. And as if that is not enough, our hall bathroom, a.k.a. our main guest bathroom, is nearing completion, and improvements on the upstairs bath are in the works! This is all so fantastic, it leaves me smiling and lighthearted.

August 9, 2011

I wrote this last week, but I was unable to post due to technical difficulties. I debated on whether or not to post it as is, and decided to just go with it. Today is a new day; we are leaving tomorrow, and we are thrilled! Warning: what follows is a bit rambly and perhaps hard to follow ....

This morning, I would like nothing better than to just lie around, reveling in the rainy, cool weather, passing the time sitting out on my porch dozing and reading. I want to be totally indulgent: ignoring things that need tending to and ignoring cancer for just a few sweet hours. The boys are at camp, so the glimmer of this reality exists, faint but present, in my consciousness. But this little fantasy will have to remain a dream. I have to head back to CMC for radiation in little over an hour. Things, you see, have changed.

Chemo, the Halaven, was stopped Tuesday. It was not working. The cancer was progressing visibly and without question. I knew this to be true, and I was both relieved and saddened by Gary's confirmation. It was and is more difficult for Joe, my parents, and Juju. You see, I've had the past two weeks to adjust to the progression I at first suspected, then later confirmed. It is the curse of IBC. I literally see my death coming, getting closer, every day. It is a horrible, cruel thing. And I have looked, as I examine my skin and watch the death march, closely and intensely for where my expiration date is stamped, but I cannot find it. Gary, it seems, can't find it either; I asked. We don't know if it'll be really quick once this stuff ventures into my vital organs, consuming and growing daily like it is currently in my chest and skin, or if it will be susceptible to chemo, and therefore we can slow or arrest its development there. It is a bit maddening. One thing is clear though: it is time to start the Bucket List.

Despite the List, we are not without some options. However, they are blatantly palliative rather than curative. We started a short course (five days) of radiation yesterday. This is to hopefully shrink the very large tumor in my left breast, give pain relief, and beat back some areas of disease that have broken through the skin. I get the weekend off and then get treated next week, including the day we leave for Tuscany.

When we return from our trip, we will retry a drug, Gemzar, that we used in the past. The good news is that it visibly beat back the disease; the bad news is that we had to stop it because of some rather horrible side effects. We'll see how it turns out this go around. Gary's tweaked the dose, and we'll be closely monitoring the side-effects so that, hopefully, it'll be livable. We hit the ground running when we return: chemo and Kindergarten. That's not really the combo we were hoping for.

As for now, my emotions and moods are all over the place. I feel intensely motivated (perhaps it is instinctual?) to get my house in order and all the little ongoing fix-ups done, but also strangely apathetic about lots of other things. I feel like a shimmery mirage: my existence seems flimsy and shifting, delicate, one foot in this world, one foot in some other. I am definitely a bit weird now, weirder than normal. And I'm tired, not sleeping well, and just plain off. Hopefully, Italy will be just what I need, what my family needs, to get back on track.

AUGUST 18, 2011

*B*uon Giorno! Ciao di Tuscano! This is the perfect backdrop for our little escape. It's truly the stuff of dreams, of Hollywood. Joe has posting some pics on Facebook. Tuscany is so gorgeous—a land with a soul. The view from our hilltop perch in San Casciano, in Val de Pesa (about fifteen minutes south of Florence, in the heart of the Tuscan countryside), is serene, timeless, enchanting. Chianti Classico vineyards and olive groves fall away, undulating, and fade out into the distance in soft hues of green and browns. Villas, some dating back 1,000 years, dot the landscape. It is magical and grounding yet inspiring at the same time.

We have been following our hearts. We have been sleeping late. We have been eating simply yet beautifully; the food does not disappoint. We have been swimming, which is a pleasure that makes my heart sing and has been denied by treatment of late, but I have been able to swim joyfully here with my sons. We've hiked amongst the vineyards. We love to feed the horses, see the chickens, and feed and play with the cats. The cats-part is amazing, because Joe and I are not cat people at all! But there is a black and white cat here, who we've nicknamed MeowMeow, that we've semi-adopted (or maybe its the other way around). She is like a kick-ass, slightly demanding, purring dog. We've been eating gelatto and pasta, and sight-seeing whenever we feel like it. Oh, and of course, napping. Italy shuts down from one o'clock to four o'clock, just like me!

We've seen Pisa, Lucca, San Gimignano, and San Casciano. Tomorrow, we go into Florence to see David at the Galleria dell'Accademia. We'll skip the Uffizi in favor of more leisure and less crowds. The pool, vino, gelato and the view are hard to beat. The boys are experiencing the culture first hand, like at the COOP (which is the Italian version of a US grocery store, but with fresher food, an insane noise level, customers moving all over the place, and pigeons that won't get out of the way), or wandering the streets and playing in the park at night after dinner. So, if we miss a few masterpieces, I don't think it's going to matter. They've learned that they don't wave or smile to passersby here, but that most Italians are very nice and love to talk, especially when you try a little of their own language, or even a mishmash of four languages that Georgie and I whipped together while bargaining in one little shop. It was brilliant, effective, and so much fun. I really do wish we had a lot more time here--time to slow and savor, time to appreciate things (art, culture beauty, simplicity, and each other), rather than contemplate the lack of treatment alternatives dread the progression, hate the unbearable side effects, and wonder just what brand of misery this disease will whip up next.

A bit of life here has been a beautiful reminder of the good things, the sweeter side of being. Reality, though, is never far away. It has burst through a few times (basically, I need all my resources to keep my shit together, so lookout, if I miss my nap!), but I guess that has to be expected. I hope to keep this somewhat tenuous grip on joy when we return to more radiation, followed immediately by more chemo (a retry), and then kindergarten.

I better stop this ramble. Got to hit the sack, tomorrow is going to be another bellisimo day!

August 25, 2011

David gave me chills. He is so magnificent, he even managed to capture the full attention of Rocco and Luca, and not just because you can see his penis. That was a giggly bonus for them, but we smartly prepped them in advance to save some ourselves some embarrassment from any loud comments they might make; and it worked. The remainder of our stay was indulgent; we spent more time appreciating the Italian art of doing nothing, and we enjoyed repeat visits to our favorite restaurant in San Casciano and to my favorite town, San Gimignano. Perfetto!!

I had a few private tears the night before we came home. I just did not want to get back to reality and, quite frankly, was not looking forward to a ten-plus hour plane ride with the boys. But the boys did great! Luca played approximately seven hours of Nintendo during the flight, which kept him perfectly happy. He has mad skills now, too, but hopefully, it didn't cause any lasting effects on his four-year-old brain. Rocco only played his DS for a few hours, but he watched an age-inappropriate movie or two, which might account for his new, sudden usage of the word" "sucks" (and is hopefully the reason he ran down the hall last night screaming, "See ya later, suckahs!" One flight attendant even commented on how great and polite they were. The only hiccup was the last ten minutes of the flight, when, just a bit before the landing gear went down, they both finally fell asleep. This prompted some hysterical crying when, it was time to deplane and work our way through customs ....

We pretty much hit the ground running. When we got home Monday evening, none of us slept much due to the time change, and the boys only slept until four o'clock in the morning. On Tuesday, we had two kindergarten functions and had to drive to pick up Sophie at the farm (it's cheap and they are sweet). None of us napped, so all of us were rather grumpy by bedtime, but we slept well, thank God! On Wednesday morning, I had an appointment with my radiation doctor and had the first dose of the second half of my split course of radiation. They were really pleased by how the tumor has responded thus far, and, bonus, I lost five pounds while on vacation (I had them weigh me twice, because I scarfed down so much cheese, Nutella, and gelato on vacay). Sweet, there is a God! The doctor said he thought a pound of the loss was due to tumor reduction (gross but good).

Today, Luca started school. He is a big boy in the four-year-old class now! And I saw Gary, who is also pleased with my radiation results and not too worried about the visible skin progression since my last chemo. The plan is to finish radiation next Tuesday (Rocco's first day of kindergarten, yay!) and then start with chemo the following day. We are going to go with Epirubicin, an anthracycline, again. That means hair loss (even though I don't currently have much to lose), whacked-out blood counts, and nausea- the big side effects with this one. I am down with the plan. Italy restored some of my *me*. I am back in the game and ready to play.

August 31, 2011

Yesterday was a huge day for us; our big bird finally flew from the coop. Rocco had his first day of kindergarten! We were up bright (okay, not so bright, because Rocco hopped out of bed, waking his brother in the process, at 5:20 a.m., eager to start the day) and early and made the bus stop with plenty of time to spare. He got on like a big boy, gave a short wave, and away he went. He chose to ride it home too, and he gave the whole day a thumbs up. Yay!!! What a beautiful, important milestone to be a part of, what bliss. I also finished radiation and had a good follow-up with Dr. Fraser, who is pleased with the "dent" we put in the tumor. Sweet!

I got Rocco and Luca both off to school, albeit with a little less enthusiasm on each of their parts, this morning. And right now I am at chemo, waiting to get shot up with five huge syringes full of red Kool-Aid, not the kind that is a sugary treat, more like the Jim Jones kind. But hopefully, it will kick some serious ass, cancer's, not mine. As Joe put it this morning when I waved to him as he left for work, "Today is the first day of the rest of my life."

We also received our official tax-exempt status for The Go Jen Go Foundation from the IRS! This is fantastic!!! And although we began, through your generous donations, providing financial assistance to breast cancer survivors (in need of monetary help from their breast cancer battles) prior to having the 501(3)(c) status, it is now official, baby (and retro-active from September 3, 2009)!

Thank you all for the unbelievable, continued love, prayers and help! Please help us support Komen (their money goes more towards promoting detection, raising awareness, some research, and a myriad of other breast cancer related services; it is an amazing organization) by signing up and raising funds for GJG's team. AND be on the lookout for an upcoming GJG Foundation fundraiser this fall so we can continue to provide financial support to those in our community struggling financially while fighting for their lives.

I hope this makes sense. I started it at chemo and finished at home with my chemo-whacked, sideways-glancing brain, and in the middle of what turned out to be not one of our better days. Rocco took the bus to school but apparently took the crazy train home.

Better go, J

SEPTEMBER 2, 2011

I am currently getting my rear kicked by the chemo today. The two IV anti-nausea meds I got with treatment Wednesday wore off this morning. The oral meds do not work nearly as well. I'm guessing I have a day or two more of this, and then I am over the hump.

Despite the nausea, I am having a very odd, intense craving for an extra-cheese pizza from Mellow Mushroom. And although I have never done this before on my site, is anyone available to pick me one up as soon as they open and can have one ready? It seems a very unlikely thing to want given how I feel today, but I can't get my mind off it.

If you see this and don't mind making the run, please text me.

Thanks!

-J

SEPTEMBER 2, 2011

Wow!! The pizza was taken care of! Thank you for all the offers. I thought this was a total shot in the dark and honestly am surprised this is on my mind given how I feel (nauseous, weak, icky, off balance, the list goes on …), but I think this is just what I need.

Thank you, everyone!
-J

SEPTEMBER 6, 2011

One chemo-crazed woman, one pizza, three days … that about sums up my weekend. I turned the corner yesterday, and I seem to be significantly on the mend now. I've just got to watch out for cooties (i.e., Rocco and Luca) and get some extra rest. If all goes according to plan, I won't have another medical appointment until next Thursday, which is insane. Who knows what I might do with all my extra time? Some thank you notes would be a really good start, or maybe I can attack that pile of accumulated and accumulating paper in my kitchen. Nah, that would take days, and time is too precious to do "the needs;" I am focusing on "the wants" as much as possible.

One in eight sums up the breast cancer story. Your mother, your daughter, your sister, your wife, your friend—one in eight will get diagnosed with breast cancer in their lifetime. Please help us, Team Go Jen Go, to help Komen fight this disease. One in eight! This is unacceptable. Help us turn the tide, promote early detection (and therefore much better survival rates!), raise awareness, and find a CURE!

"Let's get this pahtee stahted," like Luca says!

Thanks!
-Jen

SEPTEMBER 13, 2011

WARNING: Gross Burn Info. It is not for the faint of heart, but will be good reading for those who like a high "ewwww" factor.

*F*lighty, shaky, terse, agitated, not hugging, even more casual than usual (i.e., a big, soft T-shirt. This pretty much sums me up of late (just of late?). It's not the chemo. It's the radiation burns that are now just starting to peak. The burns take time to develop (don't ask me why; I can barely add, so nuclear physics are not really my strong suit). The burns are on the verge of pushing me over the edge. Cue the violins. I woke (of course that would imply sleep, which only occurs in fits and starts for me now, because I want to scream every time I roll onto either side) up this morning wanting to rip my skin off. Yesterday, I actually did; it was a big piece in a highly sensitive area that left me almost passing out and nauseous as hell. Radiation burn pain, which I did not have even remotely to this degree following the first two courses of radiation (I did have this from the Duke hyperthermia/radiation/chemo combo though), is weird. It produces more of a systemic response in me (maybe it is because of the large areas involved?) and leaves me trembling, unable to think straight, nauseous, and just a complete wreck. The skin on my chest, on various parts of my breast, and on my left armpit are in various stages of burnt mush. The skin looks like someone left a hot iron on it; it's weeping, blistering, ulcerating (yes, ulcerating), and shedding. It is a mess. I am loath to wear a shirt, but I am running through them at a brisk pace because the wounds can't really be bandaged.

So, this morning (Rocco's first day of Chess Club!), I caved and took a strong pain killer and drank a large, extra-caffeinated coffee. It made things tolerable. I managed to put and keep a shirt on (until I got home and ripped it off). The shakiness has diminished. I got the boys to Chess Club on time and even helped out. It was awesome! I even helped out with two simultaneous games, a bit of strategy on both boards. I think it might have been the Hydromorphone talking, but I felt really smart! Or maybe it was just because the oldest kid at my boards was in second grade. Anyway, it was great! I can't wait until next week. Rocco had fun, Luca did well, and it was just an all-around good morning. But anyway, if I seem a bit distracted or angry, you'll know why.

Enough of the whining. Thank you to everyone who has signed up for Team Go Jen Go! There is still plenty of opportunity to help us support

Komen! Please urge, okay, pester, everyone you know to sign up. And thank you so, so very much for your continued support, love, and prayers!

September 22, 2011

*H*ello all. Joe here, commandeering Jen's blog for a quick note.

Jen is out in Colorado, heading to one of her favorite spiritual places on earth, Arches National Park in Utah. We've been there many times, and I can tell you, she always feels closest to God when she is watching the sunrise while sitting on a remote sandstone arch. The boys and I miss her fiercely, but we know she will have a wonderful trip.

The outpouring of support as of late has been incredible. I had to post a note to say, "Thank You" to the many, many people who have offered their love and support to us. The deliveries of dinner, the cards in the mail, the phone calls and e-mails. Just yesterday, I received no fewer than six calls from different people with offers of assistance and kind words of love and concern. The wonderful, giving, and caring people at Komen are all so sweet in their concern and consideration for Jen. And thank you to all of the generous families that provide delicious dinners for us without fail. Since those meals often go straight to the cooler out on our porch, we don't get the chance give our heartfelt thanks, so thank you very much.

As we approach the Race on October 1, I wanted to say another thank you to the people near and far who have joined the GJG team. Tough economic times have kept the team roster down this year, but we still have a formidable force to war against: breast cancer. The very generous donations from families all over the US are going to go a long way in finding a cure.

September 29, 2011

*S*hort-ish and sweet … I'm post chemo (I had it yesterday), and I'm feeling a bit icky.

It was a great trip out West with my parents. I got good quality time with each of them, which has been a rare occurrence since Rocco was born. Moab was, as usual, good for my soul, second only to Jackson Hole. I hit the ground running as usual. I got back late Tuesday afternoon, I had chemo yesterday, and I have a follow-up and bone marrow shot today. Ugh! But I have great news about the burn situation: due to two fantastic new products for second- and third-degree burns, I am like a 1,000 percent better in that department. Yay!!

I want to thank everyone who has signed up and donated to our Komen team! We are 177 peeps strong at my last check. What wonderful news! Thank you!

Although the chemo will be kicking my hiney for the first time during the Komen event, I plan on being out there to help celebrate life, survivorship, and the quest for a cure! The Komen peeps have even arranged to have the boys and I toted around in a rickshaw-type thing so I can "walk" with our team. It should be big fun.

Again, thank you for your loving, generous support and for standing up for so many women effected by this disease.

October 4, 2011

I am still a bit on the fried side, so be prepared ....

I have wanted to blog since the race was over, but the dust has just now settled enough physically, emotionally, and mentally for me to do so. I went in with low expectations. I figured I would just feel too bad to enjoy and revel in anything. But the excitement, enthusiasm, hope, love, and support just carried me along. My spirit was elevated, and it brought my body right along with it. It was a definite physical stretch; I am now over the worst of the chemo side effects, except for the irritating bone marrow suppression part, and I am most definitely tired, but I am still basking in the glow of the weekend.

The T-shirt party at the Keogh's was beautiful and as fun as ever. My boys had a blast playing "tackle" with the pack of (wild) boys running all over, and I was able to enjoy, mingle, and actually carry on some conversations that I hope made sense. Toward the end, faces were literally swimming in and out of view, and a dear friend escorted me home on wobbly legs. The 5:50 a.m. wake-up call was brutal (as I am sure a lot of you found out), and it took me like forty-five minutes just to get dressed and slap on a little make-up (it's a must since I have very few eyelashes left). During my attempt to get ready, Joe ran around like a mad man, grabbing lots of last minute items and trying to get the boys and I to hustle up. And Wendy and our crew were already downtown setting up! We hit all the roadblocks, but the cancer/chemo card does come in handy; all the cops let us through, so we got a primo parking spot, which was good because I was not up for walking at that point. My efforts were primarily focused on not shaking and not throwing up—I don't know if it was the chemo or the chemo-specific anti-nausea medicine that was causing that.

But we got to the tent, and it was so incredible to see so many people (from far and wide, from our present to our past, from family to friends, and people that we don't even know but have heard about our fight) all out and showing their love, optimism, and support. It was AWESOME! Then to look around (from my chair, which I ended up not minding too much) and see the same thing, all around me—thousands of people, a sea of pink, all out for the same reasons (supporting friends, loved ones, and strangers in their quest to detect, fight, and end this disease) was beautiful, overwhelming, glorious ....

I never would have been able to actually participate in the race if it weren't for Karen and Vicki, and all the women with Estramonte Chiropratic, who so graciously toted me around in the pedicab. It was delightful. I felt like a queen, and I loved it! The tiara and the wand certainly helped. And although we took the short route back to the tent due to my nausea, I felt like I had the whole experience and then some.

I figured I would have to make a quick exit long before the end of race festivities, but I joined a good crowd from our team (GJG represents), and we heard my incredible hubby speak, along with four other people, about who the Susan G. Komen Foundation represents. He was (and is) amazing! My heart was filled with love, pride, and joy. There were very few dry eyes in the place when he was done. We have been together twenty-seven years, and I am still in awe of him.

So, thank you all for supporting us this past weekend, and every other day as well. You have made and continue to make a profound difference in my life.

Love and happiness,
-Jen

October 12, 2011

I did a few fun mommy things early last week while trying to recover physically from Komen and chemo. By Thursday morning, I was running on fumes (I was feeling a deep cardiac fatigue like I only ever get from certain types of chemo; not even the Ironman can compare), but I volunteered at Rocco's school, because I signed up in advance and because I wanted, damnit, to help teach the kids about gardening. I came home and literally collapsed into bed. I basically had to call in reinforcements because I didn't (couldn't) really get back up again for another six hours.

We had a great weekend because I woke up feeling pretty good Friday. We packed in some serious fun: school bingo night (a hot, frenzied, fun affair; they only do this once a year so it was a must do), a soccer game, a cousin's football game, we watched the Dawg's beat the Vol's, and then we even got to go see the Panther's play. Wow! I'm not sure if I could have managed all that before cancer without collapsing. Go Jen Go!

All the football, playdates, and schoolyard fun have conspired to leave Luca with football on his brain 24/7. He woke up and immediately started asking to play at 6:40 this morning. Tackle—his rules, our basement. It is fun, and it makes his day, but Mommy, Daddy, and Papa (who is now recovering from confirmed bruised ribs from taking on the little man) get worn out and generally a wee bit hurt or sore. I managed to put him off this morning; it was a "let's whip out the Playdoh at 7 o'clock in the morning kind of day."

October 21, 2011

Another week in the life of Me
Written from the CT Scan Waiting Room of Mercy Hospital

I've been basically single momin' it for a while now (hubby has been traveling for work). Major props to all the peeps out there doing this daily, because it is flat out exhausting, and I am whooped. I was actually looking forward to chemo, because I have permission to rest after treatment (obviously, I'm desperately tired), but I ended up not getting chemo at all.

My Thursday morning appointment with Gary packed a big surprise. I was WAY stressed out, had been watching and feeling the disease progress since my horrible radiation burns healed, and I was trying to not go down the "holy crap we don't have any options left" path, when Gary delivered some shocking news. There is a trial just out for a new drug for women with metastatic, HER2 Neu Positive breast cancer who have failed other treatment protocols (like moi). It is in Phase I (which is like one degree removed from guinea pig), and I just might be eligible. There are eighteen spots open countrywide. And as of yesterday, I just might be getting one of them.

Gary was excited about it, but trying to remain neutral, during the appointment. Getting into a trial is a very, very strict, specific process involving numerous people and impartial governing bodies. It involves mountains of paperwork, lots of medical tests, and a thorough review of your entire treatment history, so there are plenty of opportunities to find something that doesn't jive with the official trial requirements. Selection is a completely objective process, which is necessary and understandable, but makes it completely nerve wracking while waiting to see if you qualify and horribly devastating if you don't ….

Well, while waiting for my labs to be drawn and scans to be scheduled, two research RN's unexpectedly came in the room and reviewed seventeen pages of legalese describing the specifics of the trial and all the side effects associated with the trial drug and the other two chemo drugs given with it. I've had both chemo drugs before, and the side effects are the usual suspects: nausea, vomiting, fatigue, bone marrow suppression, hair loss, potential heart, lung, and liver problems, diarrhea, and acne. Anyway, this seemed positive (the presence of the nurses, not the super-long side-effects list), and they explained that, after scans to see if the disease has spread to my vital organs yet and a further review by one of the third parties overseeing the trial, I will find out late next week or the week after if I am eligible. WHAT?!?!

We (or, at least, I—because I don't always share my fears when I suspect the disease is in growth mode) went into the appointment stressed, struggling not to feel hopeless. And now I (we) find myself HOPING once again. While we will be waiting on pins and needles until we hear definitely whether I am in, I am soooo excited at this prospect of healing, hoping, living, and being a wife, mommy, daughter, and friend for how ever long God grants me the privilege. And despite the prospect of going through life bald, one boobed, and with the trots, I am going to be down on my knees, asking God to get me in this trial and for it to be the magic bullet we've been waiting for. So, if you find yourself with some time and a generous heart, please give a shout out to the Big (Wo)Man on my behalf.

Thanks! Jen

October 28, 2011

*A*fter much anticipation, we saw Gary yesterday. My scans are good!!! No spread into my vital organs (brain, liver, lungs, or bones). The disease is present and evident in the other usual spots, but there is nothing immediately life threatening, which is good, to say the least. Gary seems convinced that I will be eligible for the study (we still have four sets of reviews to pass), and he even scheduled me to begin treatment this coming Tuesday, November 1, bright and early in the morning. Wow!

And despite the great scan news and Gary's optimism (both about the drug's efficacy and my ability to get in the study), I am in that place where I often find myself after such a stressful stretch, even one where we receive good news (because nothing is ever black and white in the world of survivorship). I am a bit out of sorts. I'm suffering from residual stress and am worried about whether or not everything will fall into place like we need it to in order to start on Tuesday. I'm also worried about whether the study drug will actually work (earlier this year I flunked out of the TDM-1 trial in Charleston, SC faster than I did my first college math course at Georgia Tech, hence the degree from UGA—Go Dawgs!). And on top of that, I'm feeling the pressure of trying to pack in a lot of fun and check a lot of to-dos off my list before my schedule, and our lives, switch back into that strange chemo-driven, purgatory-esque existence that is life with advanced cancer.

Whew, I needed to bitch a bit to get back on track. The bottom line is that this is good news. Hope rekindled, time gained, and prayers answered! We are ready to have lots of holiday fun, watch the Dawgs beat the Gators, savor the fall weather, and stuff ourselves full of some sweets.

November 1, 2011

*Q*uick update. I started the trial today as hoped and planned for! I didn't even find out if it was for sure, all systems go, until the drive in this morning. Whew! I'm way excited, chemo hungover, and pooped from all the holiday festivities, but I am happy.

Thanks. More later ....

-J

November 9, 2011

Halloween weekend was a grand affair! There were parties galore, we made the rounds, and we had big fun. By the time trick-or-treating finally rolled around Monday night, my scary skeleton (Luca) refused to wear any part of his costume except one boney glove. He got lots of strange looks when he rang the bells (we threw an NFL jersey on him so he would at least look somewhat dressed up), but it didn't diminish the candy distribution. Rocco was my evil, yes Evil, scientist. He won most original costume at the neighborhood costume parade. He'll be the one to watch out for later. With his intellect and love of the spotlight, I am sure there are several advanced degrees on the horizon. We'll have to make sure he uses his super powers for good and not evil. And by the way, in case you haven't noticed, all the really cool super villains have their doctorates.

It was a little tough packing in all that fun whilst trying not to worry about whether or not I got in the study. I found out the morning after all the fun, while heading downtown to Gary's in the middle of rush hour. Talk about last minute! No wonder I don't have any hair. If chemo didn't make it all fall out, the stress would. I was so keyed up, even after I heard the news that I was in, it took me another thirty or so minutes, which turned out to be the rest of the drive time, just to settle down.

Yesterday, I had my one week checkup with Gary, per study protocol, to see how I was doing. I was very curious to see what he thought. I typically keep most of my observations about the daily progress of things to myself. What good is beating a dead horse? Why not watch the death march and worry in private? Don't worry, I still bitch/vent some. We are doing all we can, so I'd rather not rehash the details of my dwindling mortality any more than I have to, than I am compelled to. Plus, it sucks stressing out everybody around me too.

So anyway, I had been playing my thoughts (on how the therapy was panning out) close to the vest. I think the "death march" is actually in a state of retreat. Swelling, redness, and nodularity seem to be on the decline almost all over. Pain (which is a major pain in the ass, but only when I am wearing clothes, trying to sleep, or wearing a seat belt) has diminished greatly. The diseased area was especially sensitive along and under my collarbone (where it was growing like wildfire), and this was a real problem when it came time for bed. The time I saved in the past week from not having to perfectly arrange my covers/pajamas so as not to cause too much weight/pressure on my chest alone is staggering. Blah, blah, blah .... Anyway, Gary concurred with my assessment! The drug is visibly working on my skin, and in just one week's time. UH-MAZ-ING!!! Let's hope and pray to God it continues to kick some cancer ass! Treatment and side effects are almost pleasurable when treatment works! And God knows, it has been a long, long time since we've had this on the run.

November 16, 2011

Harumph, grrrr. TMI warning.

I am in, to quote our men and women overseas, "the suck" right now, and I probably will be until Friday evening, at least.

I had a terrible night's sleep; it was more like a series of short, fitful naps. It was too warm, too humid, and I fought with the covers all night long. My stomach was most unhappy, and my ass sounded like a trumpeter swan. I got up to pee like five times and was baffled each time, in my semiconscious state, by the reeking odor of chemicals. What the hell was causing it? Finally, on like trip number three, I realized that it was my pee. Super. What a lovely way to treat this freaky disease. Why not saturate my insides with more super toxic stuff? And then the creature (okay, it's a bug, but one I have never, ever seen before—it's brown/tan, has a four-inch long, trapezoidal body, long legs, and beady eyes) was making a racket again in the early morning hours. It would make helicopter-like noises followed by grinding sounds. Was I concerned for my safety? No. It wasn't a palmetto bug or a moth. It sent me in hysterics the night before when I discovered it on the wall in the corner behind the headboard of my sleigh bed. It was impossible to reach without major effort. But despite the fact that I was just finally getting some good sleep as dawn was breaking, I leapt out of bed after like the third grinding episode. I think the damn thing was trying to eat my bamboo blinds, and I can't have that, what with the cost of window treatments and all. So, I have thrown open all the windows in the room and am hoping its little buggy brain works at least as well as mine and he finds his way outside to freedom. If not, its going to get traumatic and squeamish for both of us if I have to rescue his ass with a paper towel.

I think my sentence structure is lacking even more than it normally is right now. I am trying really, really hard to write this, and it is painfully slow. I am definitely six eggs short of a dozen at the moment (and my usual operating state of late is more like just a couple of eggs down). Sometimes

I just stare blankly, like nobody is home. Sometimes I can't put sentences together or think of the names of things or people's names. Hardly ever can I touch my iPod without screwing something up, and I absolutely cannot remember passwords or email addresses. It is awful and frustrating, but my hubby is very, very patient with me. I think about this problem often, but then I get side tracked and never really come up with a good solution. But finally, I have arrived at the root of the problem.

"Chemo brain" is a medically documented problem occurring in chemo patients. It does not affect everyone, nor everyone to the same extent. It is permanent in approximately 15 percent (I am as sure as I can be on this) of patients. Warning: complex math to follow. Let's say the average chemo patient gets treated with two or three chemo drugs during the course of their therapy. I have gotten in the neighborhood of seventeen different chemo drugs during the course of my treatment. So, if "chemo brain" (couldn't they come up with a term that sounds less apologetic and more medical sounding, like "treatment induced idiocy"?) occurs 15 percent of the time in the average patient, and the way I figure, I have like a 102 percent (17 divided by 2.5, multiplied by .15) chance of either having permanent damage or damage to 102 percent of my brain. Either way, it's not too good, but at least my math skills are still exemplary!

Despite my bitching and moaning and desperation just to get through the next couple of days until I feel normal-ish again, things are pretty darn good. Just a month ago, it was desperate times, the disease was visibly running rampant, and the sand in the hourglass seemed just about gone. But now we have hope and continued progress on the right direction! Gary and his crew were thrilled once again. Please keep us in your prayers that we stay on this path. Thank you!

Now I've got to go see about bugsy.
-Jen

November 28, 2011

The week in review ....
    Monday: I was very, very tired but still riding the SEC football high and SUPER thrilled with the GJG Board meeting that night (despite

zoning in and out a bit) and the very exciting things we have in the works to bring more help to breast cancer survivors in our area!

Tuesday: I woke up utterly exhausted, "treatment induced idiocy" at an all-time recent high, went to CHOA for Herceptin only (it was my week off from Taxol, a chemo drug I am on along with the others), my hemoglobin was quite low, so they had booked a transfusion day for me on Saturday or Sunday. My counts might rise because it is my chemo "off" week, so I decided to skip it and not ruin the vacay time with the family. I ended up sleeping in a semi-comatose state, slumped over in my infusion room chair for four hours at therapy (even though I got absolutely no meds to make me sleep).

Wednesday: I was still way pooped, wondering if I made the right decision to wait and see what the hemoglobin is doing. I felt like I was dragging weights around. I had heavy, tired limbs.

Thursday: I woke up a bit sluggish, but my brain seemed a bit sharper. I walked the Turkey Trot (5K) with friends. It was glorious, reviving! I felt alive. We went to Gammy and Papa's, crashed, and then had a GREAT day with the whole family. Awesome!

Friday: I woke up excited. Joe, the boys, and I drove to Raleigh to see the Hurricanes play. It was totally fantastic! The guys loved the hotel, and they thought it was a fantastic adventure. The game had a great, exciting, fun, very good family vibe (I was really impressed and a bit surprised by their team moto—Pride! Passion! Community!—how cool is that?!). Hockey games are FUN! And thanks to some friends, we met a bunch of the players afterward and got autographs. We met and spoke to Eric Stahl, Cam Ward, Larosa (who are all on the Stanley Cup Team), plus several others. They were gracious and easy going, which was not quite what I expected of some of the world's toughest athletes. It was INCREDIBLE!! We are some serious Caniacs now! We can't wait to go back!

Saturday: Whew, I was tired, but my counts were definitely on the rise! I was tired in mainly a good way. We drove home, picked up our tree, got it in the door, and we all collapsed and watched the Dawgs bite the Jackets (we had recorded it while we were away).

Sunday: I was tired, but from all the fun! We decorated the tree and the kids' tree downstairs, the house was a wreck, and we went to bed happy ....

Hope everyone had a great week too! Go get your cyber deals!

DECEMBER 6, 2011

I've been alternating between grumpy and fine, feeling downright yucky and not too bad. A sinus infection paired with chemo last week was a tough one-two punch that I have still yet to recover from, but I still have a few hours on the mend before I get blasted again today. To quote Joe Walsh, "I can't complain, but sometimes I still do. Life's been good to me so far." The trial results have thus far been miraculous. I need to "keep my ears stiff," according to my German friends.

The past week was rather enlightening though. I learned to never leave the lid down on the kid's toilet at night, which is an important lesson and one I'm glad I learned while Luca still has a rather small bladder. I learned that Rocco has tried, selected, and perfected his new fake laugh. It is HI-larious (the kid is a riot; you should see his dance routine) and MUCH better than his last one. And I also learned that Rocco "broke apart" with his "girlfriend" at school (name withheld to protect the innocent). Apparently, breaking off an "impending nuptial" at age six (and a half!) is much less traumatic than it is later in life.

Well, I had intended to write more, but I'm at Gary's. I have IV meds going in, and I am about to get very stoo-pid and comatose.

Better scoot.

-J

DECEMBER 13, 2011

I am not feeling the flow, hearing my muse at the moment, and I haven't for a few days now. I'm either resting or running around, not a lot of time for reflection. I'm caught up in the craziness of the holidays and my weekly, pre-treatment, frenzied push to get things done. But right now, I'm in a chemo-forced timeout, and I have a few minutes before I go semi-comatose, so bear with me. I'm looking around and feeling the love, the positivity, acknowledging the reason for the season.

It is about loving one another and goodwill toward men. We've (the GJG Board) been working hard at this. GJG is on the move. We are actively moving toward helping more local, in-need breast cancer patients. We've got good things in the works. We're planning upcoming fundraisers, and we've recently submitted a grant application as well as a Seed 20 application, both of which will help us make a bigger impact in the lives of more people in need. It puts a huge smile on my face knowing we are helping change lives for the better. Wow!

We couldn't, and can't, do it without you. This month, GJG has been incredibly fortunate to have the privilege of helping out several survivor families find their holiday joy. I, we, want to thank you all who have donated so generously recently! GJG would not be here without your compassion, love, and support.

Feel the love, spread the joy,
-Jen

December 18, 2011

I am grumpily joyous, or joyously grumpy, not sure which. In the midst of trying to get my holiday cheer on despite my low counts, I seem to have gotten another sinus infection. I am achy, my eyeballs might pop out of my head, my ears are full, and my sinuses have shut down. Yuck. I am praying this is not an off-chemo week trend.

We continue to be in awe of everyone's generosity. Thanks to your love and kindness, four families will have Christmas this year when otherwise they would not. It is truly a beautiful thing to be a part of, this spreading of love, this grace in action....

Thank you again for supporting us in Operation Christmas Joy!

December 22, 2011

Yesterday was a mixture of elation and exhaustion. The house looked, as my mom used to say, like a bomb went off. The boys had four days of worth of toys, arts and crafts, and candy wrappers strewn from one end of the house to the other. Mixed in were bits and pieces of wrapping supplies, labels, notes, coffee cups, stray pieces of tissue paper ... all from Operation Christmas Joy. And what a JOY it was! It was such a beautiful thing. The two families we delivered to on Monday and Tuesday were loving, good, hardworking (like the one single mom with the three-year-old son who worked, prior to diagnosis, three part-time jobs with at-risk kids to make ends meet) people who just happen to be one diagnosis away from (financial) disaster. They opened their homes to us, shared their stories, and their optimism despite their challenges, and they thanked us from the bottom of their hearts.

The boys went with us for the Monday night delivery, and the folks from WBTV (CBS) joined us on Tuesday. The piece speaks volumes. It made our hearts sing! Another family received their delivery Wednesday by a new GJG supporter. Our benefactor said the four-year-old child could not wait, and he opened all the presents while she watched! Delivery for the fourth family, the mom is battling stage 4, will be made later today.

We are deeply touched to be able to support our breast cancer community in so many ways. Joe and I, as well members of the Go Jen Go Board, want to offer our deepest, most heart-felt thanks for providing us with these opportunities. We couldn't do it without you! We also understand that the need is always present, cancer never takes a holiday, and we do not want anyone to feel that they need to contribute financially each and every time we ask. Support with prayers, kind words, visits to my website, dinners and playdates—all these are just as meaningful and easier on the wallet. Do what and when the time is right for you, do it when your heart moves you! Thank you so much! Have a beautiful holiday. Enjoy your family and friends. Smile when you think of the joy you've helped spread.

Peace, hope and love,
-Jen

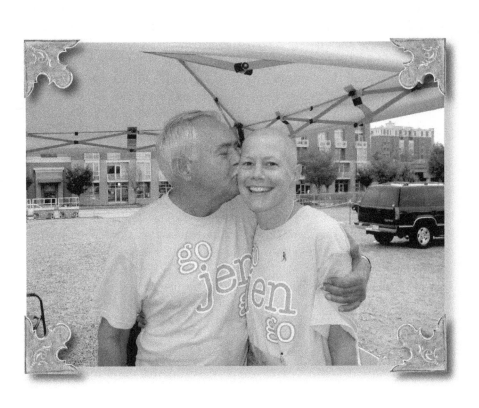

2012

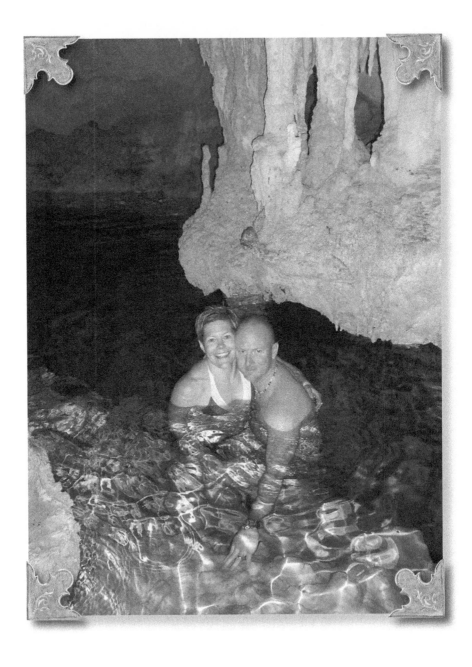

've taken a wee blog vacay and can't quite figure out where to start and what to omit ... I'll try to be brief, but brevity is not my communication strong point.

Christmas was perfect. It was the beautiful blend of family time, fun, and giving. Ahhh ... It was so tough, though, to pry myself away from my three guys, warm and snuggling in front of the fire, to slog through the rain to chemo on the 27th. It was not where I wanted to be. I hit another bump in the road around New Year's. All the thinking about times past, present, and future got a little tough to swallow. Weekly chemo, although a blessing, is a jagged little pill. I got over that bump, but I did have to power through it. I was so sad this Monday night about our vacation being over that I thought I might cry. It didn't help that I drank a bunch of coffee so I could skip my nap, for the first time in months, in order to stay up and watch the Dawgs lose.

And that brings me to today. It's a typical post-chemo Thursday, and I am nuts. Thursdays just plain suck. It's just never good to wake up shaking with a jerky motion and a slight tremor. Sometimes my voice wavers. It undermines my confidence, makes me feel weak and venerable. It's because of the neuro-toxicity. I am in a dark, irritable mood, and I don't feel well. It happens three weeks out of the month. The predictability doesn't seem to help. Add to that a mounting concern about my left breast. It's swollen and red, and other stuff is going on too .... But, am I imagining it? Am I overreacting? Am I incapable of just enjoying the newfound hope this trial is offering? My brain turned into super computer mode (okay, maybe not so super, more like one of those slow, giant models from the 1980s) calculating the odds of this or that potential outcome from the current symptom presentation, and now I can't turn it off. The whole "Is it a symptom of the treatment or the disease?" dilemma could, quite literally, drive me crazy. Inflammatory breast cancer sucks big time. I was near the red line with stress and anxiety earlier. I was close to a panic attack, had a hard time catching my breath. This has only happened a couple of times in the whole four and a half years—like the time I freaked out at Dr. White's office before like my sixth or seventh biopsy, and he and the PA walked into the room to find me standing on top of the exam table. A dear friend talked some sense into me, so I called Gary's office. They prescribed an antibiotic to rule out infection. He wants to see me before chemo on Tuesday. We'll find out more then.

On top of all that, we received news this morning that Rocco has a mouth full of cavities (Gammy took him because I was still in bed). I have many parental shortcomings, more than I would like to think I would have had if I'd stayed healthy (you follow?), but this could be the worst. It's not too early to cast your vote for me for 2012.

Mom of the Year, J

January 12, 2012

My brain is not working so well, and my body is definitely feeling this third week of chemo, especially today (Thursday), but ... great news from Gary! My current symptoms are due to an infection in my breast, NOT rapid metastasis. Thank God.

More great news: on Tuesday, GJG was able to provide additional financial assistance to another wonderful family. Thank you for helping us to continue to support families who need to focus their resources on beating breast cancer.

Lots more to write, but my brain is shutting down. I'll try again soon.

January 20, 2012

Another crazy week, Pagani style. The weekend started off with a bang, several really. The demo of my upstairs bathroom started and finished this weekend. Wow! I am CRAZY excited! My dream of a sanctuary space, something calming, restful, inspiring, and beautiful, is underway! Good bye, '60s/'70s hideousness and yucky, moldy nooks and crannies. Hello, spa-like bathroom that I can see and appreciate from my bed, and of course, savor while using. It's totally indulgent, I know, but it was a daily buzzkill, trying to focus on living and healing and keeping my mind and body in the fight while looking at the gross, crowded, icky room. A huge thanks to everyone who is helping make this happen! It is a beautiful, beautiful gift and puts a big smile on my face every time I think about it or sneak a peek at the progress. The work is going by so very quickly, and it has been really wonderful getting to know the contractors who are helping this dream become reality. Plus, the anticipated finishing date is only like two weeks away. Awesome!

The boys had Martin Luther King Jr. Day off, so they went with me to my early morning echo. They did great at CMC. They even got a little face time with the lovely RN and MD, who had not seen them since I was originally diagnosed (Luca was three months old, and Rocco had just turned two). Then the day wrapped up with a couple of birthday parties. So much for a holiday; Rocco was so tired the next morning that he was literally dragging his feet. Some yelling ensued when he refused to run and insisted on walking slowly up the street while the bus waited on him. He finally got on the bus and then refused to look at me when they drove away. Nice. I fumed for a bit and fantasized of buying a cattle prod (had the old *Guadalcanal Diary* song in my head all day) but I got over it pretty quick. Life's too short. I was a bit giddy when I dropped Luca off at school, thinking I had a day to myself, but I had this nagging feeling I was forgetting something. I gave the calendar a quick look and realized I had to go to CHOA to get Herceptin. Damnit! I am not feeling the weekly treatment deal. What kind of off week is that?

Joe's been out of town for work since Wednesday, so I've been single momin' (with some grandma assistance, of course) all week. All the wake ups, bed times, late night get-ups are exhausting. On Tuesday, at three o'clock in the morning, Rocco woke up to go potty, and Luca decided he had to go, too. Rocco made it there first, so a very angry Luca proceeded to wet his underwear and then ball them up, dripping wet. He then threw them at Rocco's face while he was still on the can. Don't mess with Luca late at night. There's also trash duty, doggy duty, laundry, meals … the list goes on. It is exhausting, especially since my bone marrow is always suppressed for my "week off." I have no idea how single women in treatment do it! But thanks to your generosity and compassion, GJG is able to make it a bit easier for a few.

On Thursday, we had the first of Rocco's dentist appointments. Rocco was very apprehensive, cried, and had a million questions when I let the news of his appointment slip at the bus stop after school on Wednesday, so we ended the school day the way we started it: with plenty of attitude and tears. But he did great. The doctor, who's great, was going to do a kiddie root canal, but they ended up having to pull the tooth because it was a bit loose. We've still got two more appointments to go to (Rocco doesn't know). But I am sooooo glad we had this taken care of and that I was able to be with Rocco for the whole procedure. Being there is what mom's do.

Today, the boys both went to school (gasp!), and I've got to catch up on my rest and my chores. I can't believe it is another long weekend! I better scoot—this house is not going to straighten itself.

January 27, 2012

*A*nother Thursday behind me, thank God. I'm off to a bit of a wobbly start today, but that'll be behind me in a few hours. I get a transfusion later today. I'm so ready to have some pep in my step (to hang with my boyz), some energy to go along with my intent to get off the couch, and some coherent brain cells to get a few things done. After two Virgin Mary's, I should be well on my way. Cocktail hour starts early this weekend.

February 5, 2012

*I*t's been a good week! The transfusion made a HUGE difference in my energy level, mindset, and just my life in general. Despite chemo Tuesday, we still have packed a lot in: playdates, lunch and dinner(s) with friends, basketball (Rocco scored again), and continued home improvement.

My dream bathroom is almost done! Initially, I was not going to peek, but I decided that life's too short. Why wait until the blossoms are in full bloom before you stop to smell the roses? I wanted to enjoy the whole transformation, and enjoy I have! Gone are the grimy nooks and crannies, the gold sparkle laminate, the horrible vanity. Gone is the extra stress it always caused me as I wondered what lurked in the corners and in the old pipes. Now it feels like the sanctuary I hoped it would: calming, beautiful, and oh so luxurious. The craftsmanship, style, and extraordinary attention to detail have yielded an amazing space. Stepping into the new bath is like taking a mini-vacation. Ahhhhh.

A big, huge hug and thanks to those of you who have worked so hard for helping to make this dream of mine happen!

Smiling, happy, and tired in a good way, Jen

February 10, 2012

*T*he one-two punch of my third week in a row of chemo and a new, raging, sinus infection have managed to knock me on my hiney. But, I am two days into some Augmentin, and I'm determined to feel better by tonight because it is the annual (and a Pagani first) Mother/Son Night at Rocco's school. This is no slack off, sit-back-and-watch affair. This is a full-on obstacle course, complete with a Velcro wall. Rocco told me Wednesday it is "game on" and that we'll probably win because he is "really fast" (and extraordinarily modest), and because I "used to do sports stuff." I will be "bringing it" no mattah what! Put me in, coach!

We did have an awesome first-time visit with our new "cousin," Bella. Gammy (and Papa) got a two-and-a-half pound bundle of puppy love and teeth. She is a Teddy Bear (half Shih Zhu, half Bichon Frise). She is a crazy little bundle, and we love her! Sophie loves her too and has been looking for her since Gammy left.

Have a great weekend!
-Jen

February 21, 2012

I feel strange, subdued, muffled—like I'm observing things from under water. It's not really too unpleasant; it's just weird. It's like I just woke up and a dream still has me under its spell, or I have a hangover that has yet to kick in. This has not ever happened on this chemo cocktail before. The side effects are generally not this noticeable yet. Maybe somebody spiked my punch? Guess we'll see ....

I finally got around to sending Joe some of my phone pictures to put online. Our favorites from last summer are of Rocco and Daddy together, Gammy and Papa in Colorado National Monument Park on the trip I took with them in October. There are also several pictures of my new bathroom, my newly-made and perfectly fab sanctuary room (my sanctum sanctorum, if you like), and a pic of Gammy and Papa's new baby, Bella. Precious.

If I'd had my act together a bit more (but alas, it was a stretch physically to even go), I would have taken some pictures of Mother/Son Night. It was totally fab. It was not what we expected. Rocco and I competed against each other, not against other mothers and sons. And even though Rocco spent more of his time running around with his friends than with me, I had a blast. There was a brief period of time when I misplaced the principal's son, though. He and Rocco are in the same class and big buds; he always calls me Rocco's mom despite my repeated attempts at trying to get him to call me by name. I cannot wait to go back next year!

For those of you going to the poker tourney tomorrow night, I hope you have some big fun.

Goodnight,
-J

FEBRUARY 29, 2012

I've been living the soccer-mom dream this week! On Monday, Rocco had his first practice of the season, and last night was Luca's very first practice, of any kind, ever. He loved it—pure boy bliss! There was running, shooting, throwing sand, tackling (he can't wait for football) with two good buds from school and a whole host of new friends. Daddy and Rocco played soccer and football on a field nearby, and I sat, watched, and chatted. It was heaven! It was the actualization of a milestone I had dreamt of for years and one I thought I might not get to see. Thank you, God. Thank you for answering that simple, beautiful, perfect prayer.

I was supposed to be post-chemo last night, but I wasn't. I went in, got stuck, was ready to go, and then that's when the subject of my latest and rapidly progressing side-effects came up. The end result was an unscheduled visit with Gary and one week off so I can heal up a bit; and then I'll be back at it. He told me not to fret and to enjoy this time, and that is my plan.

In addition to the above gifts, we've been blessed with a few others this past week as well. The All In for a Cure Poker Tournament was a huge success! Beau coup thanks to our supporters and volunteers! The GJG Foundation will use the money raised to provide financial assistance to local, in-need survivors immediately. We also went with the boys to the Checkers Pink in the Rink game on Saturday night. It was totally great. We LOVE to go to Checkers and Canes games. Hockey and SEC football are hard to beat for excitement!

Well, I've got to go make Luca's lunch. Have a great week. And for those of you south of the Mason-Dixon, go enjoy out and our early spring.

March 6, 2012

I followed Gary's advice last week. I sucked the marrow out of each day. To most, my week would have appeared mundane, tedious even, but to me, it was heaven. I did all the bus stop waiting and school drop-offs and pick-ups. I took Luca to the doctor. I did all the laundry. I reveled in some serious yard work: I am a bonafide kudzu-killing momma. 'Twas good, hearty, sweaty, tiring, gratifying work. It was glorious to let my body work hard. I caught some rays. I played some soccer and shot hoops. We ate out (twice!) and had family movie night. We went ice skating, which is my new, very favorite activity—the freedom, speed, and thrill make my heart sing. I danced around the house, disco tunes in my head, because I felt good. I did not ponder death, time, existence, or God.

It was so hard to go back today. I did not want to. It wasn't a rage-filled ride downtown or anything; it was more like a slow march toward the inevitable. Luckily (both bad and good luck, I think), Gary thought I was ready to get back at it. There was visible progression, so I knew the party had to end, but I just wasn't ready to leave the ball, wasn't ready for the illusion to end. It didn't help that it was jam packed and that I had to wait two hours to even get a seat in the infusion room. The cancer business, unfortunately, is booming. But the nurse sped up all my drip rates so I could make Luca's practice. It did not feel too good going in, but I made it. I got to practice fifteen minutes early and sat in the lot. I watched rays of light play off a car. I could see each ray as an individual beam of energy; some were visible for three feet. It was way cool, and it made me wonder how much we all miss in our daily lives. There are so many gifts, ours for the taking, if we just slowed down a bit.

While I sat, I flipped down the mirror and looked rather closely at myself. I wanted to see what my own sorrow looks like. It is so different from grief, a subtle change around the eyes, a dimming of the light within. But perhaps it was not an honest look, for I did not weep. I felt like crying then, and I still feel it now. I am mourning the loss of the old, carefree me, the one that felt good and strong, that wrestled (I'm talking about the G-rated kind) with my husband, sang loud in the shower, and danced naked around the house. The brief return to my old self was oh, so beautiful, but it makes the return to my cranky, tired, side-effected self a more difficult adjustment.

-Jens (both old and new)

March 13, 2012

I fell on dark days last week following chemo. Reality seemed just a bit too heavy. I needed to succumb to the load a bit and to acknowledge and wallow in my exhaustion, fear, and worry. With my wallowing done, I was ready by Friday evening (after dealing with two slightly hysterical, weepy, over-tired boys, a clogged potty, and locking myself out of the house...) to resume carrying my load without too much complaint. I always complain some; I figure it's my God-given right as a female.

On Saturday morning, I woke up and felt stronger but was surprisingly shaky with an undercurrent of emotion. A day had arrived (one that most parents don't really think twice about) that I had longed to see and prayed to be a part of for a few years now. It was Luca's very first team game (and it happened to be soccer, which was a huge bonus!). 'Twas a day I had been dreaming about for a long time; a hope made into reality.

We managed to get to the game on time (but with no minutes to spare, of course) despite being a man down (Joe's still out of town). The weather was glorious: crisp and cool with bright blue skies. It was totally perfect. The game was surprisingly thrilling, especially for four- and five-year-olds. Luca was the fastest guy on the field. He managed dribbling, kicking, stealing, and throw-ins, all with skill and focus. The kids were engaged and both sides took multiple shots at the goal. There were surprising breakaways and lots of goalie saves. It was fantastic! I could not bridle my excitement or enthusiasm! A referee walked over and asked if I was the coach. He said he liked my energy and enthusiasm. I literally could not help myself from sideline coaching, but our actual coach said he did not mind and welcomed the positive input. Who knows, maybe he just wanted to humor me. But I felt like I had just witnessed the US win a World Cup match (obviously, the US women's team, but that goes without saying). And Luca was all excitement and smiles. I rode the high all the way to the lake, where we had a perfect "lakation." The glorious weather continued, and we did it all with Gammy and Papa. There was football, sunning, fishing, romping with the dogs, and a delicious meal at the North Harbor Club. You name it, it was all good!

In the midst of this wallowing and then reveling, I managed a couple of meetings for the GJG Foundation. Yay! And speaking of the Foundation, we are thrilled to announce that the Charlotte Catholic Boys and Girls Lacrosse teams are going to be raising money for Go Jen Go this season! The girl's LAX team is sponsoring a dollars-for-goals drive, with pledges collected at the end of the season for each goal scored. This is fantastic, especially because they rock! And the boys are holding a BBQ this Monday the 19th at CCHS from five o'clock to eight o'clock, before the games. The boys will be in pink, and all proceeds going to GJG are in honor of Anna Strassner, a mother of one of the LAX Varsity girls currently undergoing breast cancer treatment. Our family will be there! Please stop by and join us, grab some good grub, and help us support their efforts to aid Go Jen Go in providing financial assistance to local, in-treatment, in-need women! It'll be yummy, big fun!

Thanks!
-Jen

March 16, 2012

Rated PG-13 for craziness

It will probably take me an hour to write this. I need lots and lots of time to unexpectedly stare blankly at nothing.

My hemoglobin has apparently dropped very noticeably overnight. I am lurching around the house, can't seem to get my legs under me, and I'm in a semi-stupor. It is taking me unbelievably long to do anything, that is if I manage to even try. And I am trying. I've gone from the bed to the kitchen to the couch twice now! I am surrounded by coffee cups (only thing keeping me going at all), four water bottles (I've got to stay hydrated), and several bloody paper towels that I keep balling up and stuffing in my nose, which keeps on trying to bleed. I had a very interesting thought—to me anyway, or maybe I thought it was good just because I followed the thread all the way from one end to the other without interruption—that it is a good thing that iron oxidizes in air because fresh blood is a really beautiful, captivating color, and who knows what lengths humans would have gone to get it if it did not fade into rust.

I am "working" to the best of my current ability (and my current best leaves a lot to be desired), with a lot of help from some good peeps, on some GJG collateral (bank talk for handouts and stuff). I am having a hard time with basic computer functions, like opening files. It goes like this: I'll recall I have a certain tidbits of information, I'll search three places on the computer for them, I'll get distracted by nothing or something, and then ten to twenty minutes later, I finally find said file or a promising one, and I open it. But it opens to nothing, which is a mystery to me. Where did it go? Do I dare touch those icons in the bottom corner to look further? To do so in this state is to risk permanent screw up. Stare blankly. Repeat ....

And I'm back. It's like I took a monster bong hit this morning, and my brain went on a vacay. It's not really a bad feeling. If ignorance is bliss, can't stupidity be too? And aside from a headache, the occasionally racing heart, and some tremors (not unusual), it's really kind of pleasant even.

The good news is I am scheduled for a transfusion in a couple of hours. The good juice hits fast. I will be able to focus my intent and enthusiasm on sideline coaching just in time for tomorrow's soccer games. I have a loud voice, and I get excited...but it is all positive, all good.

It really has taken a bit over an hour to write this. I should go. It will take me forever to get dressed before my friend drives me to the transfusion. Last night I had planned to drive myself, but this morning it became obvious quickly that was not a viable possibility. Don't want to get a DUIOLH on the way in. That's "Driving Under the Influence of Low Hemoglobin," for you non-cancer people.

March 21, 2012

*A*s last week marched on, I was physically hitting bottom. The transfusion Friday afternoon came just in the nick of time. I had to stay sitting in a chair alone (except for two friends for the first couple of hours). I got rather depressing as afternoon turned to evening. By the time Joe, the boys, and Sophie came to pick me up at 7:40 p.m., I felt physically like a new person but was emotionally worn thin.

I woke up Saturday feeling pretty good. Soccer was fun (Luca scored two goals), but the boys played on adjacent fields at the same time, so it was a little harder to relax and follow. We promised the boys more ice skating (okay, it was more like Rocco and I really wanted to go). Our plan was to go Sunday morning, but the rink wasn't open for public skating then, so we ended up going Saturday night. It was big fun once again. Rocco now wants to play hockey, and who knows, maybe he can this fall if he keeps improving; he's certainly got the temperament for it. He was seriously working hard and trying to count laps. Luca spent a lot of time on the sidelines pouting, but after an hour of us largely ignoring him and having fun, he went around quite a few times with Joe. I spied on the old guys (my age and older) who obviously grew up playing hockey, tried my hand at mimicking some moves, and tried to figure out weight distribution, balance, and power. The freedom and effortlessness that happens when it all clicks is heaven. There are so many parallels between swimming (my true love, God, how I miss it) and skating. I think I am falling in love ....

Okay, so I totally overdid it Saturday (and Monday). But it was okay. With the transfusion, I knew I would recover, and I did. I've got to grab for the ring while I can. The blood makes the difference in my just existing and my living. What a gift. Donate if you can!

Monday night was the Catholic HS LAX BBQ/Girls Home Opener, and it was a great event! There was a huge turnout. There were lots of peeps in GJG shirts, and lots in the new Pink LAX shirts sold for the fundraiser. How incredible that they should choose to support Go Jen Go Foundation! The funds raised from events like this one help GJG provide financial support to more in-need families. We are currently providing monthly support to four families at this time, but lots more need our help now. If you have an opportunity or an idea for a fundraising event to benefit our Foundation, please let us know!

I had a great time meeting and mingling with the parents and kids. The spirit of caring and community is so evident within this Catholic HS group, the kids, parents, and coaches alike. It is quite moving to see their compassion in action.

WSOC-TV was there too. And despite reluctance on both our parts, Anna Strassner and I were interviewed. I think they got some great shots of the kids in, too. Set your TVs to tape tomorrow night on Channel 36 at 11:00 p.m.!

Night,
-Jen

April 1, 2012

Start of Week Two of the Unofficial Pagani Three-Week Spring Break
Episode: What the Heck Happened Last Week?

O kay, in hindsight, I've been burning the candle at both ends for a while
now, which is perhaps not the best policy for someone in my shoes,
but I don't need a lecture, I need a freaking cure. Preferably a cure that
actually makes my disease go away permanently, not one that holds things in
semi-check while I pray and limp along until the next breakthrough comes
down the pike. Cue the violins. To quote Joe Walsh, "I can't complain, but
sometimes I still do." Plus, I can only sit in time-out for so long before I
go as crazy as one of my kids (yes, I'll really go that crazy). Now though,
the only things burning are my lungs (due to pollen, I hope) and maybe my
lower back a bit. I am aching everywhere. I feel like I fell off the roof, which
I did not, by the way. I haven't been stranded up on my roof in at least
two years.

Last Sunday, Luca came down with the high fever that was going around,
and he missed a few days of school. Thank God the rest of us dodged that
bullet. But I was already physically beaten down and my soul tender to
the touch by the time my chemo appointment rolled around on Tuesday.
Luckily, I managed to wrangle a last-minute counseling session on the
way to see Gary. My counselor did my heart and soul better, but my body
was still dragging. I did not feel like I could withstand treatment, neither
physically or emotionally. Usually, I can suck it up, get back on the horse,
put my nose to the grindstone, and get through another one. But not this
past Tuesday. It turned out that Gary and the nurses could see it on my face,
hear it in my voice, and of course, read it in my long list of notes about side
effects that I am required to keep for the study. To my surprise and disjoy
(that is dismay and joy all at the same time), he gave me another one-week
siesta from all three of my cancer drugs. Wow! Sounds great, right? Not. I
got the week off because I need to heal. I need a week at the Well, need to
flee to the ends of the earth, sit alone in the unmoving and quiet, and find
that place deep within myself that gives me the strength and courage to
continue treatment without an end, without a cure. I resolved to do this at
home, to find peace amidst the storm, to find my strength and solace in my
own backyard. I planned to find it despite seeing the slow creep of disease
the "vacay" allows.

Instead, Rocco came down with croup. I felt progressively worse (this happened the first bit of the last time I had the week "off"). We all got slammed, are getting slammed, by all the pollen. I usually feel better after a "workout" (sometimes it is just a slow walk around my neighborhood), but I am feeling more and more beat up, shaky, and sore. I am not sure what this means. Of course, I can't help but go *there*. Are the cumulative effects of the multitude of aggressive treatments during the last five years (five years will be in August, so humor me) finally breaking me down irreversibly? Or has this week been the perfect storm for kicking my ass? I don't know. Gary wants to see me Tuesday, and I'm not sure if he'll treat me or not. I should be feeling good by now, but I seem to be heading the wrong way ... and now Rocco is officially on Spring Break (Luca is not off until next week). Awesome sauce.

If you have made it this far, you are a trooper.

Thank you.

APRIL 9, 2012

I'm in the Sanger Heart Failure Clinic waiting room at CMC, awaiting my usual three-month echo. They are busy post-holiday, and it looks to be mainly other women on Herceptin here. I'm guessing chemo will be positively slammed tomorrow. It was light last week.

Speaking of last week, I am still recovering. On Sunday and Monday, I had a fever/virus. My chest X-rays showed bronchitis but no pneumonia, which I knew, but I guess Gary needed to be absolutely certain. On Tuesday, I was much improved, so I got chemo, and Gary was even pleased that we did not see too much spread during my hiatus. On Wednesday, I felt good enough to go on a walk with a friend, but went to bed not feeling well. Rocco came in at 3:30 a.m. because he'd had a nightmare, and I woke up to a fever of 103.3 degrees. On Thursday, my fever was 104 degrees around 10:00 a.m., so I went to the ER feeling wretched and ready to be admitted. I got fluids and antibiotics, another chest X-ray, blah, blah, blah. I practically ran (well, it was more of a slow roll) out the door that evening. On Friday, I did not get off the sofa until the evening when we shot some fireworks, thanks to a friend. The boys loved it! On Saturday, we made it to the annual Easter Egg Hunt and more fireworks. On Sunday, the bunny came with two goldfish for the boys, and we made it to Gammy and Papa's for the whole day. It was good.

I am currently on two oral antibiotics to make sure nothing else pops up. I hope nothing does. This morning, I woke up exhausted out of a telling dream. In the dream, I was constantly under pressure to do things, different types of things, but I had a very, very heavy load to carry. My bag was overflowing, and I was constantly having to stuff things in it. People were urging me on, but I knew that I could not shoulder the burden, do what was expected, get where I was supposed to be. Not the best way to wake up.

April 11, 2012

*M*y husband is amazing!

Last night after chemo, a big group of us (Joe, Gammy, the boys, Juju, Joe's brother Christopher, our sister-in-law Michelle, Britt Yett, Matt Matone, and Wendy Bentien, and I) went to the Komen Reception 2012. The event was inspirational and beautiful, and was held at the Uptown Charlotte Mint Museum. They honored volunteers, board members, grant winners, and survivors and their families. All the people who make such an incredibly positive impact on local survivors and make up the heart and soul of our local Komen chapter were honored, which according to the National Komen Board Members present last night, is one of the strongest in the entire nation.

Joe was honored as the 2012 Annual Co-Survivor of the Year! He was chosen for his selfless, unwavering, loving support of my sons and me during these five years, the stresses of which would have torn many families apart. Divorce during cancer treatment is not that uncommon, and I recall when I was getting diagnosed, one of my oncologists asked if I had a strong relationship with my husband; and at the time I found that a most perplexing question. But not only does Joe go to the ends of the earth for us, he does it every time we get a phone call about a woman or family in need, too. He is the driving force behind the Go Jen Go Foundation. He goes to bat for these families, hard and immediately. He gets utilities turned back on, coordinates with social workers, writes checks to pay rent and phone bills, finds out whatever these families need, and gets those needs met to the best of the Foundation's abilities. He is passionate, frequently teary eyed, and deeply committed to helping people with nowhere else to turn.

He does all this quietly, proficiently, without complaint, and whenever the need arises. He puts his own needs aside, and the needs of us and these other families first. He never ceases to amaze me in this. His commitment never waivers.

I am so indescribably proud of him. I love him deeply, and I thank God he is mine.

-Jen

APRIL 20, 2012

I need some extra prayers. I have not recovered from the last month of sickness and spring breaks, life and chemo. Or perhaps it is the last five years of treatment? Five years of fighting every single day.

I look fairly normal on the outside. I can even still manage to function in my life some, and by all outward appearances, I look and seem relatively okay doing it. But on the inside is another story. On the inside, I feel differently than I ever have before. I feel used up, like there's almost nothing left. Like another, even minor, health setback might derail the whole system, and create a fatal error. My body has never felt like this before—undermined, vulnerable, weak. I am not sure what to make of it. I don't know if it is a natural progression, my body finally giving in, or if it is the fallout from all my illnesses of late coupled with the weekly chemo that never, ever lets me get my feet back under me before it strikes again.

Either way, I don't feel as if this is going to be a quick recovery. I worry it is the beginning of a downhill slide. I am not sure exactly how long or what I need to recover from, but I am fairly sure whatever I do won't be enough. I feel that in the core of my physical being, not so much in my mind. My mind is still hoping for some kind of miraculous turnaround before the whole system shuts down.

Time, I suppose, will tell.

APRIL 22, 2012

*A*pparently, a soccer game and a half was my limit Saturday. I was over-served. Halfway through the second game, I finally cracked under the strain of these last years. A totally normal parenting challenge (Luca had a meltdown while in the goal and came off the field, crying) sent me over the edge. There was no coming back this time. It took all I had not to lose it in front of the boys, in front of everyone, right there on the sidelines. Sheer force of will kept the crying concealed (from the boys, not Joe, Juju, or Dad) until I got home. Then somehow, I kept it under wraps until both boys were out of the house. The levee gave way at approximately 12:40 p.m. Eastern Time.

I completely lost my shit.

It was not pretty. It was hopeless sobbing. It was anger. It was desperation; some of it still is. It was the anguished verbalization of things best only silently, fleetingly acknowledged, not said aloud. It was hell to spew forth. I would imagine it was even worse to hear.

It was a dark afternoon for both man and wife; both suffered and are suffering greatly. I was afraid to come downstairs after my nap. What is it like to gaze upon your soulmate after you have just crushed them? After you have taken their hope and optimism and replaced it with your futility, exhaustion, and sorrow? I was afraid. Not for me, but for him. What damage did I do? And what, God forbid, did I say that couldn't be unsaid?

He had left for a bit, I think. The house was silent at first. My fear grew. But in the basement, I found Joe playing Xbox games with Rocco. And Rocco was happy and excited (he had just gotten back from a laser-tag birthday party and then came home to shoot the airsoft gun with his Dad). Joe was, well, still Joe. He looked weary, and in his eyes I could see the price he paid for my breakdown. But he was still himself, still my husband. I apologized when I could muster the strength. I was still very tender and swollen-eyed myself. But he said there is nothing to forgive. It is the cancer, not me. And at that moment I marveled at his heart, his goodness, his unbelievable spirit in a way I never had before.

April 25, 2012

Hi Everyone,

Joe here. Jen asked me to post an update as she is purposely disconnected from all things electronic for a few days. She is getting some much-needed recharge time.

We wanted to give our heartfelt thanks to the outpouring of support we have received over the past five years, but especially over the past couple of weeks. They have been difficult, to say the least, as you all know.

Two very dear and giving families have shared their homes with us this week and a week in May to allow Jen to have a refuge. We have several other offers to help Jen get away, offers to take the boys, bring food, mow the lawn. The list goes on. We are so lucky to have so many wonderful people who care so much about our fight and our lives. I just can't say thank you enough. It is meaningful, and it is making a difference. And the everlasting help of Gammy and JuJu is vital to our mere existence, too.

I can tell Jen is already feeling better. The boys and I are driving down Friday morning to join her. And I can tell you, they cannot wait. Neither can I.

On another note, which I am sure Jen will expand on, the great people involved with All In to Fight Cancer handed me a large check for GJG yesterday from part of the proceeds from their fundraising efforts. I hope everyone will look for the event next year and throw some chips down to fight with us. Thank you.

So, look for our girl to be back to her fighting, feisty self next week, just in time for the next round of chemo.

We love you all.
-Joe

May 7, 2012

I arrived at the beach bloodied and broken, beaten, ready to accept defeat. But my time there was very healing. It brought me back from the brink, and back amongst the living.

The timelessness of the ocean, the infinite grains of sand, the blurring of the sky, sand, and sea on the distant horizon gave me inspiration and perspective. I did sun salutations alone at dawn. And I felt, for the first time ever, the tremendous energy of the waves and the sun and that it was mine for the taking. I filled my cup until it runneth over. I drank it in, soaked it up. I cycled leisurely on weak legs that grew stronger each day. I reveled in the soft, delicate beauty of the sea oaks and Spanish Moss. I feasted on the strength of the Low Country and did not find it lacking. I gained strength, restoration, and acceptance. Acceptance that I have perhaps entered a new chapter in my fight, that although I am rejuvenated, I am now no longer physically the same. Acceptance that while I stay on this regimen, on chemo, my life is greatly diminished, but it is still mine to embrace. Acceptance that the path ahead will be difficult no matter what way I turn.

I was ready when Joe and the boys came to join me there. We had a great time. I rested a lot, but we still had lots of fun family playtime. Both boys now love the beach, love to play in the sand and the surf, and they can play for hours. Gone are the days of packing for the beach only to return to the house thirty minutes later. Also, the weather agreed with us for a change: low humidity, breezy, not too hot. It was joyous perfection and just what we each needed.

Thanks to my restorative trip and my much needed break from chemo, I am participating in my life once more. Life is so much easier when I don't feel like shit all the time. We celebrated Luca's fifth birthday on Friday, and he had fab time at his party. We went to soccer games, out to dinner with friends, and even stopped by a get-together. It seemed a bit like a dream. Why can't my life, our lives, be like that all the time? Normal. I don't feel like it is asking too much. Acceptance is a bitch.

Tomorrow I am back at it. I see Gary at 11:30 a.m., and I'll have chemo after. Vacay time is over for me, and hopefully the cancer too. It looks like it enjoyed the time off as much as I did.

May 24, 2012

Posted from the Blumenthal Cancer Center Infusion Room

I am currently wrapping up a second unit of blood, and my brain is still struggling a bit, so I hope this makes sense! I'll be ready for the long weekend after this. The timing really couldn't be better. We are all very excited about the pool opening and are ready for some old school, family fun. Since my last post, so much has gone on. I feel less burdened with my fight. I needed to hear that we (Joe, Gary, and I) have the mutual goal of keeping me on this trial for as absolutely long as we can make the side effects livable and provide me with a good quality of life rather than just an existence.

I am now a happier, stronger version of myself. Gary marveled last week at my vibrancy and asked me what I was doing differently. I told him I had taken the "seize the day" advice to heart, and that I was taking every opportunity to pamper myself a bit. I've started yoga, got a haircut (I actually felt like I looked good, which is a big deal these days), got a massage, increased my house cleaning service from once a month to every other week, AND we just got back from the beach once again. It was glorious, cleansing, invigorating, restful, and fun. We have committed to having a fun activity/trip/whatever every couple of weeks as a "carrot" to keep me (and really all of us) focused on the positive and having fun rather than dreading, fearing, and mourning. I am now under Gary's orders to continue all these pursuits! Yes, you read it correctly: "UNDER DOCTOR'S ORDERS!"

We rolled back into Charlotte Monday just in time for Rocco's first swim team practice, a huge milestone (for me too!). It was an event I've dreamt of since I first held him in my arms. It was fantastic. I was so proud. He was a bit nervous, but he had fun and did really well. I decided not to cry. I still don't think about it fully, the emotion would overwhelm me.

I am going shopping tomorrow night with two girlfriends and then out to dinner, if I still have the juice, which, thanks to this transfusion, I just might have. Then it is a fun, relaxing weekend with all of my boys. Life to live! I can't wait!

MAY 31, 2012

Our weekend was beautiful and everything we hoped it would be. With Tuesday came a bit of a surprise. I went in to get my Herceptin IV, because it is my "off" week, and I found out I was due (surprise!) for chemo again because of my two-week respite a while back. Cue, animated discussion, time-line diagram, etc. The bottom line was this: I could refuse treatment, with consequences, but obviously, I did not. So instead of my "off" week, I got treated for the fourth week in a row, yuck. It's not been easy, but the well-timed transfusion last week has made it much more tolerable than I expected.

The change wreaked havoc on my schedule, because, had lots of great Rocco things (it's a big week for him) planned and two GJG Foundation meetings set up. Lots of guilt, frustration, and discussion later, I ended up basically forgoing all my plans and chose rest, a massage (I had that on the schedule already), and some yoga too. The yoga, by the way, is freeing. I expand and purge my mind and spirit as much as my body. 'Tis a beautiful thing that I'm starting to really crave to promote my recovery, restore my life force, and brighten my body. This morning, I woke up tweaky, jumpy, and uncomfortable in my own skin. I'm tired but restless, twitchy, pacing, volatile, and nuts. I felt like a junkie might. Yoga focused my mind on breathing and settled me down.

This afternoon, one of the things I had to miss was Rocco's first-time trial for swim team. For most (and Rocco was clueless about its significance), it's not a big deal, but for me, it is very exciting! I was set to be a volunteer timer and everything, but I didn't make it. I sat home sad and wondering how he was doing, what I was missing exactly. Then I received a couple of phone calls and text updates. It seems my little man was crushing it! He rocked the backstroke! Did well in the freestyle. What?! So many emotions at once flooded my soul. I just wanted to be there, to be part of the experience and to see the cute, funny things they do at that age, like the feet first "dive" off the blocks, the flailing arms, the stopping several times midway to lift their heads and empty their goggles. I had no expectation of an awesome swim performance. I boo-hoo'd. The yoga is actually really purging, because I was startled when my tears ran down my face and into my mouth but did not burn my checks or taste like acid—they tasted like tears, amazing really. This disease sucks! I miss so much now. How many beautiful moments will I miss out on in the future too? More boo-hooing. I tried to feel it all a bit and not stuff it back down. Be present in the moment and all that. Acknowledge, feel, and move on. Done.

Got to scoot, boys to see!

-J

June 29, 2012

Summer vacation's been flying by at warp speed. I can't believe how long it's been since my last post. The swim team finished last night and was glorious—big fun for all of us! We couldn't have asked for a better experience. Rocco looks like a totally different boy in the pool now; it must be the coaching (the assistant coaches are hands on and enthusiastic, and the head coach has an Olympic gold medal), and hopefully it has a bit to do with his genes too. Luca has turned into a fish, as well. He decided about two weeks ago that he can swim under water; and now he swims all over the place, and we don't even have to be in the pool with him! He's starting to do some freestyle and backstroke on his own too. Sweet! We've been savoring our pool time and managed to squeeze in lots of it despite my chemo schedule. I've even been back in the pool swimming laps (after a one-year absence). It makes my heart sing. The past month has been a sweet summer dream come true.

We (okay, maybe mainly me) are super psyched about the Olympic Trials, and I can't wait for the games to start. The stories of the athletes and the para-athletes are very inspiring. They remind me to suck it up and keep working hard toward my goal: living a full life despite disease and treatment. I LOVE the overcoming-the-odds stories. They really get me motivated.

We're having oodles of fun, but I still hit the occasional rough patch. The reality of constant (if I'm incredibly lucky and the study drug keeps working, or if I'm even luckier still, and a new, good trial comes out that I qualify for) treatment overwhelms me from time to time. Basically, it sucks. And cancer continues its destruction in the lives of our friends and family.

Thank you for reading, praying, and supporting us! Stay cool if you can this weekend, and cheer those athletes on!

-Jen

July 10, 2012

I don't believe it, the weather broke before we did, but it was a very close race. Swim team ended a week ago, which, unfortunately for all of us, left Rocco with lots of energy to retaliate in response to all of Luca's provocations (he's our provocateur). 'Twas a bit of a long, hot week. Add in an ultrasound, echo, Herceptin, an impromptu fireworks party the kids organized, late bedtimes, two back to back Fourth of July pool parties, and then rushing off to fireworks. As for that impromptu fireworks party—they came up with idea, posted a sign, went around and invited all the neighbors, and Rocco told me to "put snacks all over the house." I was tickled by their enthusiasm and creativity, so I humored their efforts; but folks showed up, and it turned out to be rather fun.) The result of all the excitement this week was some serious, post-fun crankiness for kids and parents.

That brings us to Thursday morning. Throw in more activities (have fun, damnit!) and weather so hot that even my kids refused to go outside or to the pool, and we proved that too much of a good thing, is, well, just too much.

My decision to keep the boys home as much as I could this summer so I could spend time with them was a great one at the time (I decided that in the spring when it was like twenty degrees cooler). But let's face it, that time is long past. We've had our fun. Time for camp! Mommy needs some peace and quiet.

I've got to scoot, swim team banquet to attend.

-J

P.S. Due to post-chemo technical difficulties, I didn't manage to post this before the banquet, but it was fun, and Rocco won Most Improved! Yay!

July 20, 2012

Last week, to paraphrase the Andy Grammer song, the heavy colors fell on me, the blues, the grays, the black. I was not in the mood for much of anything, so I spent lots of time staring but not seeing the TV, depressed and angry in that weird, uncomfortable-in-my-own-skin feeling. I took solace in eating anything salty and/or chocolatey or basically anything not nailed down. And to top it all off, I have apparently also been suffering from delusions in addition to the anger/depression. I had fooled myself into believing that the increase in size around my mid-section was due to swelling from my inflammatory disease, not because I was stuffing my head into the Nutella jar to lick the last delicious bits out. I hopped on the scale before treatment Tuesday (as if getting chemo isn't punishment enough) and I've gained almost five pounds. Grrrrr! The icing on the cake(s), so to speak. If I was a masochist, I could schedule chemo (and its inevitable weigh in), scan results, and trying on bathing suits all in one gloriously anxiety-and-suffering laden day. I'll never be a masochist.

My body feels weird, kind of toxic (food choices?), my hemoglobin is hovering just above my transfusion point (which makes me dark and stupid, not a good combo), and my disease is visibly spreading. Stressful times. I've got scans in two weeks to rule out any distant spreads. But at some point, we'll have to make the call about when to ditch this trial. The good news is, another drug just came off trial last month that would be an option for me. It's unbelievable timing, and breast cancer research is an amazing thing! The down side: like a fool, I looked up the drug to see if it would be an easier regimen. Nope. And I saw that it provided, on average, six months of "progression-free survival time." Ugh! Why did I look? My optimism bit me in the ass on that one. I guess I should stick with my normal "glass half-empty" outlook.

I'm currently out of carrots (fun travel to take my mind off the chemo/disease reality), and I'm trying to buckle down for what is usually my least favorite time of the year—late summer. The drippy dew points, the oppressive heat, the bored kids, the beaten down/browned-out foliage. Yuck, I hate it all. I long for cool, wet weather, the need for jeans and jackets, and I fantasize about snow. It's time to get a trip to a cool climate on the books for some renewal, rather than staying around here and getting hot and sticky.

For all my whining (it should dramatically decrease after I get a transfusion!), there is one cloud with a silver lining. The Go Jen Go Foundation has been busy providing financial aid to my fellow breast cancer survivors, helping to cover unexpected expenses, paying for gas to travel for out of town treatment, providing funds to help a family continue on Cobra, and helping cover the costs of medicine and coinsurance …. The Foundation is making a difference. WE, together, are making a difference! And we have several, very exciting fundraising events on the horizon! I'll keep you posted. Together we can make beating this disease a bit easier for our local, in-need women. Thanks!

July 25, 2012

I'm feeling rather like a truck ran over me, so I'll keep it short. On Saturday night, we survived Rocco's Skylander birthday party and a three hour onslaught of crazy boys. It was actually really fun.

Chemo came too fast again yesterday; the third week is always tough. Turns out, in addition to low hemoglobin, my labs are all out of whack as well. The good news is that I get blood Friday afternoon. Yay! I should be feeling a lot better by Saturday, so I can enjoy the family get-togethers planned for Rocco's (actual) birthday, and for cousin Parker too.

July 31, 2012

I've been off for a while, and I couldn't quite figure out why, but then it finally dawned on me. Tomorrow's a big day. It's the fifth anniversary of my diagnosis. Five years ago, everything changed, forever. And to top it all off, I've got scans in the morning. Lovely. I'm ready to get the day behind me and hopefully get back to counting my blessings instead of my losses.

August 2, 2012

Yahoo! Despite visible and palpable skin progression, my SCANS REMAIN CLEAN!!! Fantastic news! Now I just need to recover from the toll the last couple of weeks have taken. Thanks for holding me up with your prayers and good vibes.

Go USA!
-J

August 7, 2012

'It was a great appointment with Gary today! Despite a few spots on the move, he thought there were lots of visible areas of improvement. And the areas of pain in my left chest, side, and back were most likely caused by an infection, rather than spread. So, steady as she goes. We continue full speed ahead on my current trial! Yay!

It is also a very exciting time for the Go Jen Go Foundation! Our board has been working hard behind the scenes on ideas and strategies to further our mission, develop our community-friendly, interactive website, and plan for our future success. So many of you have expressed interest in the process and offered your assistance, and I am happy to say that we are ready for you!

At this time, we need to form committees for three very important GJG activities. We would like to have a Fall Fundraiser (this is time critical), a committee to handle our Holiday Giving, and a Spring 5K race. Make a difference in the lives of our in-need breast cancer survivors now. Be somebody; sign up with us!

THANKS! Jen

AUGUST 13, 2012

*B*ear with me, I'm pooped ... more to come later.

Abby Wambach (I'm a look-alike, or so I keep hearing), now that you've just won (um, watched on TV several times) the Olympic Gold Medal for Women's Soccer, what are you going to do? I'm (we, the Pagani's) going to Disney World! WOW!! We got "Disneyed" this weekend. At a family get-together for some of the Pagani birthdays (Joe and Tommy are both born on the same day, three years apart), we were presented with the most amazing, unbelievable gift: a trip to Disney World! Joe and I were, and are, blown away. The boys' reactions were somewhat underwhelming. They didn't quite get the gravity of the announcement at the time. I think Rocco asked for birthday cake immediately afterward, and Luca mentioned something about *Skylanders: Giants* (obsess much?). Why the luke (Luca, get it?) warm kiddie reception, you ask? Well, Joe and I might not have written the book on how to best parent, but we're both smart enough to know you don't foster and build the Disney-hype if there is no trip in the forecast. Well, now we've got a trip on the horizon, and after peeks at the parks and rides on the computer, and some time spent perusing a new *Plan Your Disney Trip* book, the boys have worked themselves into a frenzy. Today, we finally managed to get Luca out of the new Mickey T-shirt that he had refused to take off since the announcement Saturday night, and Rocco only parted with the Disney World trip book because we dropped him off at away camp this morning.

We are deeply touched, humbled, and very, very excited! Thank you all for giving us what is sure to be a Disney dream come true!

THANK YOU SO MUCH!!
-Jen, Joe, Rocco, and Luca

AUGUST 18, 2012

*B*ig bird's been fine at camp, or so we assume. It has been several days since our last update. The week's flown by, and its been fab spending time with just Luca. He's so sweet and silly and funny. We snuggled and cuddled and played. And of course, I had to watch him watching someone else play *Skylanders* on YouTube (yes, you read that right) and constantly comment on his progress, and "ohh" and "ahh" over various killer character attributes and leveling up "accomplishments" when he played. Okay, maybe some parts of the week were longish. But our one-on-one time was precious, rare, and it was sooo refreshing not to have to constantly referee the incessant sibling squabbling that constitutes the end of summer at our house.

We pick up Rocco tomorrow. I hope he's had a great week, had some incredible adventures, and made lots of friends. We'll know as soon as we see him. If camp didn't go as advertised (Mommy had to "sell" it a bit because he decided he didn't want to go as soon as we found out he got in), it will be immediately obvious, and we'll probably pay for weeks. The kid can hold a grudge with the best of them. Despite his blond hair, blue eyes, and ridiculously long, blond eyelashes, thick Italian blood courses through his veins. He is so feisty (to put it mildly). And when Rocco hears that his brother, whom he apparently threatened with death, played *Skylanders* in his absence, there could be real hell to pay! Luca confessed to me that this was whispered to him in the camp drop-off parking lot during the thirty seconds I left them in the car alone to see where to head for check-in. Ahhh, regular family challenges are (somewhat) refreshing for a change!

In spite of the sweet time with Luca, this week's been a bit rough mentally. I just finished a round of antibiotics for bronchitis, had chemo, a day or so of "reprieve," and then went straight into a raging sinus infection that has left me weak, exhausted and very, very, very tired of constantly being sick. I HATE being sick on the days I'm supposed to be "well," according to my chemo schedule! Those days are so precious, damnit, and we always plan to do things on my good days. I miss too much as it is. Now, my body aches everywhere, my chest hurts (from disease and coughing), and it has been quite hard keeping "my ears stiff." I continue to watch new disease spots popping up weekly all along my left chest, abdomen, and side. Cancer totally sucks. Treatment sucks too. Yikes! I'm getting whiney ....

But on the flip side, there have been a few carrots out there helping me to soldier on:

1. The Disney Trip. It has been dreamy planning all the fun we are going to have, and I cannot wait to see the awe on the boys' faces as they experience it all! That's been amazing to focus on, and I've just got to get through two more months of treatment.

2. The new, fabulous Go Jen Go site is live (still needs a bit of tweaking), and it is AWESOME!! We will be able to make even more of an impact in the lives of our local and in-need breast cancer survivors

and their families. That definitely lifts me up! Check out our website, and join our team for the Komen Race. The support, love, generosity, and compassion surrounding the race always lifts my spirit. Just six weeks or so until that ....

So for now, I'll just have to be content with my antibiotics and heating pad. I'll keep calm and carry on, and I'll keep reminding myself to savor all the sweet little moments and to focus on the carrots.

AUGUST 31, 2012

It was looking doubtful there for a while, but I made it! I made it through the end-of-summer doldrums (the humidity, mosquitos, and uber-bored kids), past the intense pop-up storms (mainly of the sibling variety), the continual chemo beat-down (it's now my "off" week), and two sinus infections. Whew! This week I've been playing catch-up and savoring the delicious moments of quiet. Oh quiet, how I love thee. I just need a bit of extra rest before the chemo smack-down starts all over again next week. Rest, SEC football, maybe one last trip to the pool: just what the doctor ordered! Now, I'm looking ahead to October, some cooler weather, Komen, Disney, Halloween (a Pagani family fav!), and a girls' beach weekend. The view looks great!

Have a great weekend and stay out of the DNC traffic,
-Jen

Oh, by the way, Rocco loved camp. Thank God, grudge avoided!

SEPTEMBER 4, 2012

I'm sitting out on the porch in the semi-dark, bathed in the soft glow from the little white lights we have strung up out here, listening to the rain. It's soothing, nourishing, cleansing. I want it so badly to wash away the cancer from our lives and from the lives of others who suffer as well. I want it to restore life to those who have passed, heal bodies broken by treatment and disease, rinse away tears, mend broken hearts, wash away unbearable sadness and stress. If only life was so simple.

September 20, 2012

Bear with me, my brain's a mess ….

It's been two weeks since my last confession, I mean blog. Lots of the usual has transpired, plus Rocco was sick two separate times last week. Back-to-school germs stink. It's hard to have sick little peeps when I'm post-chemo.

'Twas a bit tired by the time we were able to go to the Carolina Breast Friends' Pink Boots Ball Saturday night, but Joe and I both had a great time! It's a fun, inspiring group, and I can't wait to do more with them, both as a survivor and a Go Jen Go Foundation board member. By the way, they are partnering with GJG this Christmas to help us fulfill Christmas wishes (and needs!) to even more local and in-need survivors and their families. Yay!

Sunday, following Saturday's Ball, we had a soccer game and did several hours of yard work ('tis the great monkey-grass transplantation of 2013). I felt dreadful, whooped, heavy. On Monday, I managed to get the kids to school and then came home, sat on my porch, and stared listlessly out the window. My chest felt very odd and heavy, and I felt nauseous with any physical effort. I was very much worried I might be getting Rocco's throw-ups. On Tuesday, I wasn't looking forward to chemo, especially since it was my third treatment for the month. I felt so wobbly and fuzzy headed that I actually got a ride to and from treatment, something I rarely do anymore, but I didn't think I could safely drive home. It was a smart move; I would hate to get a DUIC (Driving Under the Influence of Chemo).

My brain's weird, off. The lights are on, but nobody's home. I have done things I have no recollection of (like taking Rocco to the bus stop yesterday morning), said things I don't remember, and I oddly had two epiphanies, which I was going to share because they were brilliant, but I actually forgot them. I'll have to write 'em down next time.

But even in my odd little fog, I do remember this: I am thankful to be here, still here. There were women, at least two quite a bit younger than I am, that should have been present Saturday night but were not, because they had already lost their battles to breast cancer or were in the final stages of fighting.

October 4, 2012

The usual game plan for a Thursday following chemo is to rest, recover, and just get through the day. Today, though, I'm just home from getting scanned. Gary wants to rule out progression as the explanation for a few things that are going on. The wait begins. The fatigue, compounded by stress and chemo, is hitting now. The lower GI distress of two barium shakes followed by an oral chemo chaser will be in full swing this afternoon. Good times. Thank God I just adore my new bathroom!

I should have results by tomorrow this time, so hopefully the T-shirt Pick-Up Party and Race will be a clean-scan celebration as well.

October 5, 2012

Let's celebrate tonight! Scans show no disease in my abdomen or liver!! Wahoo! I still have some enlarged nodes they want to check on, so we'll do a biopsy, but not until after Disney (we leave the 13th! OMG). Gary felt totally good about waiting, which is good in my book.

It's time to celebrate life/survivorship and helping others at the GJG T-shirt Pick-Up and band party, the Komen race, and the Carolina Breast Friends Party at the Pink House post-race!

And then on Saturday night, pull for UGA as we face USC! It's going to be a tight game, and the Spurrier's are tough to beat. GO DAWGS!!!

Much love and many thanks!

Jen, Joe, Rocco, and Luca

October 7, 2012

I'm trying to write this right now while the boys are singing, dancing, and generally acting bananas about two feet away from me, so please forgive .... Friday's T-shirt Pick-Up Party was awesome!!! We had a huge gathering of family, friends, and neighbors, and I think we were in the neighborhood of 250 folks or so. It was fun, festive, and a great celebration of life, giving, and survivorship! The band, Grievous Angels, rocked and totally set the tone for the night. Our boys had so much fun running around—granted some of the fun including them scaring people while decked out in hockey masks and holding knives dripping with fake blood. A sweaty, drippy Rocco announced at ten o'clock that night that it was the most fun he had ever had! Wow! The 5:30 a.m. wake-up call came a bit early Saturday morning, but it was well worth it. The new location in Marshall Park added some confusion to the morning, but it was great! There was lots of room, pretty scenery, and a good vibe. Our team was treated to a flash mob—great stuff! The only flash mobs I had seen previously were on TV. We ran into DeAngelo too, and I was happily crushed in a big bear hug (it was worth it!). Apparently, he posted a picture of us together on his Facebook page.

It took an army of people to pull this weekend off. Thank you to each and all from the bottoms of our hearts. Together, we supported Komen in their quest for a Cure, and the Go Jen Go Foundation in our mission to prevent financial disaster following a breast cancer diagnosis and treatment. Joe and I humbly thank you from the bottom of our hearts! And to wrap up an already amazing weekend in style, we have been invited to join the Panthers on the field today for pre-game practice and then watch the game from a box on the fifty-yard-line! DeAngelo told me yesterday he thinks we might get to run through the tunnel! Not too shabby!! It can't get here soon enough. Luca has asked, "How much longer until we leave?" about ten times in the last hour!

Better scoot; I've got to squeeze in a rest/nap before we leave!
-Jen

October 9, 2012

The Panthers game was AWESOME!!! We were treated to an absolutely incredible day! We arrived at the stadium early, around 2:15 p.m. for a 4:00 p.m. game. Downtown was already buzzing with all the tailgaters. I forgot about all the fun things that go on around town all the time. We were checked in (along with lots of other breast cancer survivors and the families—it was an awesome surprise to see friends!) and came in through the office. With our special passes, we went right out onto the field and were allowed to meander and watch.

Awesome! We saw players warming up, the gear they have stowed away on the sidelines for the players and coaches, the chains (oops, stepped on one), massage tables, trainer stuff, the phone bank for coaches and officials, all up close and personal. The boys were star struck, overwhelmed, and clingy. They had a chance to be interviewed or just stand next to the sideline reporter for the NFL Channel, but they bashfully declined. That was odd for kids who never stop running, yelling, and talking about penises and poop all the time, but at least no one said anything about wanting lots of cats when they grow up.

I had the opportunity to meet some very cool peeps, and then we were shuttled to the tunnel where we met up with the other survivors, and it was a beautiful moment. To see my friends and fellow survivors there, like that, was beautiful! We ran through the tunnel onto the field. IT WAS AWESOME! We lined up along the sidelines for the National Anthem. We smiled and cheered and lived! The players almost ran us over when they came off the field. They are kind of amazing up close—beautiful, strong, sculpted, focused, full of life and strength—everything a cancer survivor strives to be. It was so touching to be supported like that, to see the players in pink. INSPIRING!

The box seats were SWEET!! It was an honor and an immense pleasure to be with these women and their families, most of whom I knew. It was just fantastic! Joe, the boys, and I had the best time. We were spoiled silly, and it was so much fun! Incredible, really! Our box was on the Panther Cam for a while on the big screen. And FOX featured a picture of DeAngelo and me (full screen for like ten or fifteen seconds! I'm a star, baby!) during their half-time report and also on the NFL's Breast Cancer Awareness Games. DeAngelo was instrumental in getting the program started. Go De!!

OCTOBER 12, 2012

I needed a day and a half doing the bed-to-sofa shuffle, but now I am ready to roll. Hysterically excited boys in bed, bags packed, electronics charged, pharmaceuticals at the ready. DISNEY in the morning!!! WAHOOO! We will be rocking at the House of Mouse! Thank you!

OCTOBER 15, 2012

I really thought I would have written by now, but honestly, since we landed in Orlando Saturday, we've been packing in the activities or sleeping. We are having the most fabulous time ever!!! We've done downtown

Disney, including the Lego Store, which Luca just informed us was his favorite part of the trip thus far, and we followed up with a meal at T-Rex, which was really quite incredible. The meal included lots of heaping plates of food paired with periodic live-action animatronic dinosaurs as the ice age comes to a screaming end. It was very exciting, like being in a movie, and it was great to watch the boys' faces as they took it all in (and of course, to sneak a few peaks at some full mouthed, slack jawed, adults too). Lots of entertainment!

Yesterday, we did Magic Kingdom with a guide. We did the whole park in one go. Uh-maz-ing!! Thanks to an energy drink, I did not nap until 4:00 p.m. It was crazy! We did every ride we wanted to, and we did a couple of them several times. Joe and I did Space Mountain, and it was fun and scary and made me feel like a child again. We ended our day at Mickey's Philharmonic 3D movie, and the boys went nuts. Luca was laughing and screaming and grabbing at stuff. I had a flashback of me on a mustard/brown and orange couch watching *The Mickey Mouse Show* reruns, and I remembered just how much I loved Donald (and used to love drinking his brand of OJ out of that big can you had to open with a can opener. Sweet memory lane and making sweet memories! Ahhh, a little slice of Disney Heaven.

Tomorrow, we will go to Animal Kingdom. Thus far, the view from our Animal Kingdom room includes giraffes, wildebeests, an impala, an ostrich, giant vultures, two enormous long-horned bulls, and a menagerie of other creatures—Spectacular! Then I will take a nap, we will have dinner at the Sci-Fi Dine-In Theater restaurant and then we'll trick-or-treat at Disney. I think Rocco and Luca hit the Superfecta. I will be managing my pharmaceuticals to achieve better living (i.e., get the through the day feeling good and having fun) through chemistry. Thank God for pills!

I am almost falling asleep writing this. Time to go. We can't wait for another adventure tomorrow!!!! Thank you again, everyone!!

OCTOBER 22, 2012

*O*ur trip was a dream come true. Actually, scratch that, it was better than anything we could have dreamed up! Our hotel in Animal Kingdom was perfection. We had two rooms; one for the snorer and the boys, and one for Mommy (a very light sleeper) to catch quiet naps and sleep at night without interruption. The rooms were adjoined by a living space/ kitchenette, and all three rooms were connected by a long balcony with close-up views of UH-mazing safari animals. A truly magnificent treat and a wonderful way to stay connected to nature on our trip through the manmade fantastic.

Our visits into Magic Kingdom were just that: magical. It reawakened the inner child in both Joe and me. And Luca and Rocco were delighted and completely spellbound. One of the best things I've ever witnessed is the looks on their faces as they took in the sights, or the looks of pure joy after they just finished a favorite ride, the type only kids are really capable of, the type not tempered by reality or reason. It was priceless, perfection. Thank you!!!

When we were strolling through Tomorrowland for the first time, I asked Luca what he thought about Disney. Did he like it? And he (in all his infinite five-year-old wisdom) said, with a look of unadulterated awe, "Mom, I just didn't know it was going to be like this!" Wow!! And Rocco, after viewing our first of three(!) fireworks shows said, "That was the best fireworks I've seen in years!" We hit most of the big rides and did The Barnstormer coaster like five times (Luca's favorite coaster … we'd finish it, and he'd run through the line wanting to do it again and again), and we played the Buzz Lightyear Space Ranger Shooting Game (Rocco's favorite) probably eight or nine times. Joe's favorite was the Expedition Everest coaster, which made Mommy nauseous for like three hours after riding it despite taking heavy duty anti-nausea meds. DinoLand was a great re-creation of a Route 66 amusement park, and the boys won stuffed animals for their skills (shooting water-guns and playing basketball).

We loved Animal Kingdom too. Both boys seemed just as fascinated by the safari tour as Joe and I did. I thought that was awesome, especially since getting back to nature (even if it is an incredible duplicate of a real African savannah) could be boring to some kids craving the frenzy of the other parks. I loved the re-creation of Asia too! A visit to the temples of Angkor were on my bucket list, but now I feel as if I can check that off the box. SWEET! We (okay, maybe just me) loved the huge flying fox and fruit bats (they had a wingspan of five to six feet), and I thought it was rather amusing that the big male hanging literally fifteen feet from the viewing stand (not glassed in) was meticulously cleaning his "boy parts" the entire time we observed him. It was just like having an upside-down flying dog, and I love dogs!

We met and had pictures taken with Mickey, Minnie (Luca refused to do this part though), Donald, Pluto, and Goofy in Epcot!!! Luca and I love Donald the best! Rocco loves Mickey, and Daddy loves Goofy. We rode the "Big Ball" twice. The boys loved it because it used photos it took of you in animated, future concept cartoons that you could then email to yourself. They are hilarious and somewhat reminiscent of Tom Bergeron's head pasted on someone else's body on *America's Funniest Home Videos*. Brilliant. We had a superb dinner at the German Pavilion and loved the Oompah band show! Fireworks that night over the lake were incredible too.

I suppose I could go on and on. It was the most amazing, thoughtful, precious gift. Thank you!!!!

Our most grateful and humble thanks,
-Jen, Joe, Rocco and Luca

October 24, 2012

Well, I'm ready to run back to the fantastic House of Mouse. Reality sucks sometime. This week has been shitty. A friend of mine passed away at home Monday morning. She left behind two beautiful daughters, a devoted husband, and scores of people who were amazed and inspired by her beautiful spirit, never ending faith, and positive outlook despite five years of progressing cancer. I have been grieving a lot for her and her family. It is just so damn sad.

Yesterday morning, Dr. White shocked me a bit when he said he was certain that my nodes were cancerous. Great way to start the day. I went from the procedure to chemo and burst into tears the second I walked in the infusion room; my grief hit me like a tidal wave. The staff were all emotional too. She was well loved by all and was an old timer like me. Tough, long day.

A bit ago, I got the call confirming the nodes are positive for disease. This will be considered my first, official, distant metastases (not a first I was hoping for). The rest of the disease on my chest, arm, and back is all considered local-regional, not that the semantics really matter at this point.

Joe and I picked Gary's RN brain yesterday in anticipation of a bad biopsy result. I have one new (as of August of this year!) treatment option available. It is a chemo cocktail that I'll get every three weeks. Yay! I hate going weekly. I will probably have one icky week followed by two pretty good weeks (as long as I can stay healthy in between treatments). It will include the usual side effects and no hair, which bothers the boys a lot, and therefore, it bothers me. It also makes walking into school a bit harder too. I'm tired of writing, just plain tired.

Please pray that my new treatment works.

Thanks,
-Jen

OCTOBER 31, 2012

Happy Halloween! I can't wait for Luca's class party later and then trick-or-treating with the boys! Then, thank God, October, with all its glorious fun and sucking the marrow out of life, will be over! It's time to play catch up (I am crazily behind in thank yous, emails, phone calls, and all things for the Foundation) and to get adjusted to my new chemo.

After another fun weekend that included a beach trip with some girlfriends for the first time since college, my birthday, Rocco's kids vs. adults soccer game and party, and then a very stressful pre-appointment morning yesterday, I am pooped. But the appointment went really well! Apparently, the distant progression to just groin nodes rather than vital organs is freakishly rare. And although Gary can't say for sure what the future holds, he thinks that this is not a radical game changer and that we do not need to switch into Hyper Seize the Day Mode (thank God), because right now, I have neither the desire nor the energy. Fantastic news!

So, I am off the trial as of yesterday and will start the new chemo cocktail tomorrow. It's got the usual long list of side effects but seems to be working quite well (i.e., beating advanced breast cancer's back) in other peeps. It's every three weeks, and the first week will likely be a bit tough, but then if all goes well, I should have two pretty good weeks. Sweet!!

I've got to scoot. Have fun tonight, and be on the lookout for some upcoming information about holiday gift giving and volunteer opportunities for the Run Jen Run 5K on March 2nd of next year.

Thanks,
-Jen

NOVEMBER 8, 2012

I've had THE BEST MORNING! I woke up, for the first time since chemo last Thursday, feeling pretty darn good: no nausea, no crippling aches, no lightheadedness, minimal shakes, and a much clearer brain. I was able to get the boys breakfast, and get Rocco to the bus! Hurray!

And I just spoke with two local in-need moms and asked if Go Jen Go (along with our partners Carolina Breast Friends and 24 Hours of Booty) could fulfill their families' Christmas wishes/wants as a part of our second annual "Operation Spread the Joy!" campaign. They both graciously and excitedly accepted!! How humbling, how awesome. What a beautiful blessing. This makes my heart sing!

Thank you for making it possible to make dreams come true this Christmas for our local, in-need, breast cancer community!! This year, we are looking forward to giving a beautiful, joyful holiday to fifteen families!

Thanks!
-Jen

NOVEMBER 16, 2012

I should never have tempted the fates like that last Wednesday morning. My shiny, happy self got kicked back into submission just a few hours after my last post. Labs the next day revealed "terrible" (not a word you want to hear from your oncologist) counts, my lowest in five years. Super.

The brief reprieve: A Neulasta shot enabled me to get out in public, and Saturday we had a great meeting for our upcoming Run Jen Run 5K. We have a fantastic, committed, compassionate group. And it is so thrilling and deeply satisfying to see this dream come true. I also made a friend's fortieth birthday party for a bit. I was tired and achy, but 'twas fun. Joe and I felt like a couple of regular peeps.

The ass kicking: I have not been sleeping well for quite a while. I've been having realistic nightmares of being violently beaten, traumatically injured, etc. I'm progressively achy during waking hours. I'm slowing down, and have no motivation to move, especially for exercise, which is really rare for me. I had to ramp up to some big-time pain killers at night to dull the edge enough to sleep. Stuff was hurting enough to look up chemo side-effects again; even though this far in the game, I know the usual suspects. The new drug, Perjeta, causes bone, muscle, and joint pain. Yes, yes, and yes. Monday was grin-and-bear-it day. My daytime meds were not offering any measurable relief. Tuesday morning came and went. I hurt too much and was exhausted to boot. I did not get up for my kids. I did not even check on my kids. I just fitfully slept and hoped for the best. My entire body was a study in intense, somewhat migratory, aches. No body part was immune. The soles of my feet, my face, and parts I didn't know I had all freaking hurt at some point or never stopped hurting. I didn't crawl out of bed until 12:30 p.m., college hours.

The call with Gary: I basically asked, "What the hell is wrong with me?" Gary told me to hang in there and that it was probably the perfect storm of the Neulasta shot (which makes your bone marrow hurt kind of like the flu) and the Perjeta. Super. I should get better in a few days. Is this the way my "good" weeks are going to roll? Scary. Sad. Shit.

The reach out: I texted my friend who is on this drug. She's battling a stage 4 recurrence (she's thirty-three) and has had three rounds of the Perjeta cocktail. She's had a rough go; she had two hospital stays after the first two rounds (our progression is different). I asked her how she dealt with the aches. She did not. She had serious other problems from the Perjeta. She is now off of it, but she may try it again later. Gary cut her loose from it after three rounds because the side effects were not tolerable. Yikes for us both!

The freak-out: This was yesterday and earlier today. I've had red-line stress levels because there is so much to do before the next treatment (Tuesday). I was almost to shut-down mode, beyond acceptable, near anxiety attack. Today, I got up and got the boys to school for the first time in a week. My aches dramatically reduced. I came in and started on GJG business and worked all day. My stress levels are reducing, and my aches overall are getting much better.

The look forward: I'll be meeting Mom and a dear friend for the Christmas show. We will spend some good weekend time with the family. We have another good race meeting soon. And I've got lots of questions for Gary about how to achieve better living through pharmaceuticals to make this option livable.

Please say some prayers for me, the women GJG is helping (and those we haven't yet), and for all cancer survivors out there.

Thanks,
-J

November 29, 2012

*T*hanksgiving was a mixture of fun, family time, chemo side-effects, and occasional tears. 'Twas caught between needing quiet, stillness, and rest and wanting to be a part of the chaos with family and friends. This new regimen is still a bit of an ass kicker despite the tweaking by Gary. On Monday, when I was over the worst of the nausea, headaches, bodyaches, and lower GI unpleasantness, I was suffering from an acute onset of zero-personality disorder. I was flat, annoyed, and didn't want to be near/interact/look at another person. Lovely! Poor Gammy, she had the unenviable task of getting me to Gary's for labs. At least the blood tests confirmed there was a medical reason for my personality disorder: my labs sucked. My bone marrow was crushed, and my hemoglobin was at transfusable levels. After one quick Neupogen injection in the abdomen, we were out the door. Well, here we are several days later, and I am still a bit irritable (and have crazy fatigue), but I'm on my way back to Gary's again in a few minutes. I told you beating cancer was a full-time job! We'll see if he can fix me the rest of way ....

December 3, 2012

*L*ast week, I had two shots to boost the old bone marrow, fluids, and a transfusion. It was a un-week off—not. By Saturday, I had enough pep to enjoy several margaritas and not get an immediate hangover (Yay!!), but then I cried myself to sleep after the Dawgs lost.

Sunday was Go Jen Go Day. I had so much to do; there are so many great events in the works: Operation Spread the Joy (now), Pink in the Rink with the Checkers (February 9), and of course, the Run Jen Run 5K (March 2).

Have a great night!
-Jen

December 7, 2012

*T*his is going to be short-ish and semi-sweet. I've tried to post several times today but either get distracted, interrupted, or get thwarted by a hinky iPad. I do seem to carry electronic Ebola or something. I'm sure it's not operator error; no one could possibly make that many mistakes.

Seriously though, I want to thank everyone out there who is working, donating, or volunteering on one of our many Go Jen Go Foundation projects currently in the works!!! Just this week alone, the GJG has provided financial assistance to local survivors to help with rent, groceries, and utilities. Can you imagine using a heating pad to stay warm because you can't afford to turn on your heat? Can you imagine having to do it while dealing with stage 4 cancer? Thank you for making all that possible! You are all making a tremendous difference in the lives of our in-need survivors!! Yay!!!

Be thankful, be compassionate, and be well.

Humbly,
-Jen

December 13, 2012

*H*ola peeps! I hope the holidays are treating everyone right.

Christmas is right around the corner, and Santa has yet to kick into high gear at the Pagani house. I'm slowly doing some online shopping as I convalesce from Tuesday's chemo. I've managed to knock a couple of items off the list. Tomorrow I will wrap at least one thing (a girl's got to dream big), and the tree skirt is openly mocking me, empty, wanting ....

In fact, the boys are mocking me a bit too. Their behavior seems to have taken a recent backward slide. Some of it is just plain excitement and silliness, but Luca is entrenched in a new "let's push all the buttons and see just what I can get away with" phase that better end soon-ish. Even threats of a bad report to Santa from our Elf on the Shelf, the aptly named "Watcher," holds no sway. Luca noticed a tag on Watcher's pants a few days ago that prompted a very thorough inspection (from afar, of course, you can't touch him or he loses his Christmas magic) by him and his brother.

Daddy then stepped in and saved the day by explaining that even elves have to buy their pants at the store.

Whew! But then when Rocco asked during bedtime prayers why Santa doesn't bring the in-need kids and their families "all the cool toys too."s Basically, why is there a need for Operation Spread the Joy when Santa ought to be taking care of everyone? I felt a bit more of their wonder slip out of my reach. My kids are really putting some thought into traditions this year. I answered that question by saying that Santa has to bring those families things they need just to live: food, clothes, things we all take for granted, so he doesn't have much room for toys. The answer settled them down a bit, but I am not ready for the magic to be gone just yet. Let's have one more year of innocent wonder.

I hope your wonder continues to abound. Have a great night. Be well, be peaceful, be generous and be compassionate.

-Jen

December 16, 2012

I've spent the past three days orbiting the sofa and bed, not quite feeling like doing too much more than sit on my heating pad or nap. I'm over it. Hopefully, my body will be ready tomorrow. Despite the down time, I am exceedingly thankful to be so healthy (relatively speaking) this holiday and to have another Christmas with my sons, husband, family, and friends. Thank you, God for this gift! Speaking of gifts: huge thanks to everyone who has donated to Operation Spread the Joy! Our hearts are heavy for the children and their families in cancer treatment. May they be surrounded in prayers, healing, and love.

December 24, 2012

Operation Spread the Joy was a huge success!! All the wrapping and delivering is done. The Operation was a beautiful collaboration of the folks from the Go Jen Go Foundation, Carolina Breast Friends, and 24 Hours of Booty. We all came together to service the needs of our community of cancer survivors. It was truly a wonderful thing.

Recipients were blown away, and a few were moved to tears. Several recipients invited volunteers into their home for a visit. All were so thankful! I've heard from a few of our delivery volunteers too, and it was just as wonderful and incredible for them. Wow!

Many, many thanks to all who helped us make this holiday a joyous occasion! God bless, and to all a good night.

-Jen

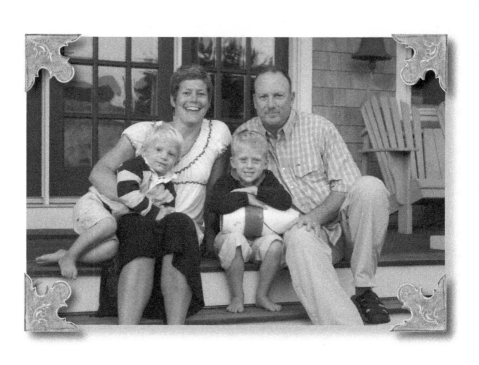

2013

January 6, 2013 8:32 p.m.

I've got a consult for radiation tomorrow. Scans a few days ago showed disease progression in my neck. Please pray for good results and not too much fatigue from yet another chemo/rad combo.

Thanks,
-Jen

January 10, 2013

I have gone down in flames. I am caught between the inevitable and the struggle to find the will to persevere despite a progressing disease and a progressively intolerable list of side effects. The neuropathy and nail problems have gone from bad to worse. We've doubled my medication, but I am still having trouble sleeping through the discomfort. To add to that, all of my fingernails are dying, weepy, and painful. It hurts to type, to do much of anything. We dropped the dose of the offending chemo drug by half to help with this, but to no avail. The disease on my right upper arm has spread like wild fire. I can see the creep of disease along my collarbones and my lower abdomen. The new node in my neck is now getting radiated, but the "juicy" nodes on the other side of my neck hurt now too. If I am honest with myself, I do not feel like I am living with cancer but rather finally dying from it now.

This feeling of death, of dying, could be from a combination of my emotional state and the side effects. I am at that intersecting point on the graph where to increase my chemo dose would possibly hold my disease stable but cause side effects incompatible with life. That point sucks.

I am spent, empty, sad. I cry every time I go by the Pink House to go to radiation. I cry at radiation. I just cry. I keep thinking, "Suck it up, be sad, and move on," because if this is the beginning of the end, then we need to find joy in every day. But yet, I cannot do this. Joe and I have had a few difficult discussions. He is still hopeful. I met him at the door last night crying. It was not fair. I felt guilty. He had just gone to our friend's funeral earlier. I don't know how he finds hope. He amazes me.

I have very little left to give, and what precious little I do have, I need to give to my family and myself. I need to show the boys things are okay despite the weird and suspicious stickers (radiation markings, not a new tattoo) on my neck. I need to spend time with them doing normal and even fun stuff. I cannot strategize, review, coordinate, request, approve, or thank. I cannot answer the phone, email, text, or even talk. I can barely get out of bed or my pj's. I have nothing left to give, really. I have many balls in the air right now, and some of them will crash to the ground, but so be it. It has gotten to the point where if they don't, I will. It's selfish, I know.

Moab is calling my soul. I don't know how I will get there, but it needs to be soon, like next week. I can't even manage daily life, let alone the logistics of planning a trip. But I need to go—to be alone among the red rocks, the timeless and stillness of the place. I need to hike quietly and contemplatively, out and then just sit and be until I almost turn to dust; until I almost fade away. Then I will know what to do, how to gather my resources, how to reconnect with my life source and my joy. The notion of it is sustaining me right now. It almost puts a smile on my face.

I will be electronically absent; I'm not sure for how long. I am dropping out of my life as much as I can and still be a little bit of a wife and mom. If you need to reach me, contact Joe.

Thanks,
-J

JANUARY 14, 2013

I want to thank everyone for reaching out to us, praying for us and supporting our family since my last post. Your compassion, prayers, and generosity are sustaining us. Thank you.

For the most part, I am in a much better place. A visit to Moab (Google Arches National Park if you are not familiar with this bit of heaven on earth) is now on the books. I leave Wednesday with my dear friend Britt. The trip holds the sweet promise of spiritual and emotional renewal. It is a place of vast horizons, endless sky, extraordinarily harsh climate, and timeless geology. It is a place where the struggle for existence is both beautiful and difficult; a perfect metaphor for my own life, and a poignant reminder of my insignificance in the grand scheme of things.

Having the trip to look forward to, even though part of this journey will likely be filled with tears, has buoyed my spirit and my mind. It is a "carrot" of the best sort.

Jen

P.S. Thank you to our mystery nativity-scene benefactor—we loved getting the pieces and reading the Bible verses! Thank you to my mystery Olive Culinary benefactor—it is the only healthy food I am eating of late! And finally, Santa brought the most adorable Olde English Bulldogge pup for the boys, her name is Vinnie.

JANUARY 30, 2013

I felt neither the desire nor the motivation to write about my trip since my return from Moab. Today, however, my muse had other ideas. Instead of drifting into a sweet, much needed nap, my muse started whispering in my ear, softly at first, so I had to strain a bit to listen. Then it became louder, faster, more insistent. Needless to say, no sleep for the weary.

I arrived expectant but a bit flat. I was trying to keep my emotions in check and savor the beauty, the cold bracing air, and the pizza. I was off. I felt apprehensive, torn between wanting to just pretend, relax, and enjoy and needing to delve deep in. I wondered if I should force things along or just let them occur organically and hope the catharsis and renewal occurred during time allotted for this "vacay." The verdict after discussing this with Britt was to go organic.

The drive from Grand Junction, beautiful in the fall, was spectacular covered in snow. Climbing out of the valley, up and over the Grand Mesa, and into the desert of Utah was a silvery, shimmery pearlescent slice of heaven. It literally looked otherworldly. The desert was almost completely covered in snow, ice crystals glittered in the air, and the temperature plummeted into the single digits. Things were looking up already.

We stopped by the Arches National Park (right outside of town) to find out if the park was open and if the roads were passable. Ice-covered roads and trails, highs in the teens, lows in the single digits, red monoliths and arches all visible? Perfect.

Britt and I managed several sunsets all at below zero degrees and two sunrises in the park. We were dressed in layers of technical gear and had no problem with the cold. I was desperately worried about my neuropathic hands and feet. But maybe God saw to it that I had absolutely no problems with the cold. Thanks, Big Wo/Man.

The vast, still beauty of watching the sunrise over snow covered, 12,000 foot peaks (La Sal Mountains) and finally cast its brilliant rays over red rocks and arches, turning the sky from pink to orange to glowing red, cannot be adequately described. You have to experience it.

I did—from a quiet, high, solitary perch, one of my favorite places on Earth. It is the perfect place to feel your fleeting insignificance, to realize you are nothing more than a bit of dust in an infinite universe. It is terrifying and reassuring at the same time. It is the perfect perch from which to look and see how life must struggle mightily, constantly, to survive in the harshest of conditions. At first, it may seem so desolate, dead, but if you look, if you open your soul, you see the most profound beauty and life everywhere. There are crows calling constantly, one-thousand-year-old pinyon trees, tracks in the snow ... The struggle for existence is extraordinarily beautiful, soothing, and inspiring.

My heart, body, and soul renewed in those quiet moments. I gathered strength and acceptance there. I tested my will to go on in those harsh conditions and did not find it lacking, no matter what the universe brings next.

Britt and I hashed out a plan. An outline to live by so I spend my time trying to stay as healthy as I can, prepare for what comes next, stay focused on the present, and enjoy time with my family and friends. I am not answering the phone, returning emails or texts, and I will be doing fewer and fewer of my responsibilities—the fun or the tedious. I am trying not to feel guilty (still do a bit) and am succeeding more in that arena, but I am just letting things drop. I have good friends, dear old friends, to call, and I just haven't. Despite this blog (which I am doing because I know many are wondering how my trip went), I just don't feel expansive, don't feel like talking. It's not out of sorrow. It just is. Please forgive me.

I have most of the Foundation business covered and will continue to do what I can, when I can, but some things are just going to pass by undone. I do this for me, selfishly but totally necessary for my continued (hopefully well-) being. I, we, continue to remain inspired, buoyed, and very, very thankful for all of you who support us during this long journey. I do not doubt for one second that without all of you, my fleeting time would have already passed.

To quote Beck, "Things are changing, I can feel it." Aside from my family, my other legacy is the Go Jen Go Foundation. Its mission, my promise to God, is now being fulfilled in a profound and growing way. I find much comfort and a sense of completion in this.

'Tis a beautiful manifestation of a dream, one that will now certainly continue long after my absence.

I really don't like to continue to plug or ask, sometimes it feels cheap. But if you are so inclined, please help the dream continue. Go to our website to see our upcoming events. Next Saturday, February 9, is Pink in the Rink. We've sold a bunch of tickets, but we are still about 125 tickets short of our goal. It is one of the balls I dropped of late. The night is crazy fun; and if you'd like to go shoot me a text, I can grab you some seats in the GJG area. The tickets are fifteen dollars each. And the First Annual Run Jen Run 5K (talk about the realization of a dream!!) is coming up on March 2.

Thanks, Jen

February 5, 2013

What a great but busy weekend! Friday the Checkers folks came by to shoot some video. They did a wonderful job, and editing is a beautiful thing. I love it! Saturday night was Laugh for the Cure uptown at the Knight Theater. It was fab! The two comics were hilarious. The vibe was really upbeat and fun, and they raised $100K! Joe (and Dr. Gary Frenette, among others) was honored as a member of the Pink Tie Guys inaugural class. They amaze me! And I was very humbled to be named the Kristy Adams-Ebel (she founded the Carolina Breast Friends) Shining Survivor Award. Aren't we the power couple? Ha!

We've got a big group going to Pink in the Rink this Saturday. Thanks, everyone! It's going be a lot of fun. I think we are all primarily in sections 101 through 104. Please wear your Go Jen Go gear/T-shirts to show our spirit and support for this great night! Thanks again to everyone! We are beau coup excited!

Jen, Joe, Rocco and Luca

February 9, 2013

*Y*ay! Tonight's the big night; Pink in the Rink is finally here! Thank you, everyone, for supporting us in such a big, enthusiastic way. We will now have an army almost 500 strong! Y'all are AMAZING!

Remember to wear your GJG T-shirts, if you have them! There are lots of fun activities pre-game and during the intermissions tonight. I will be dropping the ceremonial puck at 6:45 p.m., and Rocco is SUPER excited to ride the Zamboni during the second intermission.

I can't wait to see everyone tonight! Thank you for supporting us and making a direct impact on the in-need survivors in our community!

Jen, Joe, Rocco and Luca

February 11, 2013

*S*aturday was the most extraordinary evening, and one of the best of our lives! It was thrilling and humbling to have so many people there for Go Jen Go. The mix of excitement from families, survivors, scouts, and the vibe of the crowd was palpable, perfect. I had big fun going out on the ice and dropping the puck. It was also cool (pardon the pun) being down rink side with the folks from KISS FM and the representatives from survivor organizations. The two players who "faced off" were quite friendly and thanked us for being there, and, bonus, they were not too hard on the eyes.

It was great to watch the first period from the team area, on the glass, right behind the goal. It was so intense. And as a former athlete, it was a treat to witness such athleticism that close up. It inspired me and reminded me of what the human body is capable of doing despite the pain it sometimes must endure. We also had a super exciting moment where a Checker checked a Rampage player literally right on the other side of the glass from where we were seated and only inches from Luca's face. The check lasted a second or two, but it seemed much longer, as our whole family screamed and stared right into the grimacing, smashed-up opposing player's face. It was awesome!

The most extraordinary, shocking, and humbling moment of the evening came for us when we were asked to stand out on the ice as the Checkers aired, on the big screen, the video story of our family's battle with breast cancer and the subsequent birth and mission of the Go Jen Go Foundation.

To say it was an emotional, surprising moment when Michael and Wendy Kahn, the Checkers owners, presented us with a $25,000 check for the Go Jen Go Foundation, is a completely inadequate description. It was phenomenal!!! It was the validation of a dream, a glimpse of my legacy, a beautiful, incredibly generous, totally unexpected contribution that we can pass on immediately to our local, in-need survivors and their families. And to make a once-in-a-lifetime moment even more extraordinary, we received an enthusiastic standing ovation from the crowd. It touched and humbled Joe and me to the core. Rocco, of course, thought most of the applause was just for him, and Luca was kind of oblivious but did dance around a little bit. I can't wait to see the video!

As cool as it was down on the ice, it was also great to be back up in our seats, surrounded by our family and friends. We loved looking all around the arena and picking out the GJG shirts and various friends and supporters. Rocco would go crazy when he'd spot one of his school buddies!

Another huge highlight was when Rocco got to ride the Zamboni during the second intermission. He had been bragging all week to his friends about it, but when the team representative came to get him with just a few minutes left in the second period, he looked like a deer in the headlights. We thought for sure he was going to forget to wave, or even look at the crowd. But he came through with pure Pagani enthusiasm. He waved his arm off, and the other arm was busy clutching on to the grab bar for dear life. He had a fantastic time and was the envy of many a kid at the game. He will never, ever forget the experience!

The event was such a beautiful gift, the most amazing evening! We are so thankful to Michael and Wendy Kahn for their extraordinary donation and an incredible evening, to all of the Checkers representatives, who are kind, compassionate, and professional. And we are thankful to our family, friends, neighbors, BWE, OG and CLCC supporters, and the Girl Scouts who purchased tickets in honor of Go Jen Go and surrounded us with their enthusiastic support and love. Thank you!!! Also, thanks to all of you who posted notices, forwarded emails, and put out information on the event in newsletters.

Finally, a big thanks to Marguerite Fourqurean and Meredith McGough, without the efforts of the two of them Pink in the Rink would not have had such a tremendous turnout. And of course, thank you to the Go Jen Go board members, in particular, Britt Yett, who works tirelessly and often quietly on all things GJG.

Thank you, everyone, for supporting our family and the Go Jen Go foundation, and for helping us make a positive impact on the lives of those in our breast cancer community!

Also, please support the Checkers—it's easy to do because the games are so much fun! They are a fantastic example of a local business actively working to better our community!

FEBRUARY 20, 2013

Okay, so I am running a bit behind in the posting department. I only had a couple of glorious days to bask in the glow of Pink in the Rink and then, boom, back to chemo reality.

Gary threw me a curveball last week and changed up my regimen because of the continued progression on the drugs (supposedly the latest and greatest) that I started back in October. I am now on a three-drug chemo cocktail that was introduced in 1976 (hopefully an oldie but a goodie). I have been on two of the three drugs before, but the third is new to me. I did not know there was a breast cancer drug I hadn't been on yet! The hope is the combo will attack the cancer in a new way and therefore work. Fingers are crossed.

The side effects are basically slightly different versions of the usual, just add in more nausea and noise, motion and light sensitivity; it shouldn't be a problem unless I have kids or a puppy. Oh shit, I have boys and a four-month-old dog; and apparently, four months in dog years is the canine equivalent to the "terrible twos." Oh well.

Over the weekend, I did perk up enough to revel in the snow Saturday evening (what a beautiful surprise!) for a bit with the fam. It was wonderful and fun. Vinnie and Sophie went bananas romping and pouncing while Joe, Luca, and I made a dirty snowman (not the perverted kind, the Southern kind, with grass, mud, and sticks all in it). But I didn't get a chance to fully get my feet back under me before both Luca and Joe got sick. 'Twas time to suck it up and swing into doting-mommy mode. Luca is still under the weather, and as I'm writing this (from the pediatrician's office), he yells, "Mom, wheah ah you?" every time I leave the room. It's sweet and full of need, and on one level, I am ecstatic to be here to able to comfort him, but on the other, I am pooped and way behind in all things GJG, and just all things in general.

On a hugely positive note, the inaugural Run Jen Run 5K is only a week and a half away! I can't believe it. Sign up now! It is going to be so much fun! We've got a great-looking, sweat-wicking race T-shirt, an anchor on WBTV will be our MC, and The Matones will provide some tunes. We will also have the Pink Heals Fire Truck, Chubby Checker, the Chik-fil-A cow (with biscuits!), and loads of other stuff too.

Come have fun, keep on track with your New Year's resolutions (spring break is weeks away!), and walk, jog, or run and help out our local, in-need breast cancer survivors!

Thanks!
-Jen

FEBRUARY 25, 2013

We had a big weekend this past weekend. We reached another milestone at the Pagani house. We purchased our very first cup for Rocco. It, along with gobs of other protective gear, is a requirement for lacrosse. It was a bit confusing (there are so many options now), and was good for lots of quality rainy-day entertainment. We just had to test it out. I was genuinely curious. It is one of those member-of-the-opposite-sex things that had remained shrouded in mystery for me. Movies provided my only education on all things cups, and not a very good one at that.

Once at home, and once Rocco was securely placed in his compression shorts, we threw balls at the cup (not too hard, but boy, was Rocco nervous) to make sure he was lacrosse ready. After he felt good about it, the boys spent the better part of the afternoon testing its capabilities. I'll spare you the comments, but let's just say it was very amusing.

Sunday was a glorious day for practice! Entire families sat on the sidelines in their fold, out chairs and basked in the sun. It felt great (I sometimes go for days on end without so much as stepping off my front porch), and I am so glad I got to go. Lacrosse is totally new to all of us and seems like it's going to be lots of fun. After practice, Rocco and I went out in the backyard and threw for a while. It was such a beautiful time for me: the two of us learning a sport together. It was full of him relating the throwing, catching, and defensive tactics he picked up at practice, and me listening and asking lots of leading questions, so he had to think about and demonstrate his new knowledge. It was such a gift, stuff this mommy has dreamt about for years, stuff I always assumed I'd get to do. The only downside was that it required me to take some additional meds last night to deal with the physical fall-out from permanently tightened muscles, inflammation, and scar tissue that prevent me from doing so many things these days.

If you stop by South Park Mall this week, check out the Go Jen Go sign and race poster at Lululemon. They are featuring our race this week at the store! They are graciously and enthusiastically spreading the word about our mission. Yay! Speaking of the race, it is this Saturday, March 2nd, at 9:00 a.m. (the 5K) and 9:45 a.m. (the fun run). It's going to be great!

FEBRUARY 28, 2013

Tuesday's bone scan was clear. Yippee! Currently at CHOA now getting labs and then a shot to boost my bone marrow. So hopefully, I will stay healthy after this weekend's much anticipated, but crowded, race and festivities. Tomorrow, I have the mandatory three-month echo. Bleh. Once that is under my belt, it will be all fun and games! I, we, are soooo excited about Saturday's race! It is going to be a blast! Huge thanks and much love to all of our sponsors, supporters, volunteers, and tireless race-committee peeps!! Thank you!!

We can't wait to see you there!

Jen, Joe, Rocco and Luca

MARCH 6, 2013

Today is the first day I've had to sit quietly (the six hours at chemo yesterday does not count; I was exhausted. Besides, it is NOT quiet at chemo) with my thoughts since Saturday's race. And what a race it was!

It was one of the most memorable mornings of my entire life! I cannot believe the turnout we had: it capped at somewhere over 900 participants! WOW. The weather, although a personal favorite of mine (snow!), was a surprise and bit cold and wet, so the early morning race set-up crew, Run Jen Run Committee folks (i.e., the unpaid, insanely hard working force behind the entire event), and the Start2Finish peeps all suspected it might put a damper (haha! a little post chemo humor) on our turnout or on the mood of the morning. Nothing could have been further from the truth! We had tons of folks, amazing energy, and smiles all around! The Matones (our band), the DJ, Molly Gratham (our celebrity MC), the "not quite as famous" finish-line MC (my amazing hubby, Joe Pagani), the cheerleading crews, the enthusiastic volunteers, Chubby Checker, the Chik-fil-A cow, the Pink Heals Fire Truck, the Martial Arts University folks, the kids' game area, and all of our incredible sponsors came together to make for a BEAUTIFUL, AMAZING RACE!

I had such a joyously happy time hugging, thanking, and cheering on as many people as I could! It was truly glorious! I wanted to speak with and thank everyone. I don't think I quite managed; the crowd was simply too big. Our whole family had an incredible time (Rocco was even motivated to run both races). We felt surrounded and buoyed by so much love.

My chemo-addled brain is starting to fade out, but just know that we were, and still are, filled with overwhelming joy, excitement, and hope over how so many of you came together to joyously and enthusiastically support not only our family but, more importantly, our foundation's mission to provide financial support to our local, in-need breast cancer community. How incredible (and how very important) is that!?

THANK YOU, THANK YOU, THANK YOU!

Jen, Joe, Rocco, Luca, and the Go Jen Go Foundation

MARCH 19, 2013

"*On these bodies we will live. In these bodies we will die. Where you invest your love, you invest your life ....*"

I woke up from my nap today with this Mumford and Sons tune in my head. Poetry set to music. They are incredible words to live by, an invigorating, inspiring way to wake from midday respite. And it was a big departure from my subconscious stirrings of late.

You see, I've been burning the candle at both ends for a while now and have been "flirting with disaster" physically and mentally. In the mornings, I frequently wake with faint whispers of disturbing dreams swirling about my head and into my consciousness, sometimes souring my mood a bit. They are dreams in which I am asked, well, expected, to do an incredibly difficult task (the task itself varies), and although in my dreams I have grown so incredibly weary, everyone expects me to continue doing this almost impossible thing. I'm expected not only to do it but to do it well and without end. I wake before I ever quit, and I throw my hands up or lie my head down in exhausted exasperation before confronting the generic, relentless task masters. The dream always leaves me unsettled, worried about foreshadowing and somewhat fearful.

So, waking midday today with the lyrics of that Mumford and Sons song in my head was a blessing. Perhaps my body is feeling the renewal of the promise of spring. Or perhaps it's because, tired though I may be, I truly have been investing my life and love in the right places of late. I've made an effort to miss as little as possible with the boys. We've done playdates (there are four boys under eight running around in our basement with their shirts off right now), lacrosse practices (a new Pagani family favorite!) and games, another Checkers game, dinners out, hoops, yard football, movie nights, etc.—all kinds of cool, regular family stuff. It has been incredible! Frequently, it leaves me wiped out and so very achy at night, but it is so worth it, and I am thankful for every single second.

And I've worked hard (although far from alone!) for the foundation. Our recent events (the Run Jen Run 5K raised $62,000+!) and the usual ones have left me a bit tired, too. But what a wonderful thing it is to do for others. It makes me feel good despite the fatigue. I'm just sorry it took such a drastic diagnosis for me to figure this out.

I've more to say, but I better go. I still have wild, half-naked boys running about the house.

Jen

April 19, 2013

I'm in the throes of post-treatment side effects—unsteady feet, nausea, pounding headache, multiple body parts that feel like they've been whacked by hammers, and of course, the semi-stuporous state of mind. The house is covered in pollen and dog hair, and both Sophie and Vinnie (Piggy) are driving me crazy as they run, crash, hump, and growl really loudly (did I mention I am quite noise sensitive?) because they haven't been walked in days. And we are officially out of Chew-lottas, which seem to take the canine edge off. And in true doggy follow-the-leader-of-the-pack fashion, they can't manage to play in a room on their own (I've tried sequestering them in other parts of the house, but to no avail). They sit quietly staring out the window or at the door they just saw me close, and pine to be playing near me. How charming (not). They are literally playing on my feet right now ….

But its a glorious day, my kind of day. I haven't been outside really in days, but I can see it from my vantage spot on the porch. There's a lovely breeze in the air, the trees are bursting forth with that beautiful, sweet, vibrant color only the tenderest of vegetation has.

Dogwoods, azaleas, rhododendron, and camelias are blooming like mad. The deer have been meandering by, the birds chirping. It's a feast for my eyes, my ears, my soul. It is a living affirmation of life unfolding for me to behold. And I am drinking it in, inhaling it deeply, connecting with that living thing inside of me, the thing that drives and keeps me going.

I have been off-line a bit more of late, finally doing what I set out to do upon my return from Moab. And in my electronic absence, I've been able to quiet my mind a bit more, rest my body, play more with the boys, tend to some side effects that have required a bit of medical intervention, and delve into the world of better health through nutrition. I now have stacks of nutrition books piled up all about the place and have begun a dietary overhaul that seems to be headed, quite possibly, toward a raw, vegan approach. And thanks to you, our supporters, donors, volunteers, and board members, financial help is constantly going to those breast cancer survivors in our area who need it. Thank you, too, to everyone who has also signed up for tomorrow's Sarcoma Stop!

May 12, 2013

The past few weeks, starting with our beautiful trip to the mountains to spend spring break with friends, have been a wonderful, joyful time, and so very full of life. I've played with Joe and the boys; we've had lacrosse practices and games; we've played backyard basketball; we went on a trip to see two wonderful and beautiful souls unite in marriage; and we also reveled in the fun of preparing for (and living through) Luca's sixth-birthday party. He was three months old and breastfeeding when I was diagnosed—what a GIFT to still be here! Ahhh, times were good. The stress, worry, and fear had all melted away.

Cue Monday. The wife of a college buddy of Joe's passed away suddenly from a difficult, long battle (but one they were told was not yet near the end) from ovarian cancer. She was about my age, deeply in love, and far too young. Please pray for her soul. Please, please pray for her husband. They found each other after a long, very difficult period in his life. They were soul mates, and her diagnosis came not long after their wedding. Joe and I feel their loss acutely. Please also pray for Joe. This hits very close to home, and yet he is still there to support and be with his friend. My own soul mate never ceases to amaze me with all he does (so quietly too) for others.

On Tuesday, my grandma, Granny (just turned 96 on Wednesday), was admitted to the CCU in acute heart failure. She rallied a bit at first but has had mainly setbacks since.

Gammy has been by her side, and I was finally able to visit a bit today. Please pray for her recovery or a peaceful and quick end to her suffering.

Also, on Tuesday, Gary broke the news that it is time for another chemo change up due to new spread in the skin/lymph of my neck, upper back, and shoulders. And it is *time*: the spread is visibly noticeable. Even in the last week, it is getting to be a challenge to move my neck, and it is hurting quite a bit. Gary suggested a weekly (I much prefer every three, especially with summer coming!) dose of Adriamycin, one of the ickier chemo drugs I've been on.

Gary wanted to go with the weekly approach instead of every three weeks so he can give a more tolerable dose with less risk of cardiac damage. I said no because the quality of life would not be doable for me. So, we agreed to continue on with my current regimen for this round. He's going to consult his crystal ball/magic eight-ball/whatever and pull another rabbit (granted, a rabbit we've seen before) out of his hat for my next treatment in three weeks. Let's hope whatever is on the horizon buys some more quality time! I've really enjoyed pretending to be normal (despite having a skin infection and then shingles) lately and don't want it to end!

And in spite of my continued break from voice mails, texts, phone calls, emails, and thank yous, contributions to and fundraisers for the Go Jen Go Foundation continues! Thank you!!! We are currently providing financial help to twelve in-need families. And this weekend, a local Girls on the Run group is surprising two of our families with Mother's Day baskets! The girls raised the money for the baskets themselves. How awesome is that?!

I hope everyone had a great Mother's Day!

-Jen

MAY 23, 2013

*B*ear with me, I'm writing this poolside from Hilton Head Island, and the boys are having a very loud, fabulous time ....

Time has absolutely flown by these past two and a half weeks. My grandmother passed away peacefully last Tuesday. I raced up to Mooresville when Mom called to share the news. I came to see Granny one last time, to tenderly wash her face and say goodbye, and to be with my parents. I was able to be with and comfort my Mom when she needed it most and even helped her with the funeral arrangements. What an extraordinarily precious gift that I was able to help her, that I was strong enough for HER to LEAN on ME, and I am so incredibly but humbly thankful for that.

The gifts continued. I was able (I felt good enough and my treatment schedule permitted—how serendipitous!) to go to Virginia for the viewing and funeral. I rode to and fro with my brother, which was the most time just the two of us have spent together in many years; it was good. We stayed at the same hotel as my folks. The four of us were able to have time and meals together reminiscent of years ago, before Jeff and I left the nest and flew off in our own directions. It was incredible to see my extended, Virginia family, to reconnect with my past and my roots, to catch up, to reminisce, and to cry a bit. It was incredible to revel in old memories and that charming, Southern Virginia, accent and to see handsome cousins and so many dark Scottsmen. I had forgotten how dark complected my people are (especially since being the pale ghost I am now).

We returned home late Friday, and I had a few hours Saturday to pack us Paganis up, and we took off for the beach. Very kind, generous friends offered us their house on Hilton Head Island, and we seized the day (well, the week). It was perfect! The boys played in the pool (salt water, so even I could get in) constantly.

Luca is now a jumping, swimming machine. He was all over the place! We are finally over that hump! Yay! The boys can, for the most part, safely and happily entertain themselves at the pool and on the beach. Its a Festivus miracle! The weather was perfect, we ate good food, we spent some quality time with Big Daddy and Lillie, and we forgot all our troubles.

June 3, 2013

When we came back to Charlotte after our vacation, my stress could no longer be contained—the fear and worry about what Gary had lined up next. Also, the disease on my neck and collarbone had, of course, been spreading rapidly. But more importantly, I wondered if what Gary had lined up would work. These things threatened to overwhelm me. By the time my appointment with him rolled around, I was pretty much a mess (not the crying kind, the insanely stressed-out kind). We addressed a huge laundry list of side effects I am currently deeming as not acceptable (the list I deem tolerable is a long one, too), and then we talked strategy. We decided to revisit the drug TDM-1, which is getting lots of great press right now and is the latest and greatest for peeps (kinda) like me. Naturally, I've done this drug before (on trial in Charleston two years ago), but I only did two rounds because I failed it in spectacular fashion. Yep, you heard me—I failed it miserably.

Why try it again, then? Well, when you are out of options, everything is worth a shot .... But the main reason is because the mutations (cancer cells divide frequently and thus mutate frequently) that are causing the new, rapid growth along my neck, collar bone, shoulders, and upper back were hopefully not present in my system when I was on trial and therefore might be susceptible to this new drug.

So here we are six days post the "new" treatment. "How's it going?" you might ask. Well, today is the first day I've driven. Joe is out of town for the week, and I had to get my boy to CLCC, if that gives you an idea. Basically, it's been a blur of side effects and time spent in the dark, semi-quiet not really watching TV or putting any effort into iPad word games. It has been slow and long and painful. My skin looks much worse (mainly on my sternum, near my open wound). It is bright, red hot, and forcing me to take narcotics at night so I can tolerate it enough to sleep. My chest, collarbone, and remaining breast are so swollen (major pitting edema) that they literally might burst open. Other areas on my abdomen have gotten more red and palpable. Are these changes the result of major cancer cell death or major cancer growth? Seems like it is presenting the way it did last time. I'm spending lots of time not thinking about it or about much of anything. I'm not doing much of anything, for that matter.

I see Gary again tomorrow. We'll see what he thinks.

JUNE 5, 2013

Quick update about my visit with Gary yesterday: He suspects my issues are either an infection (I'm on an antibiotic now) or a response to chemo (which means cell death). Either of these could be the cause of the new pain, swelling, redness, fatigue, and just plain feeling icky. I had suspected this, but it was a huge relief to hear him say it.

The stress of the last week caught up with me a bit while I was still at the office, but after a few tears, I felt lighter, less foggy, and a bit more like my old self. I am still dragging a bit, but I'm carrying a whole lot lighter load (for now anyway).

Thanks for the good vibes and prayers. Please keep them coming; we need this to work.

Thanks,
Jen

JUNE 28, 2013

I've tried to write a few times, but then I hit a snag and stop. That pretty much sums me up of late: good intentions/spurt of energy (that I always think is going to last, which is odd, because at heart, I'm a glass half-empty kind of gal; apparently, I'm a pessimist and a slow learner) and then the moment/um passes. This lack of gumption is causing me mucho frustration and guilt. But the upside is that I lose interest and energy in holding onto those feelings too.

This summer's been a mixture of highlights and very trying times, a dichotomy for sure, a real trip on the emotional rollercoaster. I'll start with the challenges:

1. Our air-conditioning broke not once but four times, which is enough to try anyone's patience.
2. There was repeated flooding from the room in the basement where the A/C unit thingy is.
3. Husband was out of town for the entirety of this experience.
4. A multitude of wet, air conditioning-leak-filled floor towels that needed wringing out and washing despite a (chemo caused) germaphobe not wanting to touch them let alone put them in her washing machine.
5. The cost of replacing a new system.

6. Two boys who took a total of three, yes three, days of summer break before announcing they were bored and that there is "nothing to do at our house."

7. The fact that the new therapy hit me hard (it knocked my legs out from under me much longer than I had expected, and I've had an increase in some of the side effects, and of course, there's always the big, overriding worry about whether or not the therapy is working).

8. After our A/C was finally fixed, big storms rolled through knocking out our power for forty-eight hours. When power was finally restored, our newly repaired A/C was totally fried, and so was I: totally and completely fried. I hit another couple of bumps in the road, and then the emotional gauge flipped to rage, actual rage (a rarely experienced emotion for me, I am very happy to announce). No cell phones (can't rip my iPhone in half) or children were harmed though, and that's all I have to say on that matter.

And finally:

9. Thanks to an unusually stormy season, I missed three swim meets (due to rescheduling) last week when I was only expecting to miss one.

After my "episode," and in huge part thanks to Dominic and his crew's help with the A/C, things started looking up. Dominic came out last Monday and promised to have a new system (the outside and inside parts!) in by the time I got home from chemo the following day. He delivered in spades! He is a very kind, honest, big hearted, professional man who does great work. He saved the day (coming home from chemo feeling nauseated and with a blistering headache to a hot house is NOT an option)! Yay, thank you!!

So that's a tour of the lows, but there have been some notable highlights. Luca graduated from pre-school at Christ Lutheran. He was so proud (and kind of sad, but not nearly as sad as Mommy, because CLCC is like part of our family). Rocco started there at three months old, and they are an incredible, compassionate, caring, giving, loving group of people who have helped and nurtured and taught our boys and have been with our family every step of the way, from diagnosis to current day. It was a true gift to behold, and one I frequently did not think I'd get to see. I've also been to the pool some to play. It's been fun and fab, and my skin is doing okay (I just need to wear my sun shirt and really limit my UV exposure, which is not too hard because anything more than small doses makes me feel rather awful). I've managed to sit (in the shade) poolside and chat with other moms, and I've even swam in fits and starts (it's an exercise in pain management but a glorious one that makes me feel alive and a bit like the old me). I love it! I've seen Rocco swim at a few meets and even timed at one—wonderful.

Yesterday, I had a "great exam" at Gary's! My skin is showing (visually and palpably) signs that this regimen is working! Whew!! As to the side effects, they are most likely due to a "serum reaction" from the chemo. Basically, it's working very well in some (hopefully all!) spots, and the massive cancer cell death it's causing is resulting in its own set of (unpleasant) reactions as the body deals with the fallout. As for the fatigue/apathy, my heart rate was only 39 yesterday (normal is 60 to 100). I will have labs, an EKG, and an echo later, so that will probably explain some of it. He also thought all the stress of late, coinciding with my (now predictable) quarterly need to run away probably accounts for the rest. I will have scans in a couple of weeks just to make sure it's not something new.

I should stop now. Thanks for hanging in with me! And thanks for continuing to support Go Jen Go. We are currently providing financial assistance, on average, nine to twelve local, in-need survivors and their families!

-Jen

July 15, 2013

Cross your fingers and say some prayers, please. I have head to toe scans tomorrow, which are always stressful and tiring. And this morning, I had a routinely scheduled echo. Some new "funny little beats" (tech's words not mine; she obviously was not aware of my online PhD) have shown up. These paired with some recent cardiac symptoms (not the low heart-rate kind) have me a bit concerned. Per Gary, I know have to see a cardiologist. Hopefully, it'll be something a pill can fix and won't require any changes to my treatment regimen. I'm on two potentially cardiotoxic drugs right now and have been on quite a few over the years.

I'll see Gary Thursday, so we should know more by then.

Stay dry,
-Jen

July 20, 2013

The Good, the Bad, and the Ugly

*T*he Incredibly Good: Scans look good! Wahoo!! Thank God, and thank you for all the prayers!

The Very Good: We finished up the swim season, and Rocco qualified for, and swam in, the All-Star Meet at the MCAC uptown. I was able to join the whole family at the meet. It was so exciting to see my boy, cheer for our team, and be back in an environment that was so much a part of my life before cancer. It gave me chills! And Rocco came home with a third-place medal and a sixth-place ribbon. Sweet!

The Pretty Good: My current cardiac issues (my heart rate is koo-razy irregular) should be fixable with some meds. And any heart damage from the cardiotoxic drugs I am on should be reversible (I would have to go off of treatment for a bit, but let's not put the cart before the horse). So for now, we will make no changes in my chemo routine! Whew, I was sweating that big-time!

The Bad: It was such a long, stressful week. I HATE spending so much time, especially on my "off week," in hospitals and in doctor's offices. It doesn't help when half the appointments occur during my nap time (this baby needs her nap). You know it's desperate times when I counted the twenty minutes of shut-eye I grabbed during my bone scan as my nap for Tuesday afternoon. My body, mind, and soul were absolutely worn thin by Thursday evening. Thank goodness I slept hard and long that night.

The Ugly: The boys had lacrosse camp a week ago. Rocco went from nine o'clock to five o'clock. I finally managed to clear the gear out of my car a few days ago (all the laundry, thanks to all the help from Gammy, had largely been finished). I smelled what might have been moldering cleats and thus stuck my hand inside of Rocco's giant, black LAX bag to dig them out. I fished around in there, just to make sure I hadn't missed a sock or something, and came out with a sticky, yes sticky, pair of compression shorts and a cup. I was horrified and petrified initially. I stood staring at my disgusting find, my mind racing to come up with plausible explanations for what I had discovered. When I finally decided there was no biological reason for the stickiness, I noticed a partially opened and melted piece of gum were also in the bag. Whew, no wonder I'm having cardiac problems. I now mentally refer to the bag as "the little shop of horrors."

The Other Ugly: My brain scan, which looked good, showed "frothy" (ewww!) sinuses. "What the hell does that mean?" you might ask. Gary countered this sweet inquiry with, "Well, haven't you had any symptoms?" And to Gary, I sweetly (again) replied, "My body is riddled with symptoms, I would only consider myself symptomatic if I felt fine."

Apparently, "frothy" means I have a "significant" sinus infection that is going to require three weeks of antibiotics (I protested this mightily) to start. My GI system is really pissed.

Anyway, thank you for your support vibes and prayers! While all this has been going on with us, GJG is supporting ten families right now, helping with rent, gas, groceries, co-pays, and medical bills. We also provide help for specific, one-time items. This month, we purchased a new refrigerator for an in-need survivor whose fridge broke. We were also able to provide money for her to buy food to fill her new one back up. We can only do this because of your generosity!! Thank you!

AUGUST 4, 2013

*L*ast week was great, chock full of normal mommy stuff and only one medical appointment. Rocco started the week off losing a tooth, one that wasn't even all that loose, on a fresh ear of corn. It bled quite a bit, and he (rather oddly; he is prone to some drama) took it like a champ. He now has a great hockey-player grin. There's a big gap right up front next to a giant, relatively speaking, of course, adult tooth, with a new gap on the other side. It's cute and funny looking at the same time. Luca, who just started riding his bike without training wheels—Rocco got out the wrench at Juju's and took them off all by himself! Luca and I have been riding bikes together just about every day. It is such sweet fun, and we both love this time together!

Speaking of bikes, Friday evening we went to 24 Hours of Booty (for all you out-of-towners, it's a bike riding event, in the heart of one of Charlotte's loveliest neighborhoods, that raises lots of money for cancer research and charities). It was a fabulous time! Seeing old friends from my former (pre-cancer) life, being back on a bike, and being in the midst of so many survivors, co-survivors, and other riders committed to kicking cancer's booty was an incredible experience. I soaked it all up, took it all in. It was pure joy and a reconnection with my inner athlete that was very fun and life affirming! And the fact that I was able to experience it with Joe and both boys was just the icing on the cake!

Also, on Saturday we celebrated Rocco's eighth birthday. The birthday boy and his compadres had a blast! We had playdates all day long. On Sunday, I think I slept until nine o'clock in the morning. All the fun wiped me out!

Today is the sixth anniversary of my diagnosis. I have hardly given it a thought (unlike my fifth anniversary, which caused considerable stress). My eyes are on the horizon, not looking back. We've several big family birthdays coming up (although Joe will be out of town for his), both boys will be getting on the bus together in a few weeks (a huge milestone), and we have lots of great breast cancer events coming up, including the Komen race. Life is good.

AUGUST 8, 2013

Something crazy came in the mail this week. Joe's AARP card! My "old man" hits the big 5-0 this Saturday. I've kept it on the down low because he's been a bit grumpy about it and has refused a party and a to-do of any sort (it doesn't help that he's got to fly for work the afternoon of his big day). But we're going do it up a little, mommy and son style. It should be fun! And if you see our new senior citizen around, give him hell!

Thanks,
-Jen

AUGUST 18, 2013

I'm insanely frustrated at the moment. I just spent two hours updating my site, posting some new photos (but that opened up a whole can of techno-worms), and fairly easily wrote a post I was happy with. The photos stayed, but the post has disappeared into the electronic ether. Curses! The irony is that I had finally moved from attempting to use CaringBridge on my iPad (the two are NOT compatible) to using the much more capable, and I thought compatible, Mac. Of course, there will be a learning curve. That's assuming, obviously, that there will be learning, because right now I have been rewarded for my efforts by a mass of stress and frustration sitting in the center of my chest—or maybe that's just because I forgot my afternoon dose of Cardizem. Non-cancer related learning has pretty much been non-existent for a few years, because who gives a shit about new stuff when you are worried about being around next month for your kids. Along those lines, we (obviously not me—I have to rely on the gracious help of others) will have the gojengo.org site updated with my post, current events, and photos … by the middle of September. I have made the promise now to the masses, so it's gonna happen. Okay, sorry to vent ….

We managed to get a few good, pre-birthday celebrations (and one post celebration) in for Joe before he had to leave town. I am still teasing him a bit. He's such an easy target, I just can't seem to help myself.

Luca and I had a great week together all alone. We played, snuggled, giggled, and laughed. He was perfect, and I spoiled him rotten. Perfection! Yesterday, the whole fam (including the pups, Piggy is very fond of the car; she thinks it tastes delicious, but that's another story) drove up to Camp Kesem to get Rocco after his week away. Camp Kesem is an amazing camp where kids with families affected by cancer get to go to just be normal kids, away from the stresses of dealing everyday with the disease. It took us a few moments to locate him in the reception hall, and when we finally spied him, he had a look of pure, unadulterated joy on his face. He had a fabulous time, made a dear friend in one of his bunk mates, and loved his counselor. We also found out on the last night of camp he got up in front of everyone (I think around 150 people!) and talked about how cancer has impacted him and us. He cried. I was, and am, so proud, so thankful, and so sad. He's had a lot to deal with in his eight years.

Tomorrow morning, we will get the boys' teacher assignments. We are all soooo excited, maybe me most of all. And even though I get chemo Tuesday, I am going to go to the back-to-school activities that are planned throughout the week. I'm stoked!

This last week will probably drag out a bit due to chemo and it being the last week of summer vacay, but aside from that, the last few weeks have flown by. The Charlotte Komen Race is a mere six weeks away. Did anyone get the beautiful (because it has Joe and me on it, hahaha) sign-up reminder card in the mail this week? Help us support them in their funding of research, screening, and education, because early detection really is the best detection! Let's have another big, fun team, show some serious spirit!! Rock it old-school style. Please join Team Go Jen Go!

Thanks! Jen

August 27, 2013

*L*ast week was a bit long and quite chaotic, though I managed the week of pre-school activities with chemo and its subsequent "hangover" decently well (i.e., I made it to all the boys' events semi-coherent and not in pj's, but paid the price with a slower and more difficult than usual recovery—but it was totally worth it). Luca was a bit shy at the kindergarten playground event. He is not a huge fan of big crowds, and if Rocco hadn't come along, I think I would've had a clinger. Instead, he played football with some of the older boys and made a friend or two that way. We did get to see and talk with his teacher, and she is absolutely wonderful—engaging, enthusiastic, brimming with joy, and Luca loves her! She is also a breast cancer survivor and sensitive and supportive of our needs. He gets on the bus for the first time tomorrow, but he laid his clothes out Sunday night because he is so excited!

Rocco started yesterday (they only do staggered start for the kindergartners) and said his first day was "good." Trying to get additional info out of him at dinner was very difficult. We might try water boarding next time. He also has a wonderful teacher and quite a few friends in class. I think he'll have a great year. Hopefully, he'll look out for his little brother on the bus and include him, not treat him like a "little kid" or "just a kindergartner." If not, we really will water board. Luca thinks Rocco hung the moon.

Today, I go see Gary for skin and soft-tissue tumors/growths on my torso and back that have popped up and grown over the past five or six weeks. My left breast is even more swollen and painful than usual, the center of my chest is weeping more, and my right groin and into my thigh is swollen and sore. Sleeping is a challenge since I don't have a comfy side any longer. And I feel like I am beginning to look like some sort of monster. I'm scarred, deformed, lumpy, and swollen. It is not a pretty picture. Go ahead and add in the fact, that the stress and worry of the past six years is now permanently etched in my face and my hair is something I have decided to call a "chemo fro." Looking in the mirror causes me to feel diminished, less vital, and makes me worry. Sigh.

We'll see what Gary has to say. I think most of this new stuff began after my most recent scans, so there is no way to know what the disease is doing elsewhere at this point. I am hoping he says just stay the course, don't worry too much about this spread; it is at an acceptable level. I think that's what he's gonna say, at least I hope so. The last time we talked about another "option" it was about revisiting a chemo I had been on before, one of the worst, which would leave me without a quality of life worth living. I told him no way. I don't want to be at the "no way" point yet; I desperately don't.

Please help us prevent the "no way" point for other women by signing up for Team Go Jen Go in support of the Komen 5K! The race is right around the corner, Saturday, October 5th. It's a fun and uplifting family event. It is very empowering for women, girls, and survivors alike! And if you are feeling sassy, sign up for the Competitive 5K; the overall winners will be honored with awards in my name and Joe's! it is quite an honor for both of us, and we get to present the awards to boot!

Thanks!
Jen

September 2, 2013

Peeps, sorry for the delay in posting!! I meant to get the 411 on how to post directly to my website, because right now I go through an administrator, but that didn't happen. Good intentions and all that ....

My appointment last week with Gary was, in a nutshell, not good news, but not dire either, which was good, because Luca came along for the appointment—he did not want to, but the nurses spoiled him rotten! Basically, I got my wish: stay the course and manage the discomfort with some meds. The spread is of an acceptable sort (acceptable because we have no untried options), so we keep on truckin'. As for the new masses on my back and any new superficial masses that might crop up (i.e., not on my vital organs), I will see Dr. Fraser, my radiation guy, to decide when we want to hit those suckers with some electrons (the EZ radiation variety). Sixth time's a charm!

Luca was so excited the night before his first day of school, he could hardly sleep. He got on the bus like a champ (nary a backward glance, but I did get a wave through the window), and apparently he loves riding it. He had a great day even though it was mainly orientation type stuff. He couldn't wait for day two. He totally loves it! What a fabulous gift for us all!

I wondered a bit if I might have a meltdown after kicking birdie number two outta the nest and onto the bus, like one of my dear friends did, but I did okay, although I did keep waiting for the emotional damn to burst. It came out a bit later as a mix of elation and intense sorrow that manifested itself as a short temper (nothing new for the familia Pagani, I assure you) around the house. I didn't really have time for it anyway, I had way too much shit to do, like a summer's worth of backlog—the moms out there know what I mean.

Our website, gojengo.org, is underway. It is taking some time to get it right, but it'll pay off. My blogs will be posted on the website from now on. Thank you for following me—both my cancer journey and my transition from CaringBridge to gojengo.org!

Komen is on Saturday, October 5, and it is coming up fast! Please join Team Go Jen Go, and tell your friends, neighbor, co-workers, and random peeps to sign up too! The Go Jen Go Foundation, and the financial assistance and help it provides to our local, in-need, breast cancer community, evolved out of our very first Komen team! This year we are gonna do the T-shirt Pick-Up Party on Friday, September 27th, a week before the race, rather than the night before. This will be less taxing on moi and will hopefully allow me to actually have a cocktail or two, rather than stumbling (literally—last year I had to have two friends help get me back across the street) home exhausted and stone cold sober. Join our team!

Thanks!
-Jen

SEPTEMBER 9, 2013

Wow, today is the first day since school began that I haven't had a single appointment, pressing concern (we had a yard sale Saturday, and yes, we are gluttons for punishment), school commitment, or speaking engagement. Whew! Too bad tomorrow is chemo time again. Blech! Today I need to get some things done (always a bit of a mad, pre-treatment rush to accomplish before I get way behind again), but I'm tired, not really motivated, and am kind of in a semi-stupor my permanent state these days, some might argue. I'm also trying to rest my right leg, which is swollen from cancerous nodes. Grrrr, for having breast cancer, this disease has managed to effect just about *every* part of my body in some way, death from a thousand cuts and all that. I'm not sleeping well at all. No position is comfortable for long because there are too many active cancerous areas that flat out hurt despite pain meds. And my dreams continue to hound me; they're the usual variations of the same: there's the expectation that I must continue to perform some impossible task while a clock counts down in the background. There's no hiding from my subconscious, though most nights I pray there is. So today, maybe I'll manage to check some boxes off my list, but we'll have to wait and see how the day plays out.

But all the whining aside, last week was really quite good. The boys finally both went to school for almost a full week, and we started our first fall sport—swim team for Rocco. I was also the lunchroom helper for both boys' classes, which was precious and informative. It was good to see the boys interacting with their classmates and to put names to all the little faces. I also had the opportunity to share our cancer story and the mission of the GJG Foundation to the folks at Consolidated Planning and McGladrey. Both companies are supporters of Go Jen Go and Komen and have corporate commitments to serving our community. And Luca lost his first tooth yesterday; what a milestone! Last night, he went to bed pondering how much the tooth fairy would give him for it, saying, "It's really small but it is my first one." He made four dollars. Rocco, the stinker, tried to spoil the affair by looking me dead in the eye and saying that Daddy and I were the real fairies. I'm not sure if I should worry that my gaze never waivered when I fired right back with "that would be ridiculous" and "what would parents possibly do with all those teeth?" He said they would bury them in their back yards. I hope he's not a mobster in the making. He's already got a great name for it ....

Yikes, I'm going on and on, sorry! Race for the Cure is less than a month away! Please join Team Go Jen Go and support Komen. They fund life-saving early detection and education programs, and support breast cancer research.

OMG, I almost forgot, how bout them Dawgs?!?!

Jen

SEPTEMBER 23, 2013

These days I just don't write as often. I lack the energy and the will. I am trying to devote more time being present in moment as a mom, wife, and cancer survivor extraordinaire. In my down time, I'm avoiding introspection and trying not to ponder the meaning of things. It's a bit difficult because I'm an existentialist at heart. But why beat a horse? My consciousness has been aiming for distraction—in my down time I play repetitive, mind-numbing games on my iPad or watch a fab series (HBO, of course, where all good shows are made) on TV. Joe and I've been catching up on the past seasons of *Boardwalk Empire* and *Ray Donovan*. We'll watch one or two episodes a night. It's total immersion drama, and it's like stepping out of our own problems and into those of others. Occasionally, I even dream of the characters and of their dilemmas and dreams. It's a sweet reprieve from what generally haunts me at night.

When I finally sit down to it, I am distracted (both by own mind and the constant "Mom, Mom, Mom …"). I have too many things to say but fall silent instead. Today, though, I will put a bit out there. We're at the beach. We've been here since the middle of last week. It is the first time I've been out of town since May, and it was so very long overdue. The daily grind, which affects us all, has grown tedious for me—life measured out by the endless cycles of treatment and recovery. And its hard not to ponder things a bit here at the beach. Metaphors abound, life's rich pageant and the glorious struggle for life play out all around. It soothes my soul. For it is a gift to witness and a beautiful reminder of my own insignificance and of the interconnectedness of life and death. They go hand in hand, after all, and it's not a thing to be mourned, at least not for long; its just the way things are.

It has also given my body a chance to heal, to rejuvenate. When we left Charlotte, I was still yet to recover from chemo, and I had a sinus infection and was nursing a fractured rib (just happened, doing nothing in particular, but is the result of weakened bones in a heavily treated area). I had and have many areas (the new masses that keep popping up and growing like weeds) that are hurting bunches. Despite all that we've had great family time. The boys have been silly, and it is so fantastic for them to play together in the pool without me having to entertain, rush off for a practice, engage in the homework battle, or try and put dinner on the table. We've laughed, played, taken walks on the beach, hunted for shells, and catered to Luca's new and very pressing demands of maintaining his hair no matter the circumstances. We even made a special trip out and over the bridge for gel. He dashes to the bathroom to fix a Mohawk or another hairdo every time his hair dries and just any old time the mood strikes, and it strikes often.

When we get back to town, back to reality, it's time to hit the ground running, survivor style. I get scanned Wednesday, and then on Thursday, I start radiation on two to four separate areas of my bod. The treatment is to help with pain and edema, and I am ready for the help! But Friday evening will be a treat. We've got our annual Go Jen Go T-shirt Pick-Up party for our Komen race team. The Keogh's will host again; they live directly across the street from us. Yay! And beverages and Mac's BBQ will be provided. Yum! Come join us, get your new shirt, and have some fun!

Better scoot, the waves are calling.

J

SEPTEMBER 26, 2013

We're back from paradise (a.k.a. Wrightsville Beach) and have resumed our normal lives once again. As per Pagani usual, we hit the ground runnin'. I had my radiation set-up appointment today. We're covering a good portion of the front of my torso, up back along my right shoulder blade, and my right groin/upper thigh (yes, I have breast cancer in the tissues of my leg, go figure). It shouldn't be too horrible (feel free to remind me of this in a few weeks when it is horrible). But bonus, I don't start until Monday, because they won't have all the calculations ready in time to start tomorrow. Fab news because tomorrow evening is the pahtay! Yay!

See ya tomorrow!
-J

OCTOBER 2, 2013

Please bear with me for this post, my brain is not in peak form at the moment.

The GJG Team Party was totally fab Friday night! We had a great turnout—I'm guessing about 250 peeps over the course of the evening, with fifty to seventy-five kids running around having an absolute ball. There was great music, food, beer, and big fun. We also raised $2,850! Yay! Thank you so much to everyone who came out and supported us. I am still riding the high, feeling the love. Extra bonus for the weekend—my best friend from UGA visited, and, icing on the cake, the Dawgs beat the Tigers!!

In order to have an extra recovery day from chemo before radiation this weekend, I received treatment Monday instead of my usual Tuesday. I'm not a huge fan of starting the week that way … Monday afternoon I rushed directly from chemo to a marathon radiation set up and treatment appointment. It rocked me with pain, which I was not at all expecting. Having done five previous courses of radiation, I consider myself pretty well versed in what to expect, but it was all surprises. Lying on my back for almost two hours on the treatment table and effectively squishing the tumor over my right shoulder blade between bone and metal caused horrible pain, despite pain meds. This tumor has been hurting quite a bit anyway. Then, shocking lightening flashes of pain, but thank God only in two tumors, kicked in that night. The Hydrocodone did not touch it. After quite a few desperate hours, I put on the narcotic patch (which I totally did not think I was going to need and have never used before) at 3:00 a.m. Its effects don't kick in for twelve to twenty-four hours after application, which is also when the nausea from it can kick in as well (not what I wanted following chemo), but at that point, it was a gamble I was willing to take.

Following radiation yesterday, it all started up again, despite one patch and hydrocodone, too. After a call to Gary's, and a meeting with both of my radiology oncologists, I am now on two narcotics patches, more nerve medicine, and I'm taking Hydrocodone as needed. As I continue with treatments, and for who knows how long afterwards, cell death (tumors pressing on nerves) and swelling (stretching nerves) will continue and at some point, the pain will peak (previously this has occurred about three weeks after my last radiation). I hope it does not continue that long!!! The good news is that I was able to sleep last night, though I woke up in a total stupor. I am hoping all the meds will dull or eliminate the lightening after today's treatment at 4:00 p.m., and that I'll sleep tonight as well.

This has been a very long post, hopefully not too tedious for everyone, and I am pooped. The Race is my carrot after what is turning out to be a very long week.

-J

October 25, 2013

Komen was such an amazing experience! I was so uplifted by the support from all my team members, the crowd, all the Komen volunteers and board members, and of course, the VIP treatment. I completely surprised myself by speaking at the Jen Pagani Tough Cookie Award presentation. And I was so humbled and tickled to receive the medal.

All that fun, paired with lots of radiation, finally hit me hard, very hard. I basically couldn't do much of anything the week following the race. I was hysterically tired. I tried not to show it to the boys, tried to be present and happy and engaged when they needed me. I basically had the energy to do one "thing" a day; it was all I could do. No laundry, meals, errands, straightening ... I dropped everything else. It made me sad, frustrated, made me wonder ....

Last week ... feeling more rested but far from "normal," Joe and I left for Quebec (like old France right here in North America). It was our first trip alone in three years. On the first night there, we left dinner suddenly because I felt like a stomach bug was coming on. Rocco got big-time throw-ups right before we left (Gammy took good care of him in our absence though). We panicked a bit about what would happen if I fell ill with the flu in a foreign country, far from home, and with socialized medicine to boot. I prayed hard that first night, and I woke up feeling like I was fighting something but was gonna be okay. Thank you, God! Our vacay turned out great. We had uninterrupted time together to talk, laugh, see the sights, and rest. We even did an impromptu zip line/climbing adventure by Montmorency Falls. It was amazing, empowering, and good for my spirit, but after the thrill wore off, it totally crushed me physically. As soon as we made it back to the hotel, I stayed in bed for eighteen hours straight. I slept and slept and slept. It was obviously what I needed, but it was also concerning. I can't seem to recover. I feel like my body is failing me, and it is very worrisome.

We returned to Charlotte Monday night after a tiring day of travel. Tuesday it was chemo time again. It kicked my ass. I have been on the couch since. I have not showered, been outside, or done much of anything other than watch bad TV in the dark. I am grumpy, I feel helpless, and I feel like things are looking a bit bleak. Today is Friday, and I still feel like shit. Oh, and I have another sinus infection too. I need quiet, the dark, and time alone. But it's Friday, and we have school bingo night tonight. I will go because it is important to both boys. I want to go, but not really, just because I feel so bad. People will see me and think, "Wow, she's out, she must be doing well." I'm not, and that frustrates me too. And the rest of the weekend is full of their activities. I will do what I can and pretend to feel okay for some of it. I know I can't do it all, though.

While in Quebec, I also discovered two more enlarged, fixed, and very tender nodes. This time, they are in my left groin (right where the hip meets the torso) and exactly where my cancerous nodes were on the right side. This is not good and will most likely mean a rocky climb.

We meet with Gary on Halloween to see if he has any other chemo options to retry. Thus far, his one suggestion has been unacceptable from a quality of life stand point. I'm still on the pain patch and take additional pain meds on most days. It is controlling most of the discomfort from the radiated tumors. Additional tumors and ones that have grown since radiation now are causing quite a bit of discomfort despite the patch. It's worrisome for sure.

Thanks for hanging in through this very long post. Please pray for me: to feel better, to have less pain, for energy to get back into my life, and that Gary pulls another drug out of his hat that'll buy me some more QUALITY, time.

Thanks, Jen

November 18, 2013

I haven't blogged in forever. I'm stuck in a spiral of pain, narcotics, nausea, and sleep. There have been some great moments (UGA Homecoming weekend, silly moments with the boys, holding hands with Joe), but for the most part, it's been a struggle. I spend the bulk of each day doing the bed-to-sofa shuffle, trying in vain to get comfortable. I've been radiated again (five fields in five high dose days—high enough to cause tumors to blister and ooze after just the first treatment), and Tuesday I go in to start the chemo drug (weekly, no scheduled off weeks) I said I would not retry.

My state of mind goes from bad to despair with occasional positive breaks. I am trying very hard to focus on the good, but it is becoming comically difficult. New tumors are popping up and causing pain before I have healed from previous radiation (think whack-a-mole). My disease is painfully spreading in areas that should be freaking off-limits for breast cancer, and the swelling I have been experiencing is now increasing by the day. My lower abdomen no longer looks like my own—it's odd, not really recognizing oneself in the mirror. My right thigh, which we know has disease and was radiated last month, is now newly swollen down to my knee. It was not like this even two days ago. It now hurts to walk and bend my knee past forty-five degrees. I now walk like Fred Sanford. What the hell? Not gonna lie, these lower body issues have me freaked out. Will it continue to progress? Will I be walking around on painful elephant legs soon? What will I wear when it turns warm again? I can still pass for normal in the cold weather because all my diseased parts are hidden under clothes.

Each time I get my head around a new problem and think it can't get worse (aside from disease in a vital organ), it does. It's no longer funny. This chemo I don't want better work some serious magic, and soon.

All my complaining aside, please sign up for the Checkers 5K, uptown this weekend. The Checkers are an amazing organization, and they give back to our community, their employees, are actively involved in making Charlotte a better place. They are just darn good people! Hopefully we'll see you there!

December 8, 2013

Caution: you may need a big plate of cheese to go with all this whine!! But it's not all bad; there is definitely some reason for the season stuff too!

My motivation to blog remains a bit low. Perhaps my mind is mirroring the decline in my body. It's been a very tough few weeks since I started this "new," old chemo regimen. Ironically, the downturn in my quality of life is not due to the chemo but rather to unexpected side effects from the disease itself. Cancer has a really dark sense of humor. I've swollen up, from lymph edema, like an overstuffed sausage. It's painful, debilitating, and is putting relentless pressure on body parts that should get a pass from breast cancer. My days are spent mainly on the couch, trying in vain to position my body to minimize the edema. Unfortunately, due to where the edema is located, a position good for one area wrecks another. I get up sparingly, and when I do, I can't wait to get back off my feet and relieve the pressure. I try to "budget" my time up, weighing what I most desire doing (like throwing the football after school with the boys, which is Luca's favorite thing in the world right now to do with Mommy), with what must be done and what needs to be done. Obviously, tons of stuff is not getting tended to. Oh well.

And in the process of all this (and hopefully not due to any spread), my lower back has been destroyed. Back pain is my constant companion. Despite the narcotic patch, and despite the extra medicine I get up to take in the wee hours every night after writhing around in pain for a good hour, I can't get relief. Between the swelling, the burns from radiation (which just are super slow to heal), and my back, there are no good sleeping positions left. Grrrrr. Getting out of bed, which is usually 9:30 a.m. to 10:30 a.m. except the two days a week I get the kids off to school (and then I usually fall asleep again shortly after the bus comes), is comical. Walking is slow and awkward. A specialist I saw last week for my edema recommended checking into zero-gravity chairs. They are like weird recliners that essentially put you in an optimal, but odd, position to provide the best position for your spine. My dear friend Britt took me yesterday to a back store to check them out. She sighed like she was in heaven within seconds of sitting in the first one and tilting back. I, on the other hand, experienced chest pressure, difficulty breathing (this is also a new development—it's gotten bad, so I go get an echo Wednesday), a tremendous increase in lymphatic pressure in my abdomen, and some back relief. We sat in a bunch. Britt was in heaven, and I finally managed to find two that provided some relief and didn't exacerbate my other issues.

It was really kinda depressing. I was unrealistically hoping for a panacea of a remedy. A quick, easy, and reasonably priced fix. I hoped it would be a miracle thing that would make my pain go away, minimize my swelling, maybe even make me feel (gasp!) good. Oh, and look somewhat stylish, not clash with our other décor, and not cost an unbelievable amount of money. Too much to ask? Apparently! So, we left the store, me rather down and fighting a weepy feeling, and then Britt explained to me that the goal is to bring my discomfort down to an acceptable level, not zero. We agreed that more test sitting is definitely needed, but that's hard to do with chemo weekly and also gobs of other appointments to address all my side effects; it is an insanely frustrating spiral. We also agreed that we need to check the internet for lower prices, and because I need relief ASAP, perhaps some therapy is needed in the immediate future because I really can't go on like this for too much longer. I am worn thin. I am losing the ability to help myself when any obstacle stands in my way. I think we are beyond the point of reasonable fixes to any of my problems in terms of time, impact on my quality of life, and financial cost. I see a future of "choices" that are really just the lesser of evils.

I'm not this grumpy all the time. I still find inspiration and joy in the work Go Jen Go is doing. I still gather strength from the impact we are having on our local, in-need survivors. As many challenges as I have, I have all of you, a TREMENDOUS support network to help me along. And I am so grateful that all of you pitch in to help those women and families that don't have my incredible network of support! We are currently helping spread the joy again this holiday season. We'd love your help, so please sign up for Go Jen Go Operation Spread the Joy!

Thank you for listening, thanks to those of you who have helped our family with meals and errands, and thanks for helping GJG!

-J

December 24, 2013

Happy Holidays, everyone! Operation Spread the Joy was a huge success! Despite being in the throes of chemo, and well, not really being (or looking, but that ship sailed a while ago!) my best, I was able to go to the wrapping party for a bit last Thursday, and I got to witness this miracle of giving in action. It reminded me of Santa's workshop, everyone hustling and bustling and full of holiday cheer. It was full of smiles and joy. Thanks for the opportunity to help others and for the reminder of what the season is all about. 'Twas so good!

Thank you all for so very generously allowing (through donations of your time, money, gifts, and gift cards) us to fulfill the holiday needs and wishes for EVERY member of the twelve local, in-need families GJG is supporting that are battling cancer this holiday season. And we were able to provide a generous amount of gift cards to fifteen to twenty to other individuals. Wow! All this is in addition, the icing on the sugar cookie if you will, to the ongoing financial support Go Jen Go already provides.

And a big thanks to those of you supporting our family with playdates, errands and meals!!! It is a HUGE HELP!! I now am semi-living in my Relax The Back chair, which has had a rather profound impact on my back pain (thank God), but I am still constantly battling tumor pain and the pain from the rather profound amount of edema that has cropped up in the last six weeks or so.

I better scoot. This elf has some last-minute work to do. I can't wait to see the boys' faces tomorrow morning! Christmas is going to be great!

Happy Holiday!
-Jen

December 30, 2013

A note from the President of the Go Jen Go Foundation:
  2013 was a year of tremendous growth for the Go Jen Go Foundation, its supporters, donors, and volunteers. I am so very proud of the selfless commitment of our Board of Directors in making sure we can help every family that comes to us for support. As we draw this year to a close, I wanted share some of the important work being done.

In 2013, we have been able to help more families than ever before due to the generous contributions from individuals, corporations, and fundraising events like:
- All-In to Fight Cancer
- The Inaugural Run Jen Run 5K
- Pink in the Rink, the Charlotte Checkers and the Kahn Family
- South Park Youth Association Pink Sock Drive
- SHE 4Life and the Overlook Fall Festival
- Team Carolina Lacrosse Club
- The Pinnacle Institute of Cosmetology
- 24 Hours of Booty
- Consolidated Planning
- Smiley's 4 C's
- Sales Performance International
- Y2 Yoga
- Carolina's Hematology and Oncology
- The Plym Foundation (Charlotte Smarty Pants.com)
- All of our wonderful Run Jen Run sponsors and participants

These are just some of the events and organizations that generously support the GJG mission. And here are some of the ways in which your donations have gone to help families this year:
- A new mattress for a survivor who was in pain at night from chemo
- A trip to Africa with a survivor's ministry (a lifelong wish)

- Power bills for a survivor who was using a heating pad to avoid turning on her heat
- A train ticket for a mother to be with her daughter during her mastectomy
- Visa cards for families who have to choose between pain meds or groceries
- Three different survivors' reconstruction surgeries
- Rent for several families facing eviction
- Money to help pay for COBRA insurance after job losses
- Money for day to day expenses when co-pays wipe out the family checking
- A new refrigerator so the survivor didn't have to store her food in a cooler
- Monthly financial Support for over twenty families this year

The Board of Directors would like to humbly thank every Go Jen Go supporter for their generous gifts, their volunteer efforts, and their unending messages of love and support. As a foundation, we strive to be good stewards of the money that is donated, using very little of those funds for the day to day costs of operations. We are an all-volunteer organization with no paid staff. We are dedicated to helping women and families focus on the things that are important while they are in the fight of their lives. We know we couldn't do this without the unending support from the Go Jen Go army.

On a personal note, I would also like to thank all of the people who have reached out to help Jen in her difficult fight. The dinners, the playdates, the cards and letters, the gifts—each one is dearly appreciated and truly helpful. Jen continues to amaze me with her strength, her courage, and her grace. She inspires us all to be better people, to cherish every minute, to find the bright side, to wag more and bark less.

I could never explain how difficult it is to face our dire future, day after day, and push it aside to live for the present. It is so much easier said than done. But she soldiers on, for her sons, for her family. For me. And I try to do the same for her; I'm just not as strong. But the help from all of you is enough to keep us going. And the love we get for the love we give is overwhelming. Thank you.

Hug your family and have a very Happy New Year.
-Joe

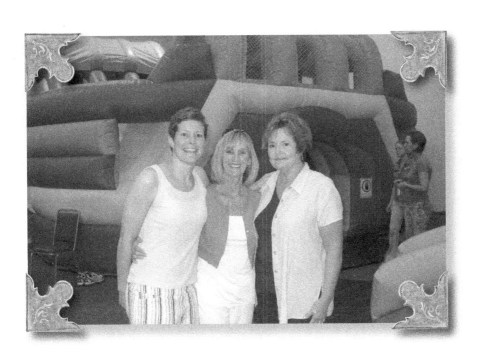

2014

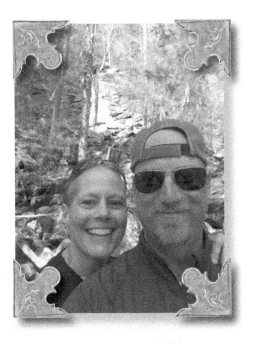

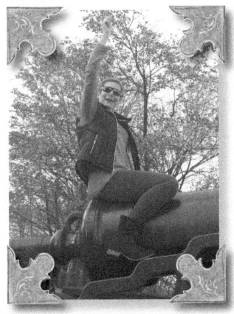

January 5, 2014

Christmas Eve and Christmas were beautiful, happy days. The boys had a blast, and Santa actually did come. Luca was semi-convinced he was getting coal right up until the last minute. It was so good to be surrounded by family and to be pampered as the celebrations whirled around me bundled up in my chair.

Post-Christmas has been a bit of a challenge. To keep the story from getting too long, I am currently not getting any chemo. Focus has instead switched to managing my breathing issues, widespread/diffuse edema, and pain. On Friday, I had about one liter of fluid drained from my right lung. It has made a huge difference in my ability to breathe while at rest. I am still struggling to breathe while up and around, which is due to the diffuse edema that is still present in both lungs. I am up and around very little, though. They can't mechanically drain this type of fluid, but I've been on diuretics to see if I can, in layman's terms, pee it out. Gary thinks it would be very unlikely that the cause of this diffuse lung edema is lung metastases, which is fab, but another potential cause is congestive heart failure.

My last echo was on December 11, and I passed it with flying colors, but tomorrow morning, I will get another one to see if my heart function has dramatically changed since then and if that could be the root of my current problems. I don't think so—I mean, I've been on several drugs that potentially cause heart failure, but my breathing issues preceded (though not to this extent) the December 11 test. We'll see soon enough, I suppose.

I hope we get these issues settled soon, because I have some serious movie-butt going on from all the sitting. I am ready to be up and participating in my life, in the lives of the boys, and of Joe and the dogs. I'm certainly not opposed to a little down time now and again, but I prefer to earn it!

Please send us some good vibes and prayers for some fixes and a return to a good quality of life.

Thanks!
-Jen

JANUARY 12, 2014

I've been out of pocket, so please accept a belated thanks for the meals, cards, flowers, and gifts. They continue to uplift and inspire.

My health has tanked of late. I'm struggling from an inability to breathe or be mobile and from high levels of pain and nausea …. At times I can't get up out of my chair by myself, turn onto my side in bed, or get to the bathroom alone. If I am up for more than a minute or so at a time, I am wracked with pain and completely gasping for air. On Thursday, my inability to get air became life threatening, and we went to CMC via ambulance. Breathing is still an ongoing, huge concern, both from fluid in the cavity around my right lung and the diffuse fluid and thickening airways inside both lungs. The emergency problem (a different one due to upper airway closing) is now gone. The doctors do not know exactly what caused it.

Early tomorrow, I will go back to the hospital for a lung biopsy. They tried to do this Friday but couldn't due to problems on their end. We will know in a few days if the dramatic differences in my lungs are due to rapid spread. We are kind of in that "wait and see" mode.

Please say some prayers for good test results, and most importantly, easier breathing, pain relief, mobility, and, well, not feeling terrible most of the time. I want more decent quality of life time, not more of what I have currently.

We'll keep you posted.
Thanks. Jen

JANUARY 16, 2014

As many of you know, Jen has been dealing with several health issues that are new and fairly serious. And you have responded in spades. As a group, you Go Jen Go fans, supporters, and friends are the most loving of people, and Jen wanted me to let you all know she is hearing your words, reading your emails and texts, and is immensely grateful for the love and support. She appreciates every gift, every meal, every playdate! Right now, however, her energy is low, and she asked that you be patient with her communications. Furthermore, while she would like to visit with every single person on this long, extensive list of friends and family, she needs to save energy for the boys and for Joe. Drop-in visits, for now, are too tiring.

Might we suggest you show your support in other ways? Write Jen a letter or support those who support us—buy tickets to Laugh for the Cure this weekend or Pink in the Rink, hug a friend, or sign up for her favorite event of the year, the Run Jen Run 5K walk/run. She is so honored you care!

Thank you,
-Britt Yett

January 17, 2014

*A*n update on Jen and the Pagani family:

Jen and Joe met with Gary yesterday. Biopsy results showed that cancer has metastasized in her lungs, and this explained the breathing difficulties she was having. Gary recommended they continue to aggressively pursue quality and quantity of life, but he thinks that Hospice & Palliative Care would be best qualified to provide that care and to monitor her closely. Jen and Joe agreed, and they are comfortable and at peace with that decision. Hospice is setting up a team that will provide them so many levels of support.

This certainly marks a new stage in Jen's journey, but it is one she is meeting head on with determination, confidence, and grace, much like she has every step of the way. She will share her thoughts and feelings with you again ... as she has every step of the way ... but she needs some time to rest and get her house and her family organized after this very busy week. She asks for a couple of things:

- This is as much a journey for the Pagani/Burnette family as it is for her. Please be respectful of their need for quiet as they adjust. Jen will be available for calls and visits soon, and she will let you know when that is. For now, be patient.
- Please be careful when communicating this news. As adults, we understand its implications, but young ears and mouths are not so understanding or delicate. Jen's concern is that Luca and Rocco get information too soon and aren't able to understand the situation in a time and manner Joe and Jen deem best. Please help protect that process as you speak to your own children and in any interaction you have with Luca and Rocco.

- Finally, Jen is well. Her health is not ideal, but her head and her heart are safe. She is quick to smile, quick to laugh, and quick to love. She is, as always, a blessing to us all.

Go Jen Go!
Thank you,

-Britt Yett, family friend

THE AFTER

"'For I know the plans I have for you,' declares the Lord, 'plans to prosper you and not to harm you, plans to give you hope and a future.'"

(JEREMIAH, 29:11, NEW INTERNATIONAL VERSION)

IN MEMORY OF
Jennifer Burnette Pagani

God came for Jennifer the other day
Gently caught her by the hand and they walked away
Long will I remember the smile on her face
Jennifer is in a far, far better place

Her battle is over, her journey is done
Jennifer is now wearing the crown she won
We grieve her passing, we wipe away the tears
But we thank you, God, for all of her years

So many things we can't truly understand
One day all shall be revealed to man
And what a reunion it's going to be
We all will be there, Jennifer, you wait and see

Three cheers for Jennifer, no more pain, no more tears
Yes we know all so well, it's a known fact
When you leave this world, you're not coming back

Jennifer is with her Jesus now, the story is now told
Praising her God, she walks the streets of gold
Lord, Lord, help us to somehow understand
Jennifer is now with her Savior, in that promised land

O gracious everlasting God, eternity shall now begin
Such is God's masterpiece, his legacy to all men
Alleluia, Alleluia, we shall all meet again
For Jesus is our ticket for that glory train

We live for Jesus' promise, all hail, all hail
Jennifer, Jennifer, our Lord will never fail
And when the roll is called up yonder in the land of the fair
Thanks be to our God, praise his name,
Jennifer, we'll all be with you there.

BY JIMMY OLGERS, FAMILY FRIEND, FEBRUARY 3, 2014

MAY 14, 2014

Jennifer went to heaven at about 1:30 a.m., February 2, 2014. Her family and three close friends who tended to and carried out her every wish were at her bedside at the time. She was ... is ... a diamond in our family and Joe's—her husband's—family. Over 1,000 family and well-wishers attended her funeral service and celebration of life reception. The location was changed three times to find a church large enough. Jen is remembered for her intelligence, determination, athleticism, her great smile, and a willingness and desire to help others.

Jen's Go Jen Go Foundation 501(c)(3), based on helping mothers with young children who are fighting breast cancer, has helped numerous women and children in the Charlotte area. Recently, the owner of the Charlotte Checkers (ice hockey team) made a large donation to the foundation, additional funds are raised each year at the Jen Run Jen 5K race now held annually in Charlotte.

Sorry, I know this is more than you asked, but I could write extensively about Jen ....

We pray all is well with you and your family.

Jan and Howard*

*Excerpt from email sent by Jan and Howard Burnette, Jen's mother and father, to a family friend, three months after Jen's passing

JANUARY 7, 2020

On February 2, 2014, Jennifer Burnette Pagani succumbed to breathing problems caused by cancer that had metastasized in her lungs. She was survived in life by her loving husband, Joe Pagani; her sons Rocco and Luca; her parents, Jan and Howard Burnette; and numerous friends, family members, and loved ones.

Over the past three years, the Go Jen Go Foundation has raised over $323,500, providing financial assistance to more than 400 families affected by breast cancer.

The Run Jen Run race continues to occur every March, and each fall Jen's friends, family, and supporters of the foundation gather for Cheers Jen

Cheers, an annual Panthers football tailgate party and silent auction. These are the major fundraising activities of the foundation, events that Jen loved so much.

Jen is remembered for her kind spirit, her unwavering faith, and the beautiful legacy she left behind in her boys, her foundation, and this book.

For more information about the Go Jen Go Foundation and how to get involved, please visit www.gojengo.org.

Praise and Gratitude from Go Jen Go Foundation Beneficiaries

"Thank you so much for approving me for financial assistance. Every bit helps to pay for the bills. I want you to know that this is truly a blessing and that I really appreciate it. It just helps to know that people understand the struggle that goes with cancer, not just the physical fight for health, but the emotional fight to keep life moving with work, family, and some normalcy. Your financial assistance really does help me with accomplishing that goal. You are an amazing organization."

Local breast cancer survivor

"I'm writing to thank you guys again for all your support and assistance. DJ had the best X-mas ever and I was able to use the donations, gas cards to get around and take care of some important things. I'm feeling great and doing well emotionally/physically and can't wait until doctors release me to return to work. DJ will be turning four this Sunday and I still have some of the gifts from you guys saved to give him on his birthday."

Young, single mother of a four-year-old and local breast cancer patient

"Once again, thank you so much for the check you sent last month. Since school has been closed, I have had a chance to go over all of my medical bills and was able to pay my surgeon and radiologist—almost the exact amount you sent."

Charlotte Mecklenberg School System teacher and local breast cancer patient

"I received your package yesterday and cannot tell you how shocked and appreciative I am. I am speechless! I certainly did not expect that amount of help. I cannot thank you enough. You certainly helped out more than I imagined you could. Again, thank you so very much."

Mother of a daughter with special needs and local breast cancer patient

In Loving Memory
October 28, 1969–February 2, 2014
"A diamond in our family."

CPSIA information can be obtained
at www.ICGtesting.com
Printed in the USA
FSHW011615070420
68909FS

9 781734 707540